www.greenandawake.com
Photo and Recipe: Nazli Develi
Design: Nazli Develi
ISBN: 9798987853627
Hardcover Edition - Second Printing: December 2025, Sweden

# PLANT BASED UMAMI

100 RECIPES TO TASTE THE DEPTH OF PLANTS

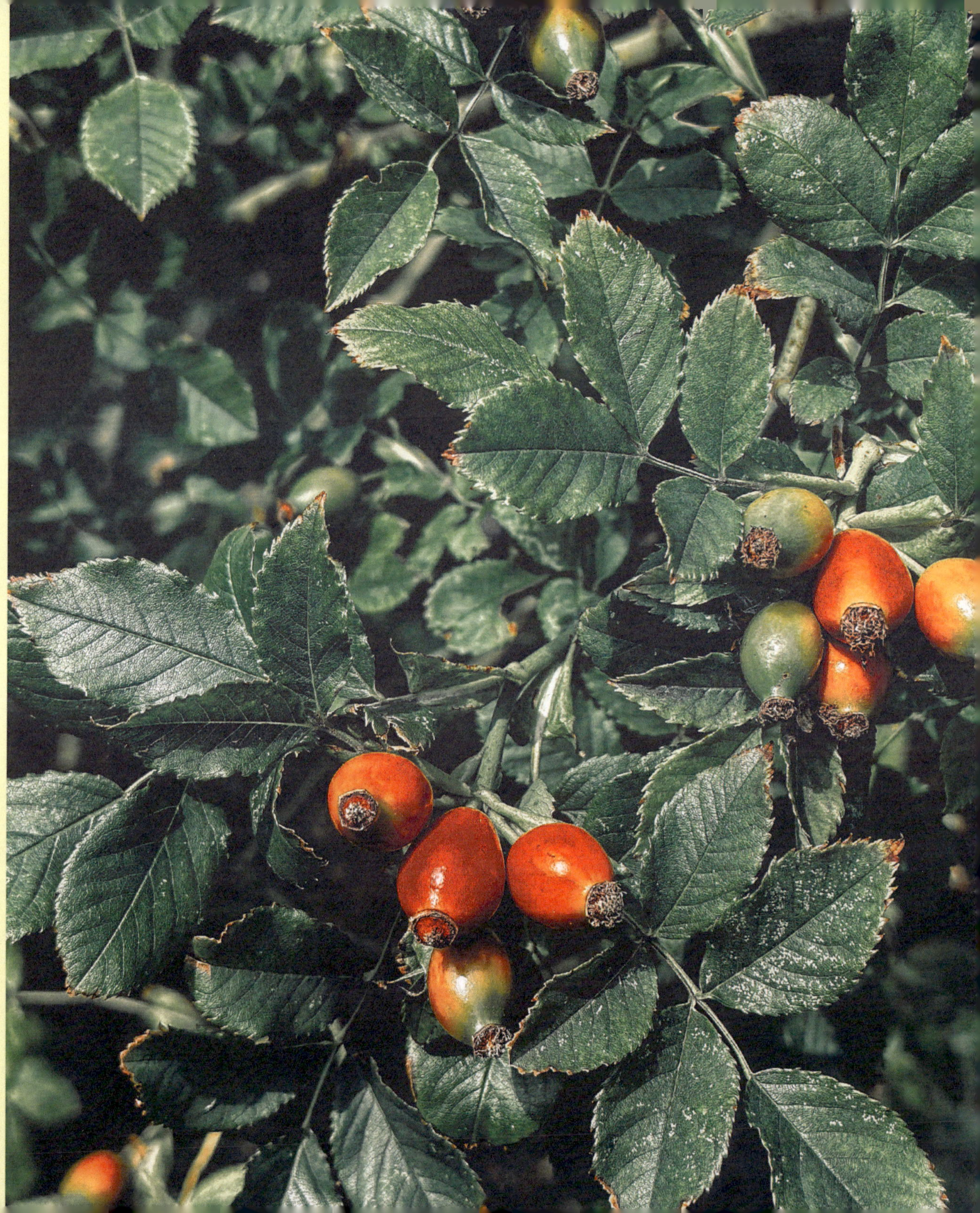

# content

# INTRODUCTION

The fifth dimension of taste, also known as umami, is subtle, complex, and transformative. It's a flavor that can be hard to define, yet its presence—or absence—is unmistakable. The Japanese term "umami" literally means the essence of deliciousness or savoriness, and it was first identified by Japanese scientist Kikunae Ikeda in 1908. But umami is not just a Japanese concept; it exists naturally in ingredients across the globe. For centuries, people have intuitively used umami-rich foods to enhance their cooking, long before the word existed.

Umami is often misunderstood as something achievable only through MSG, the artificial flavor enhancer created by Ikeda to replicate the taste in foods lacking natural savoriness. While MSG is chemically synthesized, glutamates, the compounds responsible for umami, occur naturally in many plant-based foods and are completely healthy. In this book, I focus exclusively on natural umami sources—ingredients like sun-dried tomatoes, capers, olives, mushrooms, seaweeds, coconut aminos, fermented vegetables, and roasted legumes, nuts—that allow you to create deep, rich flavors without additives.

Harnessing vegan umami is about more than just taste. It's about understanding how umami works and how it interacts with other flavors. It's about creating dishes that feel satisfying, layered, and memorable. By combining techniques like roasting, fermenting, and careful seasoning, plant-based ingredients can deliver flavors that are rich, comforting, and surprisingly complex. Even simple weeknight meals can be transformed into culinary experiences that linger on the palate.

I wrote this book because, during my travels in Asia, I realized that many plant-based dishes while nutritious and visually appealing in Europe, were often missing something essential: that lingering, savory depth that makes a meal feel complete. The solution was the fifth basic taste—umami—alongside sweet, salty, sour, and bitter. It became clear to me that achieving this naturally, without relying on processed sauces loaded with sugar, soy, modified starches, glucose syrup, citric acid, and artificial flavors, is entirely possible. In fact, it is both simple, nourishing and deeply satisfying.

"Plant Based Umami" is designed to help you unlock the power of fifth dimension of taste from the plant kingdom. The recipes in this book balance elegance and accessibility: some are inspired by casual fine dining, where presentation and layers of flavor create a refined experience, while others are spontaneous, everyday dishes designed for comfort and practicality. Each recipe is built to be flavor-forward, so that even the simplest ingredients shine.

After exploring main courses, the book moves into finger foods—small, playful bites that are perfect for sharing or enjoying in a more casual, relaxed setting. These recipes show that umami doesn't just belong in a dinner plate; it can shine in snacks, appetizers, and creative miniatures.

Next, we delve into raw desserts, highlighting the sweetness and texture of ingredients without heat, while still using umami to bring depth and contrast.

Finally, the book concludes with a gluten-free dessert chapter, proving that indulgence doesn't have to compromise health, flavor or accessibility.

Throughout this journey, you'll find inspiration from a mix of Asian and Scandinavian cuisine, along-side global influences that celebrate umami's universality. The book is both educational and practical, offering guidance on which ingredients bring umami naturally, how to layer flavors, and how to trans-form simple plant-based foods into rich, satisfying meals.

"Plant Based Umami" is playful, dynamic, and full of potential. It shows us that vegan cooking isn't just about substitutions—it's about unlocking flavor, creativity, and joy at the table. With this book, I invite you to explore that dimension, experiment with techniques, and discover how vibrant and laye-red plant-based cooking can truly be.

Nazli Devrili

Food Designer, Chef & Author

# PANTRY

# plant based umami sources

Understanding and using umami in plant-based cooking is a game-changer. Full flavor without compromise. It helps take your cooking to new heights and simply can be achieved with the addition or combination of umami rich ingredients.  I listed our favorite natural umami sources below.

### OLIVES

Olives are packed with a distinct salty and tangy flavor and a wonderful source of umami in vegan cooking. They are versatile, adding depth to salads and pastas, and can be used as a flavorful topping for vegan soups, salads, pastas, and more.

Their unique blend of saltiness and subtle bitterness can also be utilized in spreads like tapenades, enriching a variety of dishes with an explosion of umami.

### SEAWEED

Seaweed is one of the richest natural sources of L-glutamate, the amino acid responsible for umami, the fifth taste. Kombu (Saccharina japonica) can contain over 2,000 mg of glutamate per 100 g dried. Other seaweeds such as nori, dulse, and wakame also add depth. It is excellent in vegan sushi, soups, or as a flavouring in breads and crackers , offering a taste of the sea without the fish.

Not only fresh one, but dried seaweed has such a deep flavor that it can add new, bigger dimensions to a tomato sauce. Even desserts can get a boost. A little seaweed adds saltiness and umami, bringing out even more flavors than sugar alone can. Try seaweed with berries in desserts.

### KIMCHI

Kimchi is a traditional Korean side dish made from fermented cabbage and has a unique combination of slightly sour, vinegary, spicy, and umami all rolled into one. Honestly, there's nothing quite like it, and we're obsessed with it.

### SAUERKRAUT

Sauerkraut, a fermented cabbage dish, is often considered to have umami flavor, a savory flavor that deepens the overall flavor profile of the food. While not all fermented foods contain umami, sauerkraut's fermentation process enhances its natural umami amino acids.

### PICKLING JUICE

I like to use the pickling juices from sauerkraut, kimchi, preserved lemons, jalapeños, and capers to build complex layers of umami flavors—especially in sweet soups such as pumpkin. They also can be used in nut cheeses to give them a more complex sourness than what lemon juice does.

### JERUSALEM ARTICHOKE & CELERIAC

They both have a very powerful umami flavor, which makes them perfect for making a vegetarian broth or a crunchy topping. I love them dehydrated and use as a topping both on my cinnamon buns, rice and pasta dishes.

### CELERY

Celery contains fairly modest amounts of umami, but it also has aromas and substances that enhance the taste of umami in food. Celery as a base in soups and stews – preferably in combination with tomato – adds zest and aroma.

### NUTRITIONAL YEAST

Nutritional yeast can be used as a plant based substitute for cheese. Sprinkle it on pasta instead of Parmesan, or mix it into casseroles and sauces. It also works well in cheesecake fillings. Some people have sensitivity to it, in this case use a mix of cashew flour and freeze dried lemon powder.

### VINEGAR

Black rice, brown rice, balsamic vinegar and sherry – Combining vinegar with other umami-rich ingredients is one of the simple keys to increasing the richness of a dish.

### VEGETABLE BROTH

Make a broth with kombu and dried mushrooms to get an umami-rich base.

### MISO

Fermented bean paste (can be made from any type of bean or pea) that comes in several shades from mild to strong.

It can be used in everything from savory dishes to sweet desserts to enrich the flavor. I love adding chickpea or pea based miso in the bottom of raw cakes to increase the richness of savory flavour.

### DARK CHOCOLATE & CACAO

Adds a bitter, earthy umami quality to savory dishes. I like using it in my gluten-free rye bread.

### COCONUT AMINOS & MUSHROOM SAUCE

Coconut aminos are often compared to soy sauce. They have a mildly rich, salty umami flavor that is sweeter than soy sauce, but not quite as salty. One tbsp of soy sauce contains 878 milligrams of sodium. Compare that to a tbsp of coconut aminos at about 198 milligrams of sodium. And even though they are made with coconuts, they don't taste like them at all. You can also make your own soy sauce alternative from the peas or any legume rich in protein. However it is a long process and takes 6-12 months. Another alternative can be mushroom sauce which is quicker and easier (recipe on the page 22) Recipes in this book uses chickpea miso, fava bean miso, coconut aminos or mushroom sauce in the place of soy sauce due to soy sensivity. But soy sauce or tamari(for gluten-free) can be used in those recipes if desired.

### SUNDRIED TOMATOES

Sun-dried or cooked tomatoes are a fantastic source of umami. Their sweet yet robust flavor enhances pasta sauces, vegan pizzas, and soups, adding a richness that deepens the overall dish's profile.

### GREEN TEA

Green tea is known for its umami flavor, often described as a savory taste. This umami is primarily due to the presence of glutamate, an amino acid, and theanine, which is chemically similar to glutamate. The umami flavor in green tea is often complemented by other flavors such as sweetness, astringency, and bitterness. Use green tea as a stock to add more flavor to your dishes.

### ROASTED NUTS

Walnuts, cashews, pecans, Brazil nuts or almonds can be roasted to give a nutty and umami-rich flavor.

### ONION, GARLIC & BLACK GARLIC

Caramelized onions, garlic, especially black one contribute to a sweet and umami-rich base flavor.

## MUSHROOMS

Mushrooms – whole mushrooms – especially porcini, portobello, shiitake and button mushrooms – are high in glutamate. Dried mushrooms are even higher in concentrated amounts of glutamate, and don't forget the liquid used to reconstitute dried mushrooms. One of the best methods is to dehydrate mushrooms (or buy dried ones) and grind them in a mini blender or coffee grinder. I use this mushroom powder liberally in soups, stews and when I want to make a recipe as a meat substitute.

## HERBS

Spices like green cardamom and herbs like bay leaves have bold, bright profiles and pair well with a variety of umami dishes. You can experiment by combining sweet paprika, cumin, allspice, tamarind, parsley, cocoa, or cinnamon with umami-rich foods. Bay leaves add a subtle, earthy umami flavor to dishes, enhancing and rounding out other flavors rather than being a dominant flavor on their own. They contribute a complex aromatic profile, including notes of pine, cloves, flowers, and eucalyptus.

## HEMP HEARTS

Hemp, especially when combined with ingredients like nutritional yeast, can contribute a delicious and savory umami flavor, making it a valuable ingredient in plant-based cooking and as a cheese alternative. If you avoid yeast, hemp hearts can be mixed with freeze dried lemon, garlic and mushroom powder.

## LEGUMES

Slow-cooked lentils and beans develop deep flavor, especially with spices like bay leaves, tagetes, thyme and pepper.

## VEGAN PARMESAN

A Parmesan cheese with truffle mushrooms, nutritional yeast, freeze-dried lemon, hemp or cashew flour, garlic and onion as a topping can elevate any dish and give the sauce a thicker and creamy consistency.

## COMBINATIONS

Combine multiple umami sources, such as miso, mushrooms, and coconut aminos, to create a complex flavor profile.

Not everyone experiences umami in the same way. Eating habits affect umami sensitivity, meaning some people perceive it more strongly, while others need higher concentrations to fully perceive it. If a dish doesn't taste spicy enough, try adding more umami boosters. For example: A simple bowl of peas and rice can be loaded with too much flavor with miso sauce, sesame oil, carob-truffle-mushroom mix, furikake, or seaweed!

## BITTERNESS

Bitterness is often misunderstood. While many people are naturally drawn to sweet or salty foods, bitter flavors add depth, balance, and complexity to a dish. Bitterness is one of the five basic tastes, along with sweet, salty, sour, and umami.

In plant-based cooking, bitterness plays an important role—it enhances contrast, adds depth, and flavor to dishes. Bitterness isn't something to avoid—it's something to embrace. By incorporating bitter vegetables, cacao, and fermented foods, you can create bold, flavorful, and deeply delicious plant-based meals.

Common bittering ingredients: kale, radicchio, mustard greens, Brussels sprouts, cabbage, cacao, kombucha, tempeh, matcha, bitter melon, fenugreek, turmeric, hemp butter, and tahini.

# pickled, fermented & cultured

Pickling and fermentation preserve flavours and enhance umami in dishes. Below we go over the differences between these methods and give you the most common pickling and fermenting recipes for an easy start, made with only clean ingredients.

Pickling, fermentation, and culturing are three related but distinct areas of food preservation.

Pickling is like the quick version of canning. You put your ingredients in a vinegar-based brine, and the acid does all the heavy lifting, killing bacteria and preserving your food with a sharp, acidic kick. It's quick, easy, and you can have pickles ready in just a few hours.

Fermentation, on the other hand, is more like a slow-cooked love story. Instead of vinegar, fermentation relies on wild microorganisms (like lactic acid bacteria) that convert sugars into acids over time. We're talking about a process that can take anywhere from a few days to a couple of weeks, depending on what's being fermented. And you get more complex, sour flavors that build up naturally. No vinegar here—just good bacteria doing their thing.
This is a natural process where microorganisms like bacteria, yeast, or fungi break down sugars into acids, gases, or alcohol.
This method has been used for centuries to preserve food and add flavor, creating treats like kimchi, miso, and kombucha. It's why these foods taste sour and complex, and in some cases, it even makes them easier to digest.

Probiotics are live, beneficial bacteria that support your gut health. They're found in some fermented foods, but not all fermented foods. Foods like sourdough bread or beer, while technically fermented, don't contain live probiotics because they go through processes like baking or brewing, which use high heat. This heat destroys the live microorganisms, including probiotics.

Probiotics help keep your digestive system running smoothly when you eat them in the right amounts. These beneficial bacteria or yeasts are similar to the good organisms that already live in your gut. Think of them as your gut's friendly troops that keep everything in balance.

## How to Ferment Vegetables?

*A Step-by-Step Process*

1. Prep: Choose your favorites—carrots, kohlrabi, bell peppers, onions, cucumbers, cabbage, radishes, whatever you have on hand.
2. Peel and chop them into sticks, rounds, or slices. Keep it simple, or mix things up for a little variety.
3. Make the brine: Stir 1 tablespoon of sea salt into 2 cups of non-chlorinated water. This is the magic that helps the veggies ferment to perfection.
4. Pack the jar: Pack the veggies tightly into a clean mason jar and pour the brine over them until they're completely submerged, leaving just a little space at the top.
5. Weight down: Keep your veggies submerged using a fermentation weight, or fill a small ziplock bag with extra brine and place it on top.
6. Loosely cover: Screw the lid on loosely or use an airlock system to let gases escape while keeping the good bacteria in.
7. Let it ferment: Find a cool, dark place and let the veggies do their thing. Start tasting around day 5 – fermentation can take anywhere from 5 to 15 days depending on how sour you like it.

Note: Remember that fermentation is affected by temperature, so warmer conditions can speed up the process.

There's also another method called cultured, which is a more specific process. Like fermentation, cultured uses bacteria, yeast, or mold to change food (think yogurt or sourdough), but the key difference is the use of a starter culture to guide the process. With cultured, you add a known strain of microbes to control the outcome, making it a more precise and predictable method compared to fermentation, which lets nature take its course.

So, in short: pickling is the quick fix with vinegar, fermentation takes its little time with wild bacteria, and culturing gives you more control by using a starter to guide the process.

In the next chapter, you'll find recipes in these categories for making your own pantry staples.

# pickled things

Here is a list of some of our most commonly used ingredients in the recipes.

### Pickled Mustard Seeds (Mustard Caviar)

A magical ingredient that adds bursts of sweet and sour flavor to every bite, also perfect for garnishing.

#### Ingredients

2 dl yellow mustard seeds
2.5 dl white wine vinegar or mirin
2.5 dl water (for boiling)
1 dl light agave syrup (or maple, coconut nectar etc)
2 cloves garlic, halved
1 bay leaf
2 g salt

#### Instructions

1. Boil water in a saucepan. Add the mustard seeds and boil for 2-3 minutes, then pour the water into a fine-mesh sieve.
2. Boil the new water and then boil the mustard seeds one more time. Repeat for a total of 5-6 times to get rid of their bitterness.
3. Place the mustard seeds in a clean glass jar.
4. Pour white wine vinegar or mirin, water, coconut sugar or agave, bay leaf and salt into the saucepan, bring to the boil.
5. When the mixture boils and the sugar has dissolved, pour the hot mixture over the mustard seeds and screw on the lid. Let cool. Remove the bay leaf.
6. Leave the seeds in the fridge for a couple of days so that the mustard seeds can ripen. To prevent them from becoming too thick, you can stir in more white wine vinegar or mirin, about 1 tablespoon at a time.

### Pickled Red Onion

The best way to give almost any dish a bright pop of flavour with tangy and sweet twist. Make a big batch to use later, they add an irresistible extra dimension of flavour so you will want to use them in almost everything from salads to tacos, bowls, pizzas, open face sandwich and more.

#### Ingredients

2-3 red onions
1 dl light agave syrup
1/2 dl vinegar (12%)
1 dl water

#### Instructions

1. Peel, split and thinly slice the onions, preferably with a mandolin.
2. Boil the vinegar, agave and water until the sugar dissolves, remove the pan and let cool slightly.
3. Add the onions to the mixture, stir and pour into a jar with a lid.
4. Leave in the fridge for at least 1 hour before serving, preferably overnight.

Your red onions will be ready to eat when they are bright pink and tender. This can take anywhere from 1 hour to overnight, depending on the thickness of your onion.

This is a base recipe for the pickled red onions, you can also add a few peppercorns or garlic cloves to the jar along with the onions to make the flavor a little more complex and the slightest hint of heat.

You can also use any type of vinegar or sugar you like.

## Takuan (Pickled Daikon Radish)

Takuan is a popular traditional Japanese pickle, a deliciously spicy and flavorful pantry ingredient that goes very well in sushi or poke bowl. It is one of my absolute favorites in sushi and poke bowls.

### Ingredients

1 daikon radish
1 tbsp salt
85 g light agave
120 ml water
120 ml rice wine vinegar
1 tsp ground turmeric

### Instructions

1. Peel your radish and then thinly slice it into long strips as desired. Add a little salt and keep it aside for 2 hours. This will help drain all the moisture.
2. Now take a pan and add salt, agave, vinegar, water and turmeric. Let it all come to a boil.
3. Turmeric is added here to give the dish its typical golden color. Make sure you keep stirring the coating mixture and wait until the salt and agave have completely dissolved.
4. Remove any excess moisture from the radish and place it in a sterile, airtight storage container. Transfer the pickling liquid to the container containing the radish and make sure that all sides of the radish are completely covered.
5. Now keep it aside for at least 2 days and wait. If possible, wait for about 1 month. This will ensure that the ingredients soak up all the flavors and enhance the taste of the salt even more.

## Pickled Sakura

### Ingredients

2 tsp ume su seasoning (a traditional Japanese seasoning made from ume plums, salt, and shiso leaves)
1 dl cherry blossoms

### Instructions

1. Clean the cherry blossoms in salted water and dry with a kitchen towel. Make sure the petals are clean and dry before continuing to the next step.
2. Sprinkle some sea salt in a clean jar or container and place the cherry blossoms, continuing to add salt so that the blossoms are covered with sea salt. Once everything is in the container, drizzle ume su - as if seasoning it.
3. Press the blossoms down so that they are covered with salt & Ume Su. Seal and refrigerate for 3 days.
4. Once marinated, remove from the refrigerator and place on paper towels or kitchen towels to dry.
5. Once it has dried on one side, turn it over and place it directly on the strainer or sushi mat. Let it dry in an airy room for 1-2 days.
6. For storage – place the dried petals in a container with plenty of sea salt and store in the refrigerator until ready to use.
7. Before using, soak them in water for 20 minutes, then drain the sakura blossoms to use in your sushi. Don't waste the liquid, it can be used as a tea.

# creamy basics & sauces

## Your Clean Mayonnaise

110 ml oat milk, unflavored and unsweetened, at room temperature
250 ml olive oil or other neutral oil
2 tsp rice vinegar or white wine vinegar
1/2 tsp fine sea salt
1/4 tsp dijon mustard
1 tbsp olive oil - not extra virgin (see notes) or use avocado oil

### Instructions

1. Place all ingredients in a cup or small bowl.
2. Blend with a hand blender until thick and creamy. Alternatively, blend in a high-speed blender until thick and creamy.

**Note**: If your milk is refrigerated and your oil is room temperature, the mixture will refuse to emulsify, which is the process that makes mayonnaise thick and creamy. Be sure to let all ingredients come to room temperature before you begin.

**Note 2:** The type of oil used in this recipe is super important. Oils vary in acidity, and varieties like extra virgin olive oil are high in oleic acid, a healthy fatty acid. This is good for health reasons, but bad for mayonnaise making because it makes the mixture less stable and more likely to split, resulting in a failed mayonnaise that refuses to thicken. That's why avocado oil or non-virgin olive oil is recommended in this recipe.

## Ketchup

2 yellow onions
700 g tomatoes
1 piece of ginger, large (like two thumbs)
1–2 cloves of garlic
3 tbsp coconut sugar
1 tbsp Worcestershire sauce (page 20)
0.5–1 dl white wine vinegar depending on how much acidity you need
1 tbsp olive oil

### Instructions

1. Cut the yellow onion into pieces and sauté it in olive oil in a saucepan until it becomes glossy.
2. In the meantime, chop the tomatoes, peel and cut the ginger into pieces and chop the chili.
3. Put the tomatoes together with the ginger and chili in the saucepan to simmer in their own broth (the tomatoes will release their water).
4. Peel the garlic, finely chop it and add it to the saucepan, stirring occasionally.
5. Let it simmer for about 20–30 minutes.
6. Blend everything into a smooth sauce. It is advisable to keep the skin on the tomatoes for both color and flavor. The ketchup will turn light yellow from mixing in air but will soon regain its clear yellow color.
7. Bring the ketchup to the boil carefully and pour in the coconut sugar, Worcestershire sauce and white wine vinegar while stirring. Taste for how much white wine vinegar you want.
8. Simmer until it is thick enough, about 5 minutes, cook a little longer if it is too thin.
9. Pour the ketchup into a well-cleaned bottle or jar. Refrigerate. Ketchup will keep for about 6 months in the refrigerator.

### Fermented Sriracha

1 kg mixed red chili peppers
900 ml water
3 tbsp sea salt
4 chopped garlic cloves
1 tbsp coconut sugar
2.5 dl rice vinegar

### Instructions

1. Process your fresh peppers in a food processor. Pack them into a jar, leaving at least 1 inch (2.5 cm) of headspace. The peppers may ferment a little during fermentation.
2. Mix some water with 3 tablespoons of sea salt. Pour just enough brine over the peppers to cover them, pressing them down slightly as they ferment. It is important to keep the peppers covered with brine to prevent them from spoiling. Check daily.
3. Screw on the lid and place the jar out of direct sunlight to ferment for at least 1 week. Ideal temperatures are between 60-75 degrees Fahrenheit (15-24 degrees Celsius). The most active fermentation period is between 1-2 weeks, so be sure to monitor it during this time. The peppers must be submerged in the water to avoid mold growth. If the peppers are not submerged in the water, they may not ferment properly.
4. After 1-2 weeks, the fermentation activity will decrease and the brine will become cloudy and sour tasting.
5. Strain the fermented peppers, but save the brine. Place the peppers in a large saucepan with the garlic, coconut sugar, and vinegar. Add 1 cup of the brine plus 1.5-3 cups of fresh water, depending on the desired thickness.
6. Bring to a boil. Reduce heat and simmer for 10 minutes to allow the flavors to meld.
7. Let cool slightly, then place in a food processor or blender and blend until smooth.
8. Strain the mixture through a fine-mesh sieve to remove any solids, if desired. Pour into bottles.

### Cultured Oat Yoghurt

600 ml homemade oat milk
1 tsp locust bean gum (made of carobs)
1 1/2 tsp agar powder
1 sachet of yoghurt starter or 2 tbsp dairy-free yoghurt (If you don't have a yoghurt starter or dairy-free yoghurt, you can also use probiotics. For this recipe, you will need 3 capsules)

### Instructions

1. Mix the oat milk, locust bean gum and agar in a saucepan.
2. Heat over medium heat until it reaches 80°C, whisking constantly to make sure all the gum is completely dissolved and does not stick to the bottom.
3. Pour into a large glass bowl and leave to stand for about 20-30 minutes or until the temperature reaches 42°C. This is important. If the milk is too hot it will kill the culture. Using a thermometer is highly recommended.
4. Once the milk has reached the correct temperature, stir in the yoghurt starter. At this stage the oat milk has already thickened and may look gelatinous, this is completely normal. Whisk it well to break up any lumps and make it completely smooth again.
5. Pour into glass jars and close the lids, or cover with a wrap.
6. Place the jars in a baking dish filled with hot water; they should be half submerged in water. If you have a yogurt maker, skip this step and just place the jars in the machine.
7. Place the baking dish with the jars in a preheated oven at 40°C for 6-7 hours.
8. Transfer the yogurt to the refrigerator and let them cool overnight.

The yogurt will keep for up to 4-5 days in the refrigerator.

### Cultured Almond Ricotta

A good ricotta, vegan or not, is all about texture and balance. It should be creamy but not heavy, tart but not too intense, and smooth with just the right amount of fluff. This version fulfills all of those.

#### Ingredients

240 grams raw almonds, soaked in water overnight and shells removed
1–2 probiotic capsules (50–100 billion CFU) - or use 50 ml rejuvelac
3/4 tsp garlic powder
3/4 tsp onion powder
1 tsp salt

#### Instructions

1. Place the almonds in a high-speed blender.
2. Add just enough water to barely cover the almonds (about 1 cup).
3. Blend until completely smooth, adding 1 tablespoon of water at a time if needed.
4. Add the probiotic powder and stir the powder into the mixture.
5. Pour the mixture into a clean glass container.
6. Cover loosely with cheesecloth, secure with a rubber band, and let ferment in a warm, dark place for 24-48 hours.
It will develop a mildly sour flavor after 24 hours, so continue fermenting if desired!
7. Once it has grown to your liking, stir in the garlic powder, onion powder, and salt.

### Multifunctional Cashew Cream

It is a versatile condiment that easily functions as a sauce, condiment, yogurt, or dressing.

#### Ingredients

200g raw cashews
5 cloves garlic, roughly chopped
1 tbsp lemon juice
1 cup water + more as needed
1 tbsp extra virgin olive oil
1 tsp pink Himalayan salt

#### Instructions

1. Soak cashews in warm water for 1-2 hours, then strain through a sieve.
2. Drain cashews and place in a blender (preferably high speed) or food processor. Add garlic, oil, lemon juice, salt, and 1 cup water. Then mix until smooth.
3. Make Ahead: Cashew cream can be made 5 days ahead. Transfer to an airtight container and refrigerate or freeze in a resealable freezer bag for up to 3 months.

We use this basic recipe in most of our dishes as a refreshing creamy finish. Feel free to add a bit miso paste or pickling juice to get a more intense taste if desired.

## Cooking Techniques to imrove umami

Unleashing the full potential of umami in cooking involves more than just choosing the right ingredients; it's also about how you cook them. Techniques like slow roasting, caramelizing, dehydrating, sundrying and fermenting can significantly elevate the umami flavor of plant-based dishes.

Each method plays a big role in deepening and storing savory flavors. Here are some key cooking techniques that will help bring out the full umami in your ingredients.

**Caramelization**: When you brown ingredients like mushrooms or onions, it enhances their natural umami. Caramelizing vegetables adds a rich flavor and adds a piquant depth to any dish.

**Slow cooking and simmering:** Cooking ingredients slowly and at a low temperature enriches the umami flavor.

**Fermenting**: These ancient techniques not only preserve food but also increase umami. Fermented foods like homemade kimchi or pickled vegetables add a sour touch to your meals.

**Sun drying and Dehydrating**: Sun drying increases umami by concentrating naturally occurring glutamate and other umami compounds through water removal and by potentially altering the structure of proteins and other substances, enhancing their flavor contribution. Additionally, the slow drying process allows for enzymatic reactions that further develop umami flavors.

**Layering the flavours:** Combine multiple umami-rich ingredients in the same dish. For example, these miso-glazed mushrooms double the umami, creating a more complex and delicious flavor profile.

## How to balance umami with other flavours?

Balancing the five basic flavors—sweet, sour, salty, bitter, and umami—is key to creating dishes that are satisfying and complex. Here's how they work with umami:

**Sweet**: This flavor counteracts bitterness and enhances umami. For example, the sweetness of carrots or yellow peppers can soften the bitterness of vegetables like cabbage, while complementing the umami in mushrooms.

**Sour**: Acidic flavors, like those from citrus fruits or vinegar, can alter and balance both the intense umami and the heaviness of sweet ingredients. A squeeze of lemon can brighten up a rich, umami-heavy Thai soup.

**Salt**: Salt, seaweed, celery root, fennel, and cucumber, for example, enhance all flavors, especially umami. For example, a pinch of salt or celery in a tomato sauce can heighten the natural umami of tomatoes while balancing the acidity.

**Bitter**: Bitter flavors, such as those in dark leafy greens or cocoa, can provide a counterbalance to the richness of umami. For example, the bitterness of kale can contrast nicely with the salty depth of a miso.

## Vegan Fish Sauce

A deep-flavored ingredient. In a stew, a pasta sauce, add all slow and long-cooked braises early to allow the obvious aroma to dissipate while it integrates.

### Ingredients

350 ml water
10 g dulse
6 g shiitake mushroom powder
1 1/2 tsp chickpea or pea miso
30 ml coconut aminos
2 tsp pink himalayan salt

### Instructions

1. Add water, dulse, shiitake mushroom powder, and salt to a small saucepan. Bring to a boil, then reduce heat and simmer for 10 minutes.
2. Remove from heat and let cool.
3. Pour liquid through a fine-mesh strainer into a bowl.
4. Transfer to bowl, add miso and coconut aminos.
5. Taste and adjust as needed, adding more sea salt for saltiness, miso for umami flavor, and/or coconut aminos for depth of flavor.
6. Store in an airtight container in the refrigerator for up to 1 month, shaking well before using. Or pour into an ice cube tray, freeze, and store in a freezer-safe container for up to 2 months.

## Worcestershire Sauce

This vegan Worcestershire sauce recipe is super easy and the perfect vegan alternative that is anchovy-free but tastes exactly the same.

### Ingredients

2.5 dl apple cider vinegar
0.75 dl coconut aminos
3 tbsp coconut sugar
2 tbsp grape molasses
1 tsp tamarind paste
1 tsp ground dulse
1.5 tsp allspice
1.5 tsp garlic powder
1.5 tsp onion powder
1.8 tsp ground cloves
1.8 tsp freshly ground black pepper

### Instructions

1. Add all ingredients to a small saucepan and stir well. Bring to a boil, then reduce heat and simmer for 5 minutes.
2. Remove from heat. Let cool completely.
3. Strain into a glass bottle. Can be stored in the refrigerator for up to 3 months.

Note:
Simmer the sauce: Worcestershire sauce is a thin condiment (slightly thicker than water - not syrupy). A slow simmer reduces the water content and thickens the sauce slightly. It also concentrates the flavors and infuses the spices nicely.

Note 2:
Once you've strained the sauce, gently press the spice into the strainer with the back of a spoon to remove excess liquid. What's left in the strainer is a super-concentrated, ultra-flavorful spice bomb. Don't throw it away! Store in an airtight container in the refrigerator or freezer. When you need a flavor boost (much like when using vegetable broth), you can add one or two teaspoons of this flavor concentrate to stir-fry sauces, soups, and sauces.

## Kimchi

4 dl coarse sea salt
2 Napa cabbages (about 1.8 to 2.8 kg)
1 1/2 dl coarsely chopped apple (or Asian pear)
1/2 dl coarsely chopped onion
1/2 dl coarsely chopped green onion
1/2 dl garlic cloves
2.5 dl ginger
1/2 dl vegan fish sauce (page 20)
1/4 dl maple syrup
3 dl julienned carrot
3 dl green onion, chopped into 5 cm thick pieces
3 dl Korean radish (or daikon), sliced and cut into 0.6 cm thick pieces
4 dl gochugaru

### Instructions

1. Add 2.5 dl salt to 1.8 dl water. Stir and set aside until the salt has dissolved.
2. Remove any heavy stumps on the ends of your cabbage heads. Then, use a sharp knife to make a 5 cm cut in the middle of the root end of the cabbage heads.
3. Cut the cabbage quarters into large, bite-sized pieces.
4. Place a quarter of the cabbage pieces in a very large bowl. Sprinkle a quarter of the salt over the cabbage, then pour a quarter of the brine over the cabbage. Repeat with the remaining cabbage, salt, and brine. Set aside until the cabbage leaves begin to wilt, about 2 hours later.
5. Turn the cabbage leaves with your hands so that the ones at the bottom of the bowl are now at the top and vice versa.
6. Set aside until the cabbage leaves are very wilted and quite salty, at least 90 minutes but up to 4 hours, depending on the thickness of the cabbage leaves.
7. Then rinse thoroughly before tasting. If it tastes very salty, it's done. When your cabbage leaves are sufficiently wilted and salty, pour off any excess water and rinse the leaves thoroughly with cold water.
8. Meanwhile, place the apple (or pear), onion, scallion whites, garlic, ginger, and maple syrup in a blender and blend on high speed until smooth (about 1 minute). Mix the blended garlic mixture, scallions, carrot, radish, fish sauce, and gochugaru.
Pour the sauce over the rinsed cabbage leaves.
9. Using your gloved hands, spread the mixture over the cabbage leaves to make sure they are evenly and well covered.
10. Place the kimchi in airtight containers, pressing down with each scoop to remove air pockets. If you have a lot of space left at the top, sprinkle a handful of salt over the top; this will prevent yeast growth.
11. Store the kimchi at room temperature for the first 24 hours. Then, refrigerate it. Your kimchi will be ready to enjoy on the fourth day, but it will mature and taste even better if you wait a couple of weeks.

## Yellow Pea Miso

Miso is a fantastic product that adds such a nice depth to food.

As a soy-free alternative, I sometimes use Clear Springs chickpea miso or make my own. For those who want to experiment with something different, you will find a yellow pea miso below.

### Ingredients

500g dried yellow peas soaked overnight
500g koji rice
240ml water
175g coarse salt

### Instructions

1. Drain the dried yellow peas and place in a pressure cooker. Cover with 2 liters of water and pressure cook for 5 minutes.
2. Let the pressure release naturally for 20 minutes before opening the Instant Pot and draining the water from the peas. Set aside and let cool to room temperature.
3. Add 2.5 cups of water to a small saucepan. Heat over medium heat for 2-3 minutes. Do not boil. Remove from heat and let cool until it reaches about 50°C.
4. Add the koji rice to a medium bowl and pour in the hot water. Stir and let stand for 1 hour.
5. Place the cooked peas, koji, water and salt in a food processor. Process until a paste forms. It should be almost smooth and all the peas should be pureed.
6. Prepare two 1-liter glass jars (make sure your jars are completely clean). Bake your empty jars at 150°C for 20 minutes to kill any bacteria, then let them cool completely.
7. Using gloves or with a really clean hands, form mixture into balls and pack them very tightly into each jar, working one layer at a time to make sure there are no air pockets. Repeat until your jars are 3/4 full.
8. Flatten the top of the mixture and sprinkle about 1/2 tablespoon of fine salt on top. Cover.
9. Close your jars with the lids and store them in a dark place at room temperature. Your miso will be ready in 6 months, you don't have to do anything but wait! Do not open the jar in the meantime, otherwise mold may grow.
10. After 6 months, pour the miso into smaller jars and store in the refrigerator. Miso will keep for months! Use in soups, marinades, sauces and dressings.

## Mushroom Sauce (Soy Sauce Alternative)

### Ingredients

500 g sliced shiitake
1/2 cup dry-packed sun-dried tomatoes
1/2 cup water
3 garlic cloves, sliced
2 tablespoons balsamic vinegar
1 tablespoon molasses
1 teaspoon peeled, grated fresh ginger
Pinch kelp granules

### Instructions

1. In a large saucepan over medium-low heat, combine the mushrooms, tomatoes, water, garlic, vinegar, molasses, ginger, and kelp. Cover and simmer for 30 to 40 minutes. Strain.
2. Store in an airtight container in the refrigerator for up to 1 week.

## Parmesan Topping

This easy vegan parmesan is always my favorite pantry items. There is always a big jar full of it in my pantry. The cashews are a sweet, neutral, buttery base for the parmesan. Nutritional yeast is what gives the cashew parmesan its "cheesy" flavor but completely optional. If you have any allergies to cashews, use sunflower seeds, pepitas, tiger nuts or make it with hemp hearts.

### Ingredients

100g cashew nuts
30g hemp hearts
60g nutritional yeast (optional)
1/2 tsp garlic powder
1/2 tsp freeze-dried lemon powder
(or dried lemon peel powder)
1 tsp truffle mushroom powder
1 tbsp dried tomato powder (optional)
1/2 tsp pink Himalayan salt

### Instructions

1. Add all ingredients to a food processor and blend/pulse until smooth.
2. Store in an airtight container in the refrigerator for up to a month or longer and use as a vegan parmesan replacement for any meal!

## Umami mixture

Make this umami blend and sprinkle over soups, rice, pasta, vegetables and potatoes. This would also make a fun gift. For optimal flavor, make this in small batches and use within 6 months.

### Ingredients

1/4 cup shiitake powder
2 tbsp parsley powder
2 tsp sage powder
1 tsp garlic powder
2 tsp salt

### Instructions

1. Place all ingredients in a bowl, give it a good stir, or place in a small food processor and blend well. Transfer to a spice container.
2. Store in a spice container for up to 6 months and in most cases it lasts longer.

# CASUAL FINE DINING

PLANT BASED UMAMI

# BLOOMING TEMPEH

## WITH PEAS & SUNFLOWER SEED CREAM

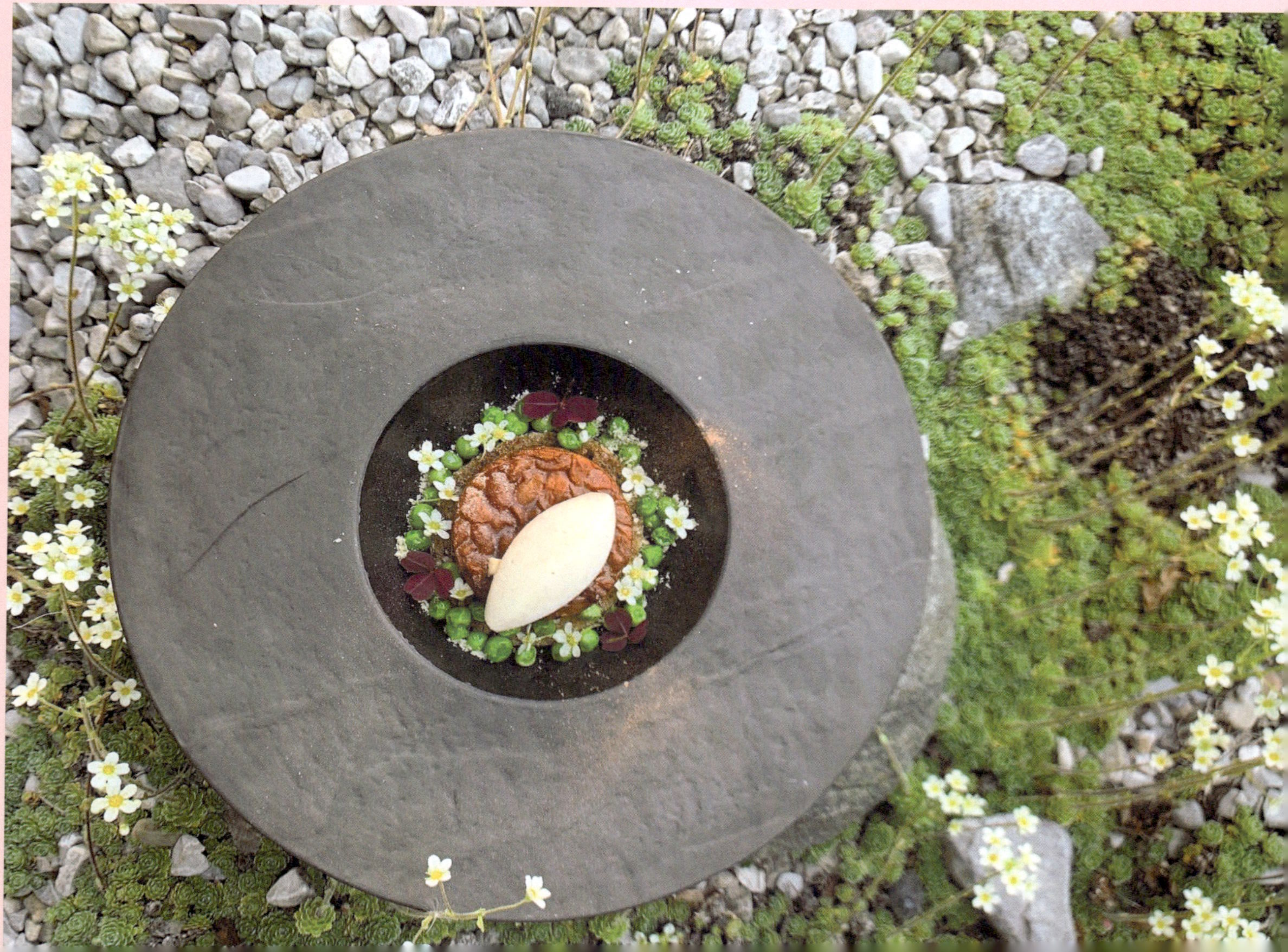

*A layered plant-based delight: tender tempeh, vibrant peas, and nutty gluten-free rye, finished with a luxurious sunflower seed cream. Simple ingredients, extraordinary flavor.*

**Serves: 4**

**Ingredients**

400 g black bean tempeh
40 ml coconut aminos
4 gluten-free rye bread slices (page 158)
1 cup green peas
2 tbsp olive oil
1 tbsp ginger minced
4 garlic cloves minced
Red oxalis
Lifelong saxifraga flower

**Cream Cheese**

130 g sunflower seeds
70 g cashews
40 g nutritional yeast
30 g miso paste
120 ml water + more as needed
60 ml lemon juice
50 ml extra virgin olive oil
50 ml coconut oil melted
6 garlic minced
1 tsp salt

1. Start by making sunflower seed cheese cream. Soak sunflower seeds in water for 1-2 hours, then strain and transfer to a blender, along with the rest of the ingredients. Blend on high speed until smooth.
2. Then transfer mixture 4 quenelle molds. Freeze for 2-3 hour until thicken enough to unmould. Then keep in the refrigerator until serving time. Alternatively you can use the spoon if you don't have quenelle molds.
3. Using 7cm round cutter (alternatively you can use glasses to cut them), cut the tempeh into 4 circles. Place them in a container, add olive oil, minced garlic, ginger and coconut aminos, let them marinate overnight.
4. Using a 9 cm round cutter, cut the bread slice into 4 circles.
5. In a pan with little olive oil and minced garlic, fry the both side of bread rounds. Set aside.
6. Then fry the black bean tempeh circles in the pan with the marination sauce until they absorb all water content and get soften.
7. Transfer bread circles on each plate, place tempeh rounds on them.
8. In the same pan, on medium-high heat cook green peas along with olive oil and some minced garlic until a bit soften and gets vibrant green color.
9. Add some green peas around the tempeh circle. Decorate with oxalis and edible local flowers. I used saxifraga flower.
10. Gently remove cream cheese quenelles from the molds. Top on the tempeh circles. Serve!

# ARCHIPELAGO MOSAIC

## NORI WRAPPED LEEKS, MUSTARD & TAKUAN

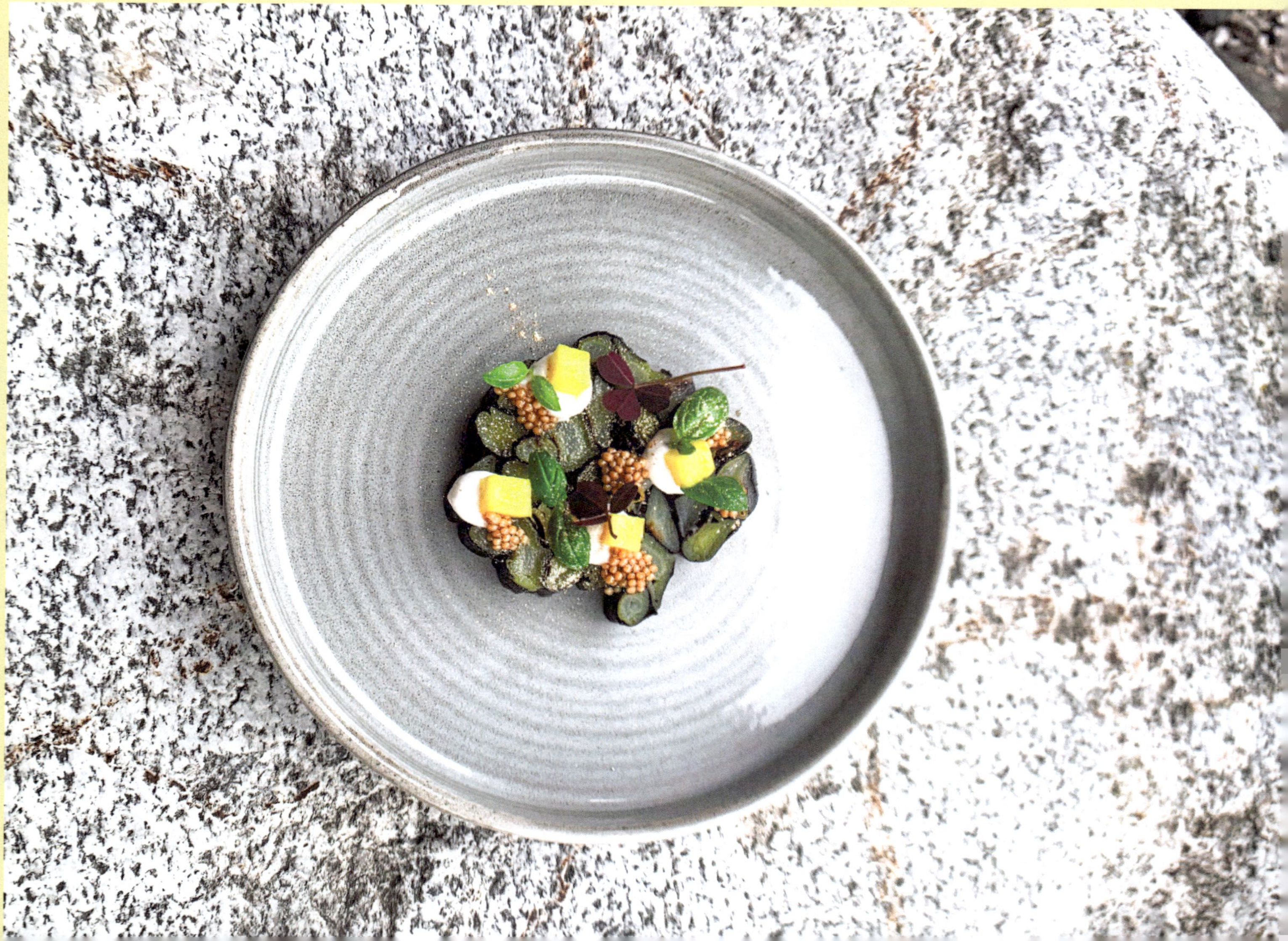

*A mosaic you can eat! Tender leeks, mineral-rich nori, tangy taken, pickled mustard seeds, and creamy cashew—plant-based elegance in every bite.*

**Serves: 2**

**Leeks**

4 leeks
4 nori leaves
Peelings from a whole lemon
5-6 springs thyme
1/2 tsp salt
2 tbsp olive oil

**For Serving**

1/2 cup cashew cream (page 18)
2 strips takuan cubed (page 15)
8-10 fresh small basil leaves
2 tbsp pickled mustard seeds (page 14)
Red oxalis

1. Cut the tops and ends of the leeks, wash and clean them. Cut in two.
2. Place in a large pyrex. Using a small knife make incisions on the leeks.
3. Drizzle a bit olive oil. Add the lemon peelings, salt and thyme.
4. Cover the pyrex in order to prevent leeks burnt. We want them soft and juicy.
5. Bake in the oven at 175 C for 1 hour.
6. Once done, let it cool at least 20 minutes. Then remove the first layer of leeks.
7. Place the leek on a nori sheet, roll it all around, cut the nori sheet in two. Use the other half for another leek.
8. Repeat the process until all leeks are rolled in nori. Place 4 of them on a plastic wrap, lay another 3 on the top of 4 leeks, then 2 and lastly one. Cover it completely with the plastic wrap and roll it up tight. Make a knot on both sides, make sure they are right enough.
9. Let it sit in the fridge at least 5-6 hours.
10. Once time is up, cut the roll in 7-8 equal thin pieces. Divide between plates.
11. Brush with some olive oil and lemon juice.
12. Transfer cashew cream in a pipping bag. Decorate with cashew cream cheese.
13. Add some pickled daikon cuts, small basil leaves and pickled mustard seeds. Decorate with red oxalis leaves.

# SUMMER PANZANELLA

## WITH SUNFLOWER SEED SHARDS

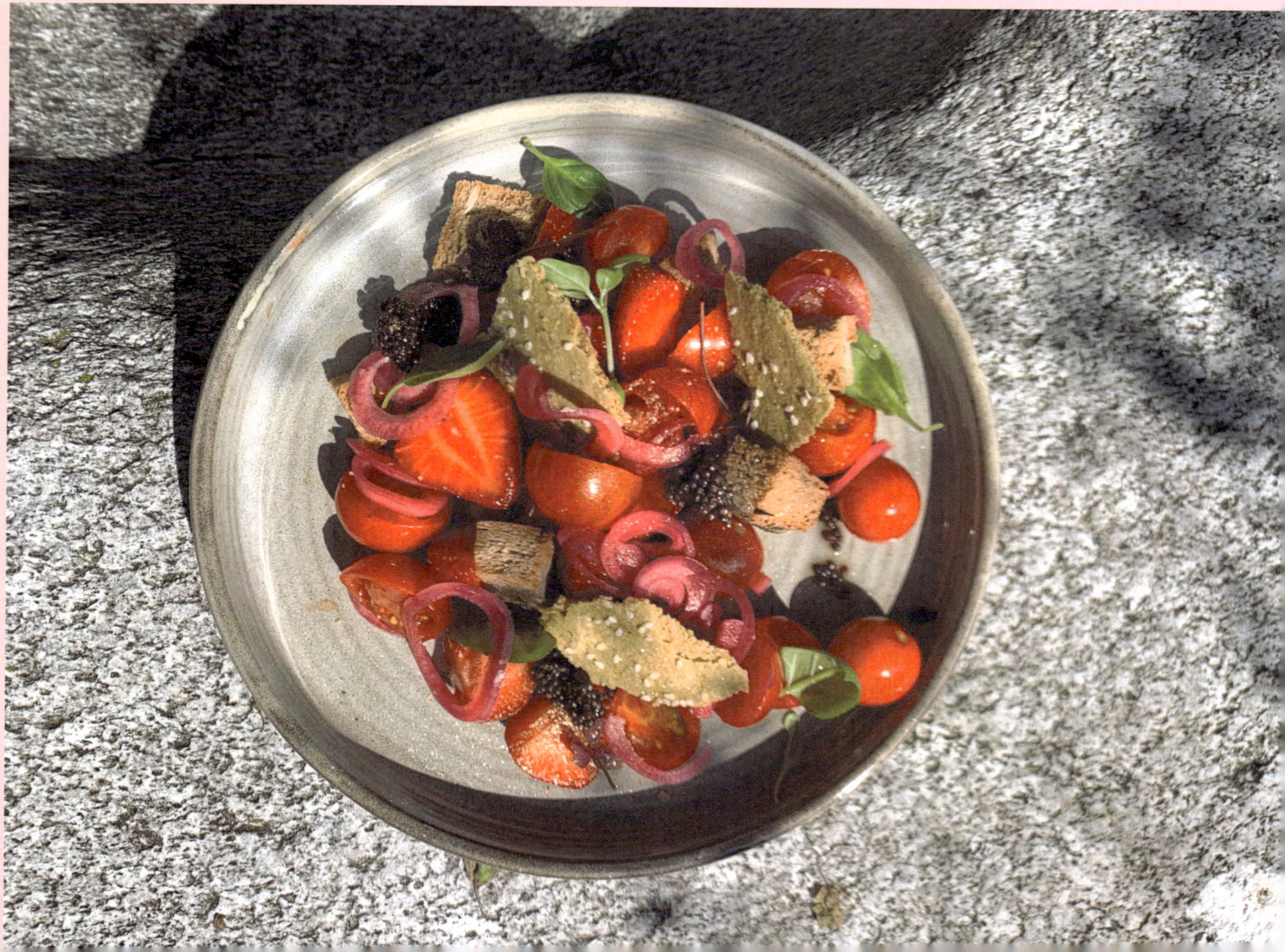

*Sun-soaked tomatoes, sweet strawberries, tender sunflower seed chards, and tangy pickled red onion, layered with fragrant basil and pops of black mustard caviar. A playful, vibrant salad that celebrates the colors and flavors of summer in every bite!*

**Serves: 2**

**For the Panzanella**

1 cup cherry tomatoes
1 cup strawberries halved
1/2 bunch basil
1/2 cup pickled red onions
1/4 cup pickled black mustard (follow the instructions on the page 14, use black mustard seeds instead of yellow)
1/4 cup balsamic
1 cup sunflower seed shards
1/2 cup roasted old day bread cubed

**Sunflower Cheese Shards (optional)**

140 g. sunflower or cashew (alternatively almond and sunflower seeds can be mixed together)
5 tbsp of nutritional yeast
3 tbsp of lemon juice
1 tsp of chickpea miso
1 tbsp of apple cider vinegar
A pinch of turmeric powder
1/8 tsp red pepper (optional)
1/2 tsp pink Himalayan salt
1/2 tsp garlic powder
5 tbsp of water

**Panzanella**

1. In a large bowl, mix the tomatoes and strawberries.
2. Add the bread cubes and toss with the vinaigrette.
3. Season liberally with salt and pepper.
4. Allow the salad to sit for about half an hour for the flavors to blend.
5. Arrange with pickled red onion, black mustard, sunflower seed shards and fresh basil, serve.

**Sunflower Cheese Shards**

1. Soak the nuts in the water for 2-3 hours, then rinse and drain, transfer to the blendtec twister jar.
2. Add the remaining ingredients to the blender. Mix at high speed until you get a smooth mixture.
3. Place a non-stick paper to a dehydrator tray. Spread the cheese mixture very thinly using offset spatula. Bake it in the dehydrator at 42 ° C for about 10-12 hours.
4. After 6 hours, flip the cheese using a new dehydrator papper, transfer to a new paper. Then cook back side of the cheese for another 6 hours.
5. When your cheese is baked, cut it into small pieces and keep it in the jar.

# POTATO DUMPLINGS

## WITH TOGARASHI MAYO & MUSTARD CAVIAR

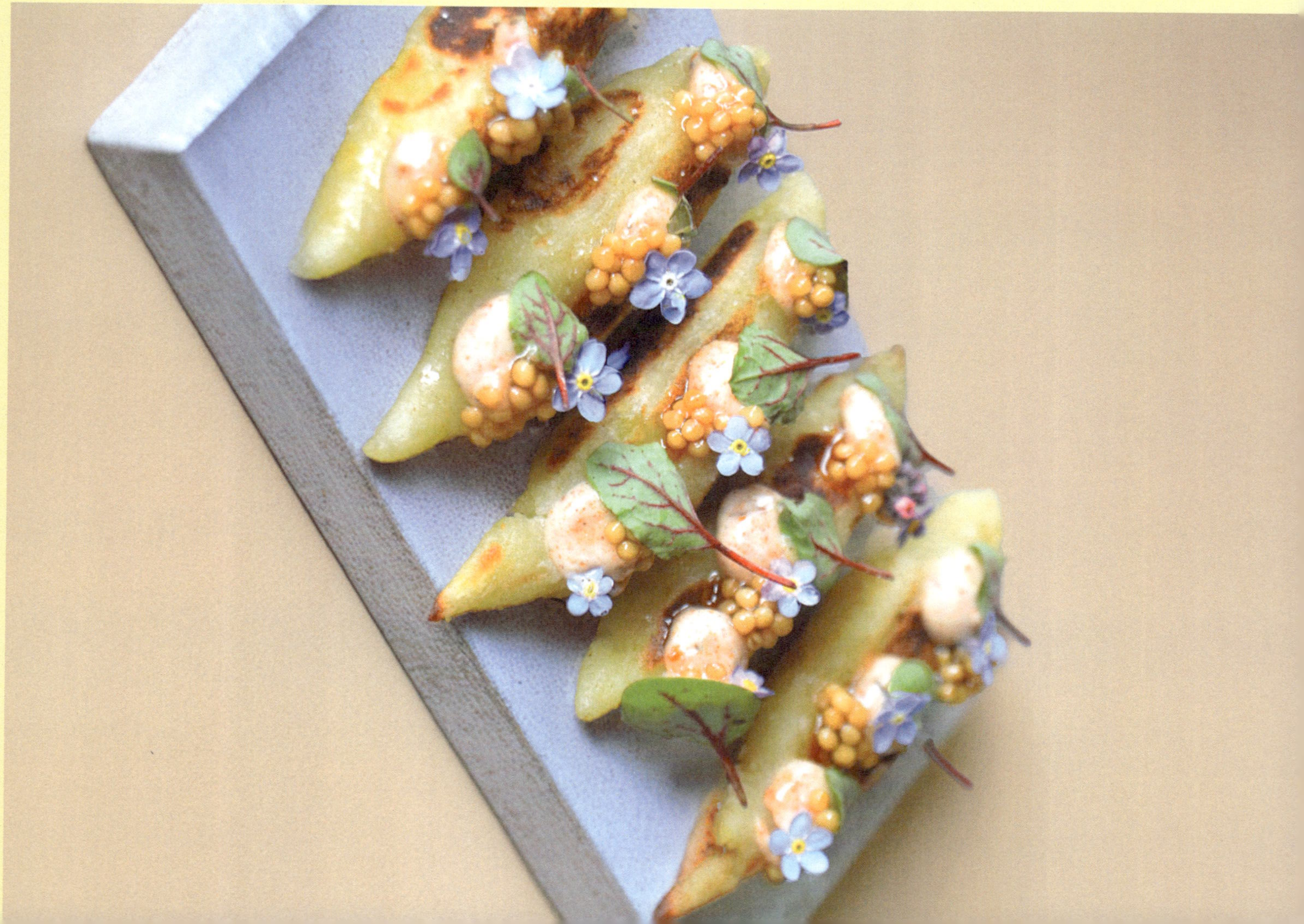

*Schupfnudeln with togarashi-infused mayonnaise and pickled mustard seeds. Versatile and flavorful, also be served as an elegant finger food.*

**Serves: 4**

**Ingredients**

500 g potatoes boiled, peeled, cut into pieces
1 tbsp mushroom powder
120 g chickpea flour
60 g tapioca flour
1/2 tsp sea salt

**For mayonnaise**

2 dl plant-based mayonnaise (page 16)
3 tsp togarashi seasoning

**For serving**

Forget-me-not flowers
Pickled yellow mustard seeds (page 14)
Baby salad leaves

1. Peel the potatoes, cut into small pieces and boil in salted water for about 15 minutes or until soft. Drain, put back in the pot and mash with a potato masher.
2. Add the chickpea flour, mushroom powder, tapioca flour and salt and then knead into a dough with your hands.
3. The dough may still be a little sticky, but should be easy to handle. However, if the dough is too sticky, add more chickpea flour and knead again.
4. Cut the dough into equal-sized pieces and dust with a little tapioca flour.
5. Roll each piece into strands with your fingers. Use a knife to cut the dough into 3-4 cm pieces and shape them into finger-shaped pieces of dough with your hands.
6. Cook them in boiling salted water until they float to the top, about 2 minutes.
7. Heat the oil in a pan and add the Schupfnudeln. Fry on one side until nicely browned. Then flip and fry on the other side.
8. Mix togarashi spice mix and mayonnaise in a bowl. Transfer to a piping bag.
9. Place small mayonnaise dots on top of the dumplings, spaced slightly apart.
10. Place a little pickled yellow mustard seeds between.
11. Decorate with forget-me-not flowers and small lettuce leaves or micro-greens.

# SPINACH KNÖDEL

## WITH PAPRIKA AND CREAM

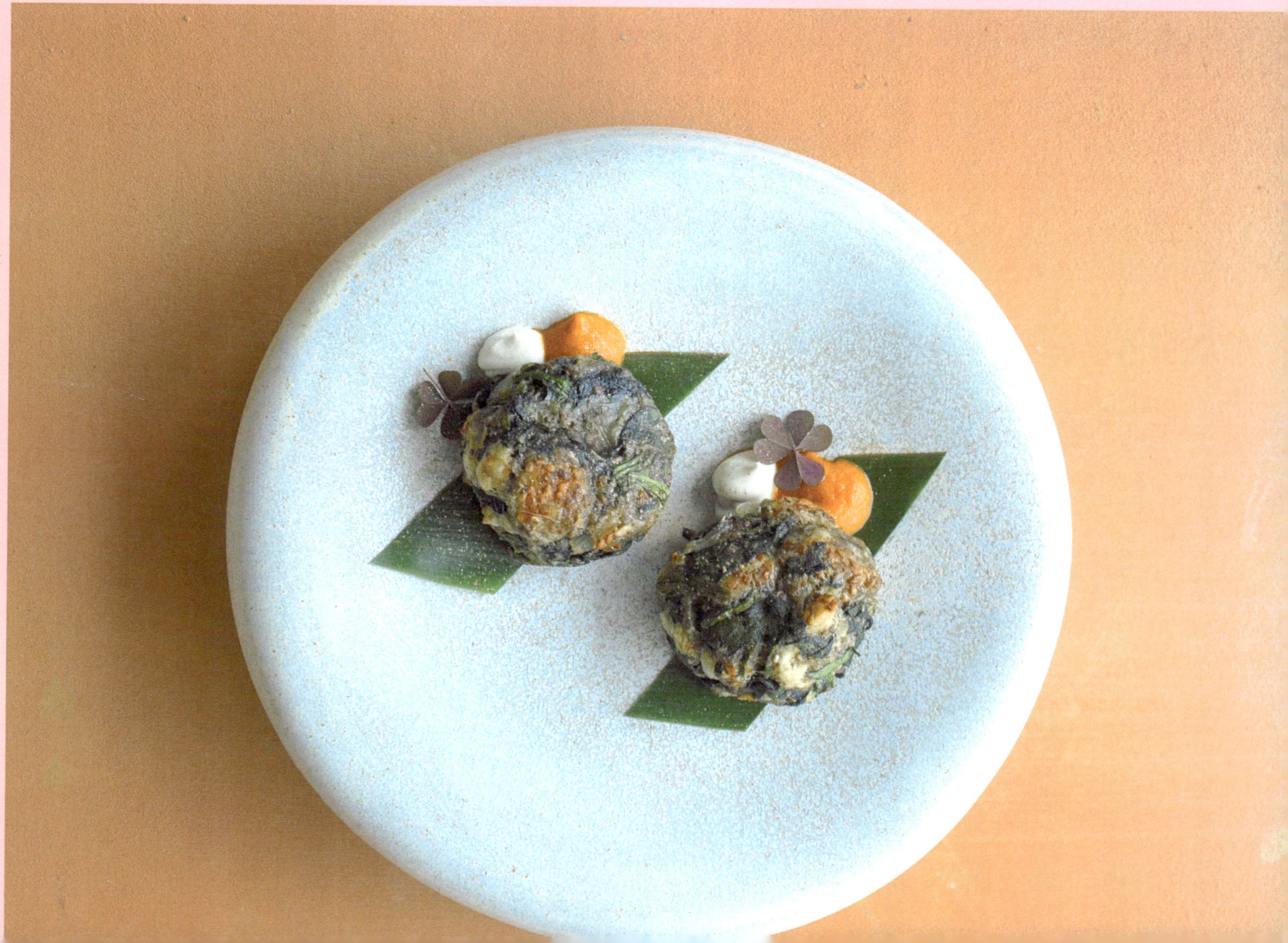

**Serves: 2**

*Soft, tender spinach dumplings meet a silky, vibrant red paprika cream. Each bite is earthy, savory, and bursting with color.*

### Dumplings

250 g stale bread rolls
200 ml almond milk
350 g spinach
1/2 onion
1 clove garlic
1 pinch nutmeg, ground
3 tbsp psyllium husk powder
Olive oil
Salt and pepper to taste

### Red Pepper Cream

1,5 red peppers
1/2 onion
1 clove garlic
2 tbsp tomato paste
2 tsp paprika powder
200 ml cashew cream
300 ml vegetable broth
1 tsp tapioca or carob gum
Olive oil
Salt and pepper to taste

### Cashew Cream

1/2 batch of multi-purpose cashew cream (recipe in pantry chapter)

### Serving

Bamboo leaves
Oxalis

### Dumplings

1.Thaw, squeeze, and chop the spinach.
2.Mix psyllium with a splash of almond milk and let swell.
3.Cut bread rolls into cubes and place in a large bowl.
4. Finely chop onion and garlic; sauté onion in oil, then add garlic and spinach.
5. Add remaining almond milk to the pan and heat briefly.
6. Pour warm milk over bread cubes and soak 10–15 minutes.
7. Prepare the red pepper cream sauce.
8. Add psyllium and spinach to the bread mixture, season with salt, pepper, and nutmeg, and knead. Adjust with breadcrumbs or milk if needed.
9. Form 4–6 dumplings with wet hands.
10. Cook in simmering salted water 15–20 min (or steam 30 min / roast in oven). Serve with red pepper cream sauce and cashew cream.

### Red pepper cream

1. Finely chop the onion and garlic. Core the pepper and cut into thin strips.
2. Fry the onion and pepper in a large pan with a drizzle of olive oil over medium heat. As soon as they start to color, add tomato paste. Roast everything for about 1 minute.
3. Pour in the broth and cream and season with miso & paprika powder. Mix the tapioca with cold water until smooth and add it into the mixture.
4. Let everything simmer for about 5 minutes until the peppers have reached the desired softness. Season with salt and pepper.
5. Transfer to a blender, blend until smooth. Pour into a piping bag.

### Assembly

Line a few small cut bamboo leaves on the baking sheet. Place the dumplings on the bamboo leaves. Use two different piping bags filled with paprika cream and cashew cream and drop sauces next to the dumpling. Decorate with oxalis.

# GREEN RIGATONI

## WITH ZUCCHINI AND TARRGAON PEARLS

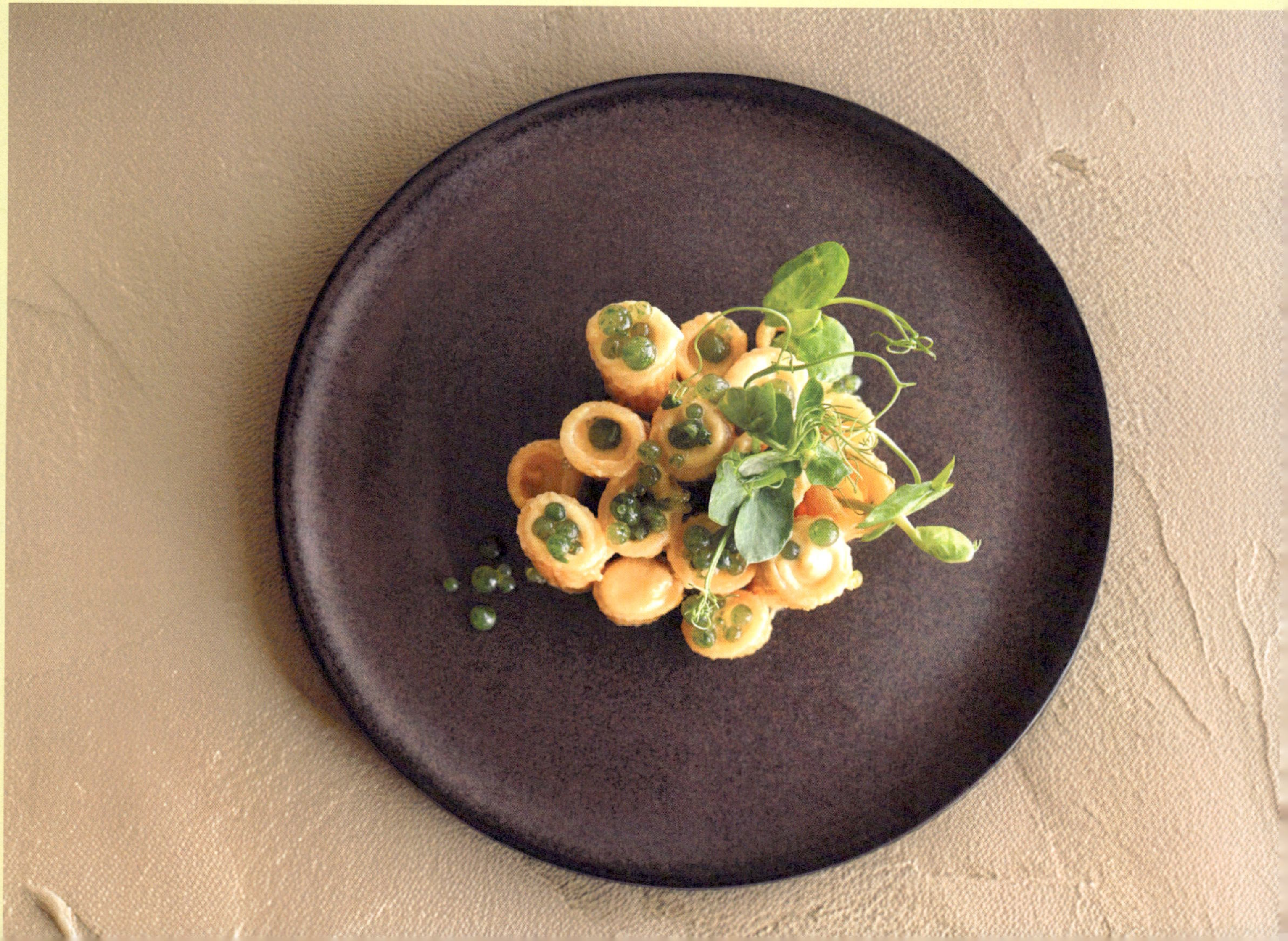

*Silky, fresh, and aromatic. Rigatoni meets zucchini cream, dotted with tarragon pearls and crowned with pea sprouts—a feast for eyes and palate alike.*

**Serves: 4**

350 g gluten-free rigatoni

**Zucchini sauce**

1 large zucchini, chopped (approx. 300 g)
3 shallots, finely chopped
2 cloves garlic, chopped
2 tbsp lemon juice
1/2 tsp salt
1 bay leaf
1 dl pasta water
1 dl vegan parmesan
Black pepper

**Dragon pearls**

15 g fresh tarragon
300 ml olive oil
1 g agar agar
80 ml water

**Serving**

Pea sprouts

1. To make the zucchini cream, fry the garlic, onion, bay leaf and zucchini in a frying pan with olive oil until soft enough. Then remove from the heat transfer to a high-speed blender and mix with lemon juice, pepper, salt and pasta water. Mix together. Then transfer to the pot. Cook until bubbling. Taste it and season with salt and pepper if you need to, then transfer to a piping bag.
2. To make tarragon pearls, put a saucepan of salted water on the stove and bring it to a boil. Clean the tarragon bunch and wash the leaves well. Boil the leaves in boiling water for a few minutes and quickly put them in ice water to keep the green color bright. Then blend the leaves with a blender adding a few drops of cold water to make it liquid. (You may need to strain it to have more smooth consistency) Once the cream is done, pour 1 g of agar-agar per 80 ml of water, bring to the boil. In the meantime, put the oil to cool in the refrigerator in a narrow, tall container.
3. Get a syringe without a needle, draw the tarragon cream and drop it into the cold oil. When the drops touch the bottom of the container, they will have become perfect pearls.
4. Boil the pasta in plenty of water. Then drain it and continue cooking in the pan with a little olive oil. The pasta will release the starch and absorb all the olive oil. Stir in a sprinkle of vegan parmesan and a drizzle of extra virgin olive oil.
5. Place the rigatoni on the plate as shown in the picture. Place the courgette cream in the center of each rigatoni with the help of a pipping pag.
6. Decorate with basil flowers, pea shoots and tarragon pearls as shown in the picture.

PLANT BASED UMAMI

# ZUCCHINI SOUP

## WITH ZOODLES & GINGER GEL

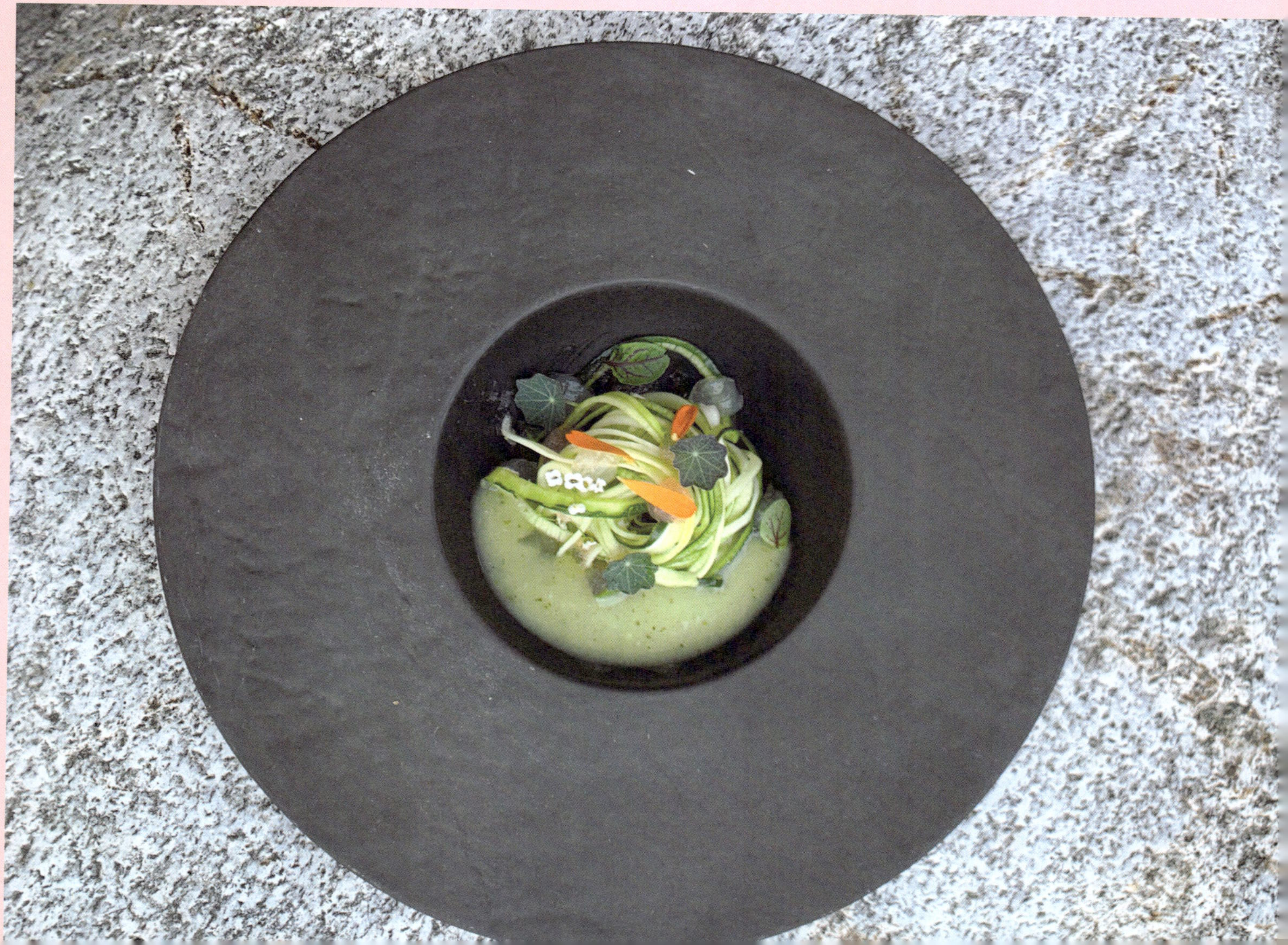

*Crisp zucchini noodles meet velvety zucchini soup, drizzled with aromatic ginger pearl syrup. A refreshing, light, and flavorful plant-based creation that dances between fresh, silky, and subtly spicy—pure summer on a plate.*

**Serves: 2**

**Ingredients**

3 black zucchini
2 large onion
4 garlic cloves minced
4 cm ginger grated
2 tbsp olive oil
Nasturtium leaves to decorate
Alyssum to decorate

**Ginger Gel**

100 ml pear syrup
60 ml ginger syrup
4 g agar agar

1. Using a zucchini spiralizer, spiralize outer parts of your zucchini. Set aside.
2. Cut inner parts of your zucchini into chunks, place in a pot. Chop the onion and transfer to the pot along with grated ginger and minced garlic.
3. Drizzle some olive oil, cook on medium heat stirring constantly for 2-3 minutes. Then cover them with water and bring to boil until soften enough.
4. Next, transfer to a high speed blender, blend until smooth puree.
5. Serve your puree along with spiralized zucchini and ginger gel. Decorate with edible flowers and leaves.

**Ginger Gel**

1. Place ginger and pear syrup in a pan, add agar, whisk together. Bring to boil for 1-2 minutes.
2. Then immediately transfer to a piping bag. It is ready to use.

# ROSEHIP SOUP

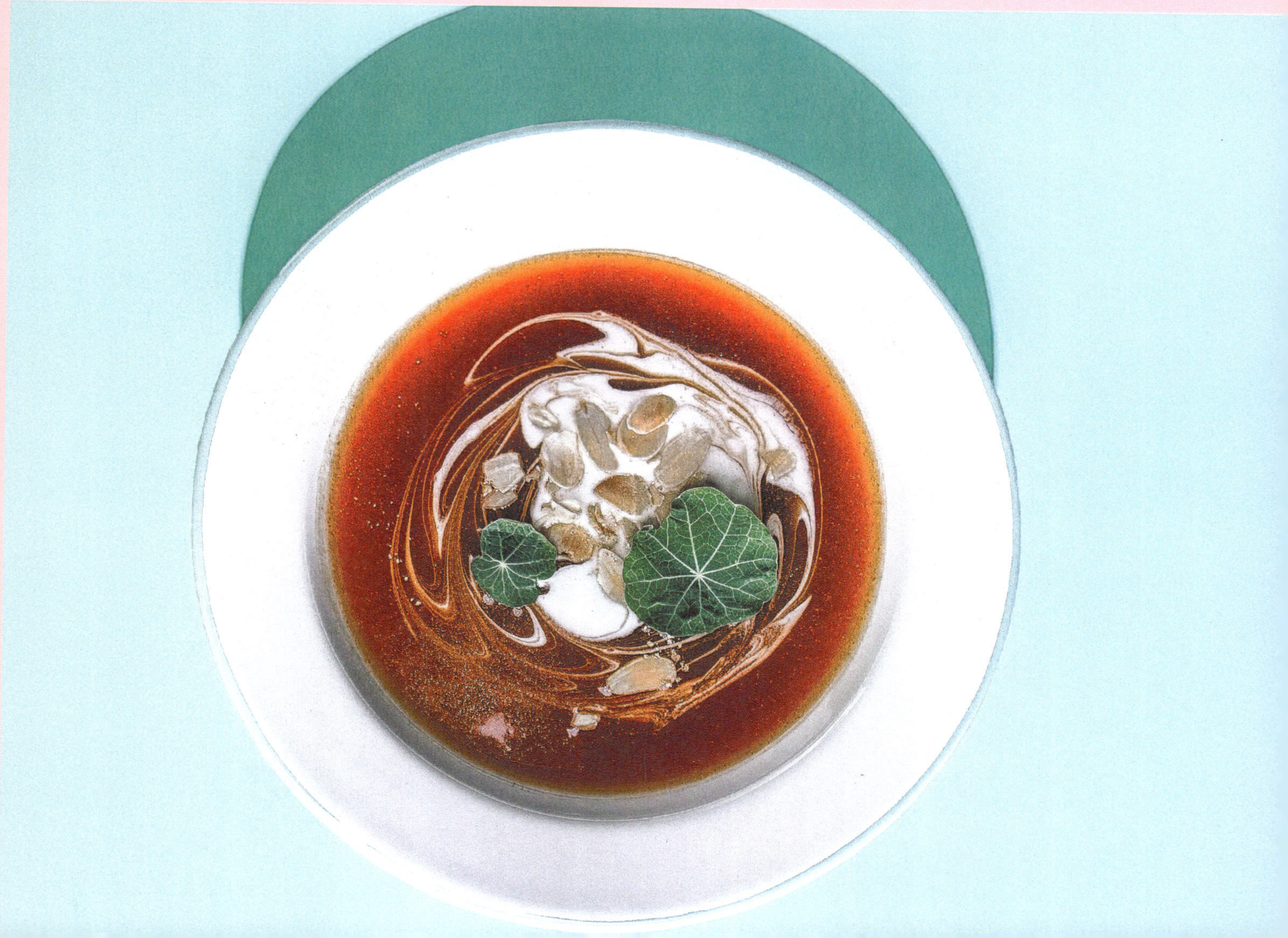

*Vibrant rosehips meet velvety coconut cream, crowned with toasted sliced almonds. A tangy, creamy, and nutty delight that celebrates Nordic flavors in every spoonful—light, elegant, and seasonal.*

**Serves: 4**

**Ingredients**

400 g fresh rosehips
900 ml of cold water
Zest of 1 orange
Zest of 1 lemon
1 fresh lemon juice
1 tsp red vinegar
1 tsp cinnamon powder
1/2 tsp nutmeg powder
1/8 tsp clove powder
2 tbsp maple syrup
3 tbsp sweet, white dessert wine
2-3 tbsp tapioca flour
Whipped coconut cream
Toasted almonds

1. Trim the top and end and cut in half. De-seed and remove fine hairs.
2. Roughly chop and dry in the dehydrator at 46 C for 5 hours or at 50 C in the oven for 3 hours.
3. Use a sieve to separate the shells from the seeds and most importantly from the fine hairs.
4. Add the water to a deep pot, transfer the rosehips, add the orange zest, lemon zest, cinnamon, clove and nutmeg.
5. Bring to a boil, then simmer for at least 5 minutes for the flavours to develop.
6. Add the maple and wine and reheat to a simmer.
7. Add the tapioca, and keep stirring until the soup thickens.
8. Then add a generous splash of fresh lemon juice and more vinegar to taste. Simmer for a few more minutes.
9. Let the soup cool a bit before serving with the whipped coconut cream and toasted almonds.

# MAKI SAKURA

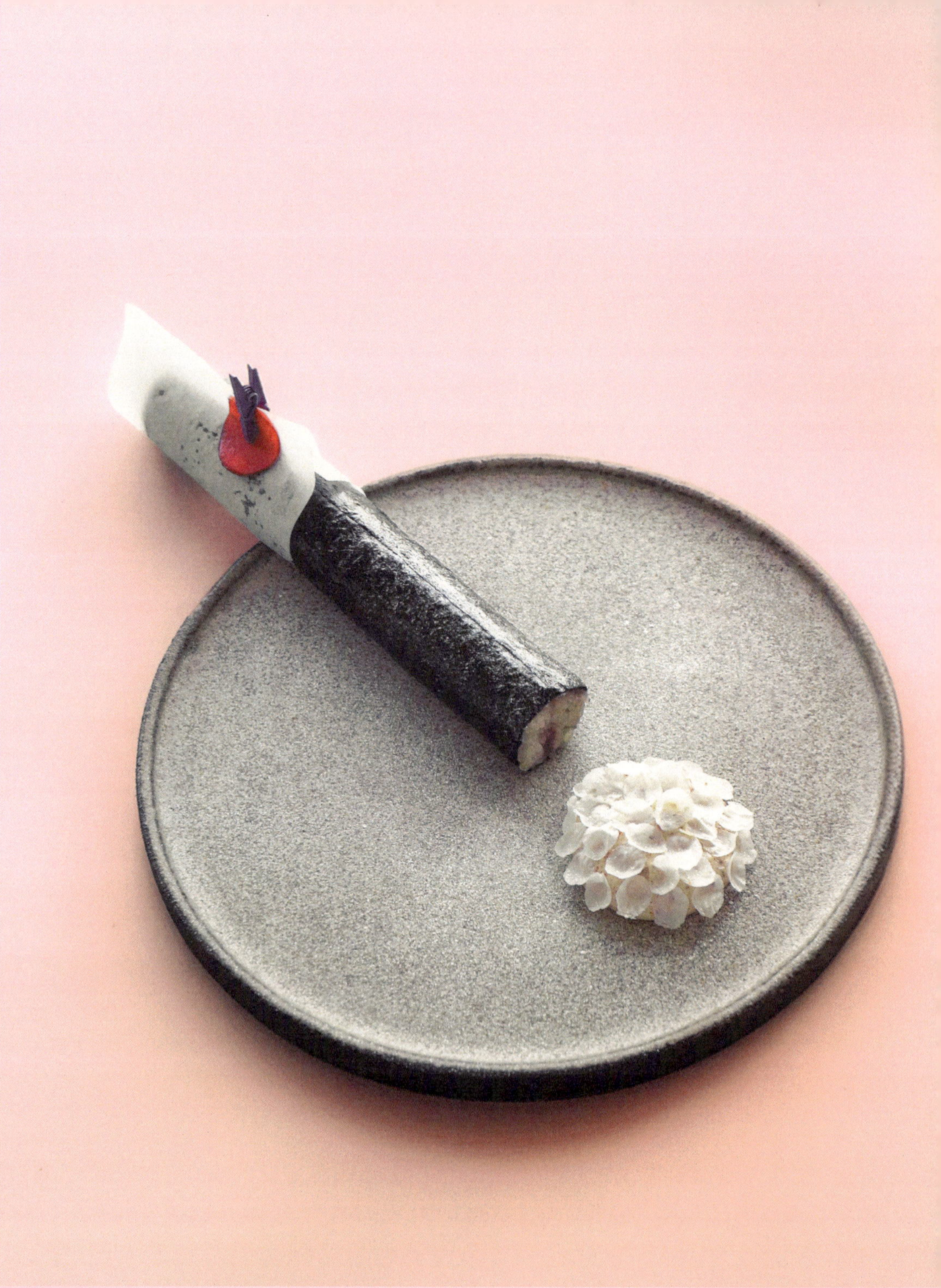

*Delicate pickled sakura provides a subtle floral tang, perfectly balanced with creamy, mildly spicy togarashi mayo. Garnished with aromatic cherry blossoms, each bite is light, fragrant, and layered, offering a refined, seasonal twist on a plant-based maki.*

**Serves: 6**

**Ingredients**

6 nori sheets
1 cup sushi rice
1 1/4 cup water
1 tsp salt
1 tbsp coconut sugar
3 tbsp mirin
1 cup pickled sakura (page 15)
1 cup caramelized red onions
1 cup vegan mayo (page 16)
2 tsp togarashi
Cherry blossoms to decorate

1. Wash your rice, leave to soak in water for 30 minutes.
Cover the pot and bring to the boil and simmer for 10-12 minutes or until all the water have been absorbed.
Remove from heat and leave covered for 10 minutes before serving.
2. Using a spatula spread rice gently over the base of a large bowl. Pour the rice seasoning evenly over the rice and make cutting and folding movements with the spatula to mix it well.
3. Place the nori, spread the sushi rice. Place some caramelized red onions and pickled sakura in the middle. Roll the sushi once (you can also use maki roller to make it quicker).
4. Cut the nori with a sharp knife.
5. Brush your roll wih sesame oil.
6. Place vegan mayo in a bowl, mix with togarashi. Serve your sushi along with togarashi mayo.
7. Decorate with fresh cherry blossom leaves if desired.

# TEMPEH INDO SAMBAL

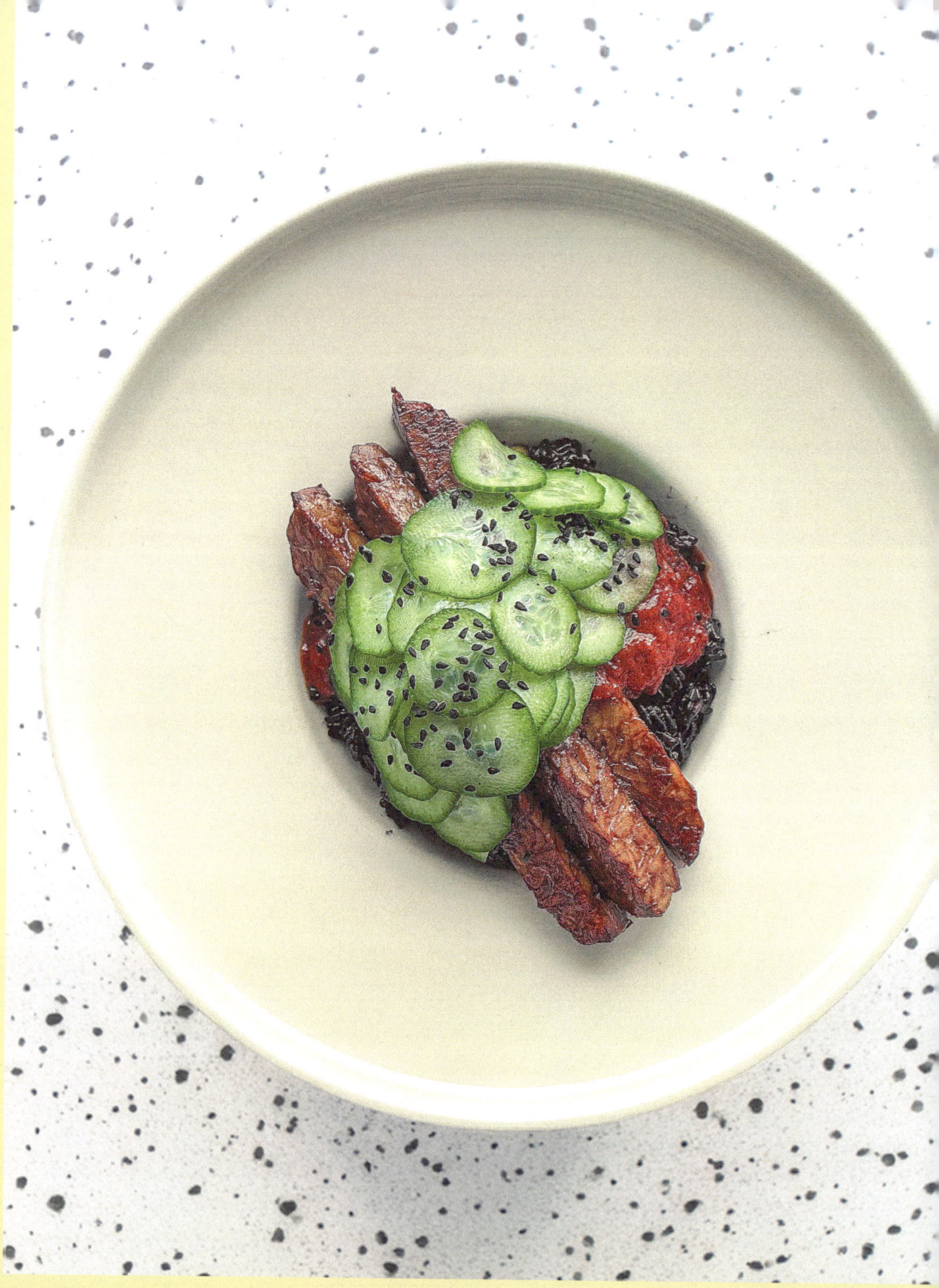

*A vibrant plant-based dish featuring spicy Indo-style tempeh sambal, perfectly balanced with fresh, crisp cucumber for a refreshing crunch. Nutty sesame seeds add texture and depth, while hearty black rice provides an earthy, satisfying base.*

**Serves: 2**

**Ingredients**

1 cup black rice
200 g tempeh cut in 6 pieces
3 tbsp coconut aminos
1 tbsp pomegranate molasses
1 tsp seaweed powder
2 tbsp olive oil
1/2 cup water
2 cucumbers
1/2 tsp pink himalayan salt
2 tbsp black sesame

**Indo sambal**

2 tbsp olive oil
2 shallots chopped
1 red bell pepper diced
1 tbsp vegan Worcestershire (page 20)
1/2 lemon juice
1 tbsp cashews toasted
2 garlic cloves
1 chili pepper chopped
1 tsp grated fresh ginger
1 tsp coconut sugar
1/2 tsp salt

1. In a rectangle container, mix 2 tbsp coconut aminos, 1 tbsp olive oil, 1 tbsp pomegranate molasses, seaweed powder and 1/2 cup water together.
2. Cut your tempeh into long strips and put into marinade liquid. Let it sit in the refrigerator overnight.
3- Cook 1 cup black rice in 3 cups water until absorbs all water content and tender. Then add 1 tbsp coconut aminos and 1 tbsp olive oil, Mix together. Set aside.
4. On a medium heat, cook your tempeh along with marination liquid in a pan. Once it absorbed all water content, add some more water to cover the tempeh, continue to cooking until absorbs all water. Then flip your tempeh strips, drizzle olive oil and fry for 1-2 minutes both sides until golden.
5. Using a mandoline slice, thinly slice your cucumber, place in a bowl, add salt and mix together. Refrigerate for 30 minutes. Then strain the water in the bowl. Set your cucumber aside.
6. To make indo sambal, except lemon juice, place all ingredients in a mortar and pestle until roughly textured thick sauce. Alternatively can be processed in the food processor. Then transfer sauce into a pot, simmer for 5-6 minutes on medium heat. Add a little bit more olive oil and Worcestershire sauce. Adjust the salt if necessary. Lastly add lemon juice and stir together.
7. To serve, place black rice, add tempeh on the top, pour indo sambal. Top with mandolin sliced cucumber and sprinkle some black sesame.

# GLÖGG SPAGHETTI

## WITH BELUGA & CELERIAC SAUCE

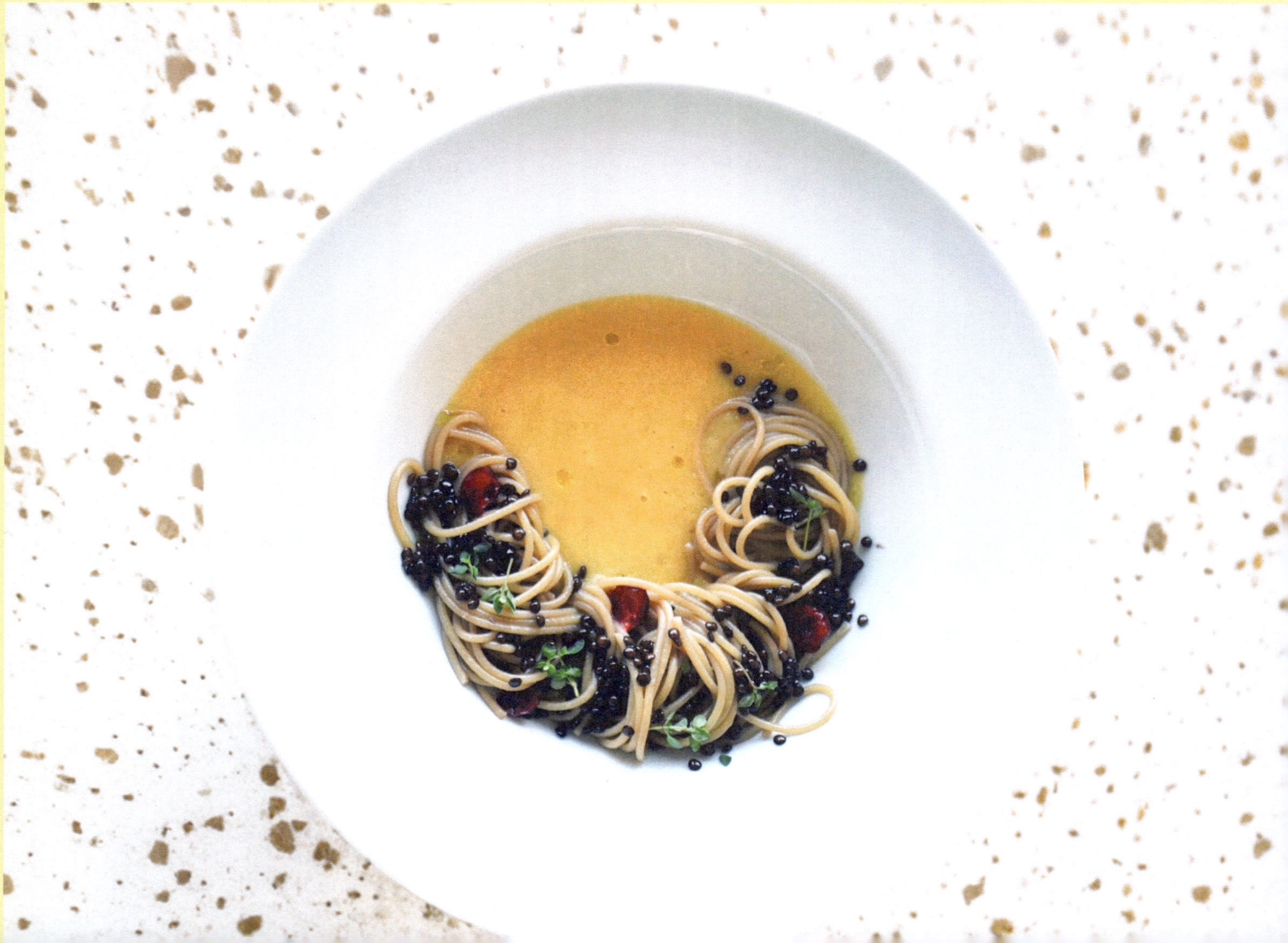

*Featuring spaghetti gently infused with glögg, coated in a silky celeriac cream sauce. Earthy beluga lentils add texture and depth, while vibrant cherries provide a subtle tartness that brightens the dish.*

**Serves: 4**

**Ingredients**

400 g buckwheat soba noodles

**Marinated Beluga**

65 g beluga lentils
130 ml warm glögg (mulled wine)
65 ml water
2 tbsp olive oil
1 tsp salt

**Apple Celeriac Sauce**

45 g carrot
100 g celeriac
50 g onion
100 g red apple
1 tsp yellow pea miso

**Serving**

Fresh thyme
Halved fresh cherries
Vegan parmesan (page 23)

1. Place the mulled wine in a container with the cooked beluga and leave in the fridge for 12 hours.
2. When the time is up, strain the lentils, set aside.
3. Pour the mulled wine sauce you strained into a saucepan. Simmer over medium heat until thick. Set aside.
4. Add a drizzle of oil to a large pan, place over high heat and add the beluga lentils, fry all over until they are a deep golden brown. Season with salt when coloured and remove from the pan. Set aside.
5. Add another drizzle of oil and miso to a new saucepan and add the carrot, celeriac, apple and onion. Cover with water. Cook until soft but not coloured, then add some fresh thyme.
6. Once softened, transfer to a blender with a pinch of salt, lime juice and water if needed. Blend until smooth.
7. Transfer the mixture to a saucepan, cook until bubbling. Then pour into a deep plate.
8. Add your cooked pasta to the mulled wine sauce, drizzle with olive oil and salt, mix well.
9. Transfer to a plate and shape into a crescent shape on the sauce.
10. Top with beluga lentils.
11. Garnish with fresh thyme and halved cherries. Serve with vegan parmesan.

PLANT BASED UMAMI

# GIMBAP

## WITH QUINCE PURÉ & GINGER PEARLS

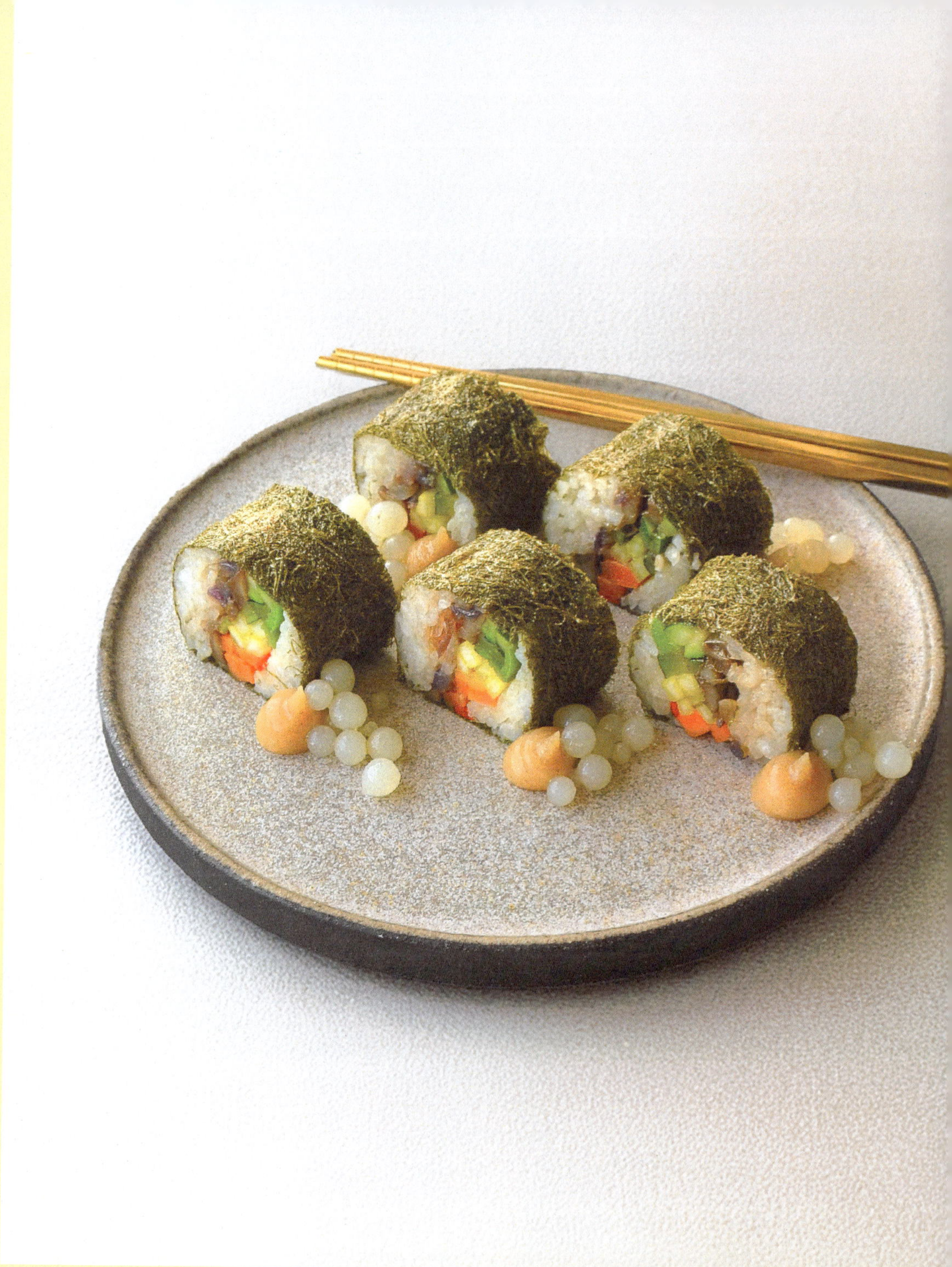

**Serves: 4**

**Ingredients**

4 dl sushi rice

4.5 dl water

1 tsp salt

2 tbsp sesame oil

**Filling**

8 gamtae

1 garlic clove

1 red onion

2 tsp sesame oil

2 tbsp coconut aminos

1/2 takuan cut into long strips

0.5 cucumber

1 carrot

1 red bell pepper

Sesame oil, extra for brushing

2 tbsp sesame seeds

Salt and black pepper

**Quince puré**

500 g quince

250 g coconut sugar

1/4 to 1/2 tsp pink Himalayan salt

**Ginger Pearls**

160 ml pickled ginger juice

4 g agar agar

300 ml cold olive oil

*Savory gamtae paired with seasoned rice and crisp vegetables, creating a bite-sized umami-packed roll.*

1. Prepare the rice. Place the rice in a bowl and let it cool slightly. Add salt and sesame oil and mix well but gently.
2. While the rice is cooking, cut the carrot, bell pepper, onion and cucumber into long strips.
3. Cook the sliced garlic and onion in a pan with a little olive oil and 1 teaspoon of coconut sugar until caramelized. Set aside.
4. Then add long carrots to the pan, add a little water and coconut aminos, cook together and until they are soft enough. Set aside.
5. Repeat the process for the red peppers as well.
6. Cucumbers will be used raw in the recipe, so cut them into long sticks and set aside.
7. Cut the takuan into long matchsticks  and set aside as well.
8. Place a sheet of nori on the sushi mat with the short side facing you and the matte side up.
9. Place a thin layer of rice on the nori sheet, leaving the top 4 centimeters without rice.
10. Place onion, carrot and pepper along the short side, top with cucumber and takuan. Press firmly and roll up the roll.
11. Moisten the rice-free part of the nori sheet with a little water and press to hold the roll together. Brush with sesame oil and sprinkle with sesame seeds. Do the same with all the rolls, then cut into bite-sized pieces.
12. Serve immediately with quince puré and ginger pearls.

**To make ginger pearls,** Place pickled ginger juice in a small pan, add agar powder, bring to a simmer. Transfer to a syringe or dressing bottle. Drop the pearls into cold olive oil in a tall, deep jar.
Then strain the pearls and transfer them to cold water. Then strain and store in a small jar, will keep for up to a week in the refrigerator.

**To make quince puré**, cut them in two places in a pressure cooker. Cover with water. Cook until soft. When cooked, core in the middle. Remove. Place the fleshy part in the blender, add coconut sugar and water as needed, blend together. Add a little salt for a balanced taste.

# TEMPEH

## WITH CHERIMOYA HIBISCUS SAUCE

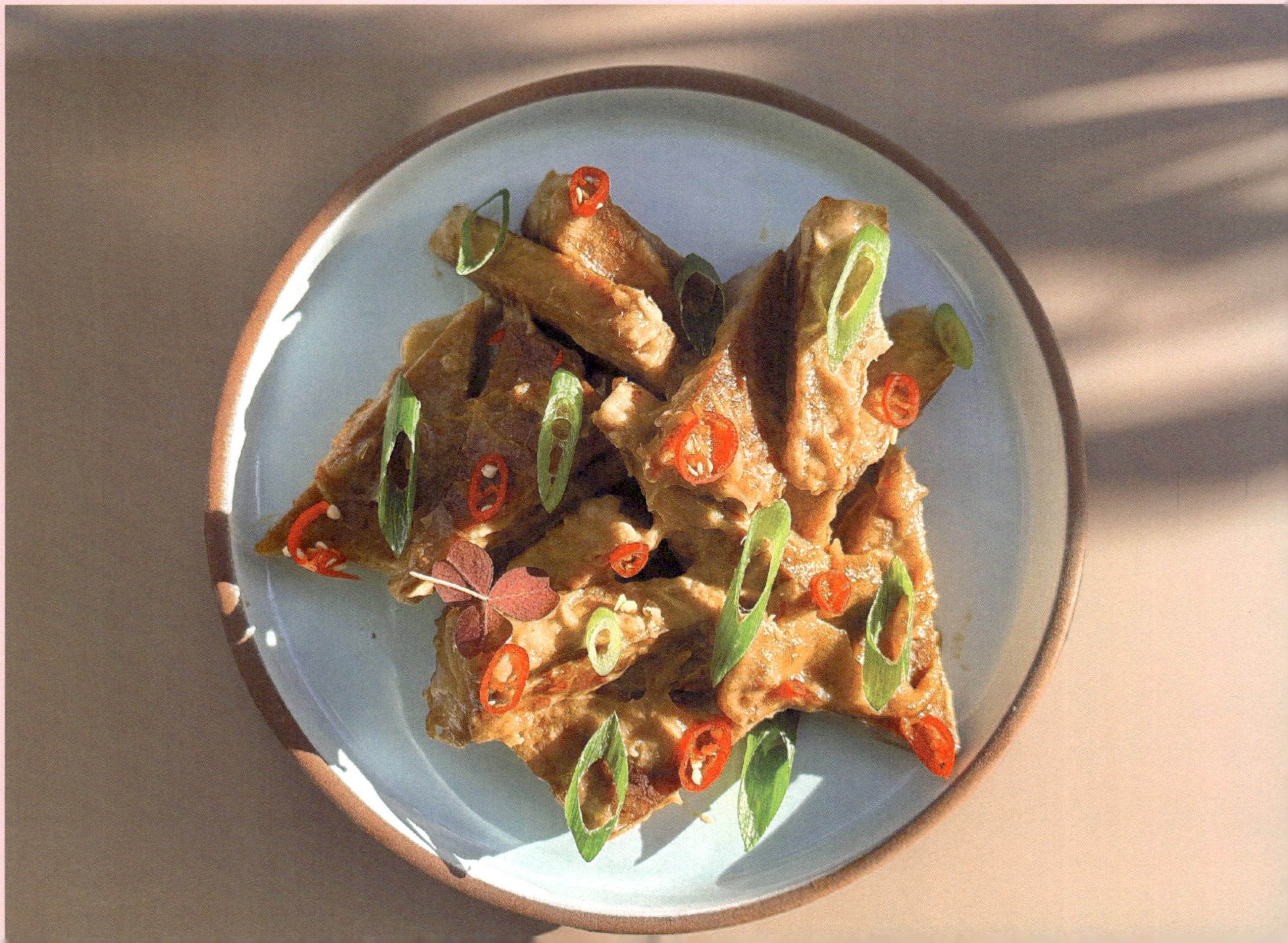

*Imagine biting into tender, golden tempeh that's been given a little extra love. It's coated in a silky, dreamy sauce made from sweet, tropical cherimoya and a touch of floral hibiscus. Fresh chives pop in here and there, adding a crisp, green brightness, while a whisper of spicy chili sneaks in to wake up your taste buds and keep things interesting. Every bite feels like a little adventure on your plate.*

**Serves: 3**

**Ingredients**

300 g yellow pea tempeh cut in small triangles
1/2 dl coconut aminos
1 dl water
1 tbsp olive oil

**Cherimoya Sauce**

300g cherimoya
1/2 cup hibiscus flower
1 large red onion
4 cloves garlic, chopped
2cm grated fresh ginger
1 tbsp coconut aminos
2 tbsp olive oil
1 tsp chili pepper
1-2 cups water to mix
1/2 tsp salt

**Serving**

Green onion, sliced
Fresh chili, thinly sliced
Sorrel to garnish

1. Cut your tempeh into triangles or desired shapes. Place in a container. Add coconut aminos, olive oil and water. Marinate for 3-4 hours or overnight.
2. Clean your cherimoya, remove seeds and skin.
3. Add chopped onion, hibiscus, chopped garlic, shredded ginger and chili over medium heat. Drizzle with a little olive oil. Cook for 1-2 minutes then add a splash of water and continue cooking until all the water has been absorbed. Fry until caramelized.
4. Then add cherimoya flesh and cook for another 2-3 minutes.
5. Add a little water and salt. Transfer the mixture to a blender. Add 1 dl water, plus more if needed to get a smooth consistency. Blend until you get a smooth puree.
6. Place the tempeh on a non-stick pan, add the marinating water. Cook until it softens and absorbs all the marinating liquid.
7. Pour cherimoya sauce over fried tempeh. Mix together.
8. Transfer to a plate, top with sliced green onions. fresh chili and oxalis. Serve with rice or salad if desired.

# POTATO DUMPLINGS WITH COCONUT

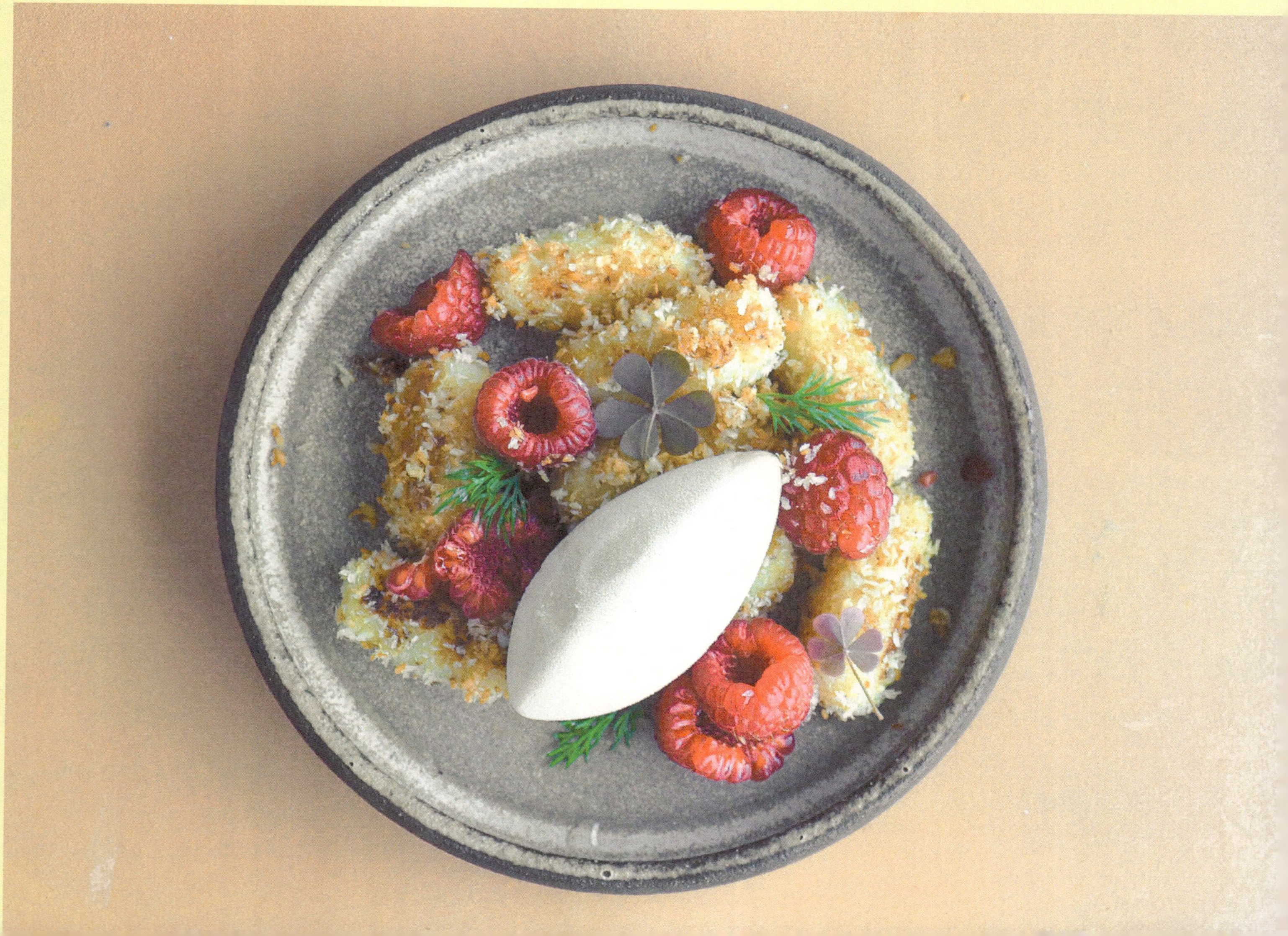

*Soft, pillowy potato dumplings coated in toasted desiccated coconut are paired with creamy, indulgent ice cream and vibrant, juicy raspberries. Each bite delivers a playful contrast of textures and flavors—sweet, creamy, nutty, and fruity—creating a light, yet decadent dessert that is both comforting and visually inviting.*

**Serves: 6**

**Ingredients**

500 g potatoes boiled, peeled, cut into pieces
120 g chickpea flour
60 g tapioca flour
2 tbsp coconut sugar
1/2 tsp sea salt
4 dl desiccated coconut

**For serving**

6 dl icecream
2 dl raspberries
Oxalis
Dill

1. Peel the potatoes, cut into small pieces and boil in salted water for about 15 minutes or until soft. Drain, return to the pot and mash with a potato masher.
2. Add the chickpea flour, tapioca flour, coconut sugar and salt and then knead into a dough with your hands.
3. The dough may still be a little sticky, but should be easy to handle. However, if the dough is too sticky, add more chickpea flour and knead again.
4. Cut the dough into equal-sized pieces and dust with a little tapioca flour.
5. Roll each piece into strands with your fingers. Use a knife to cut the dough into 3-4 cm pieces and shape them into finger-shaped pieces of dough with your hands.
6. Cook them in boiling salted water until they float to the top, about 2 minutes.
7. Heat the oil in a pan and add the dumplings. Fry on one side until golden brown.
8. Then add little bit desiccated coconut on them and toast together.
9. Serve with dill, oxalis, fresh raspberries and vanilla ice cream.

# POTATO PAVÉ

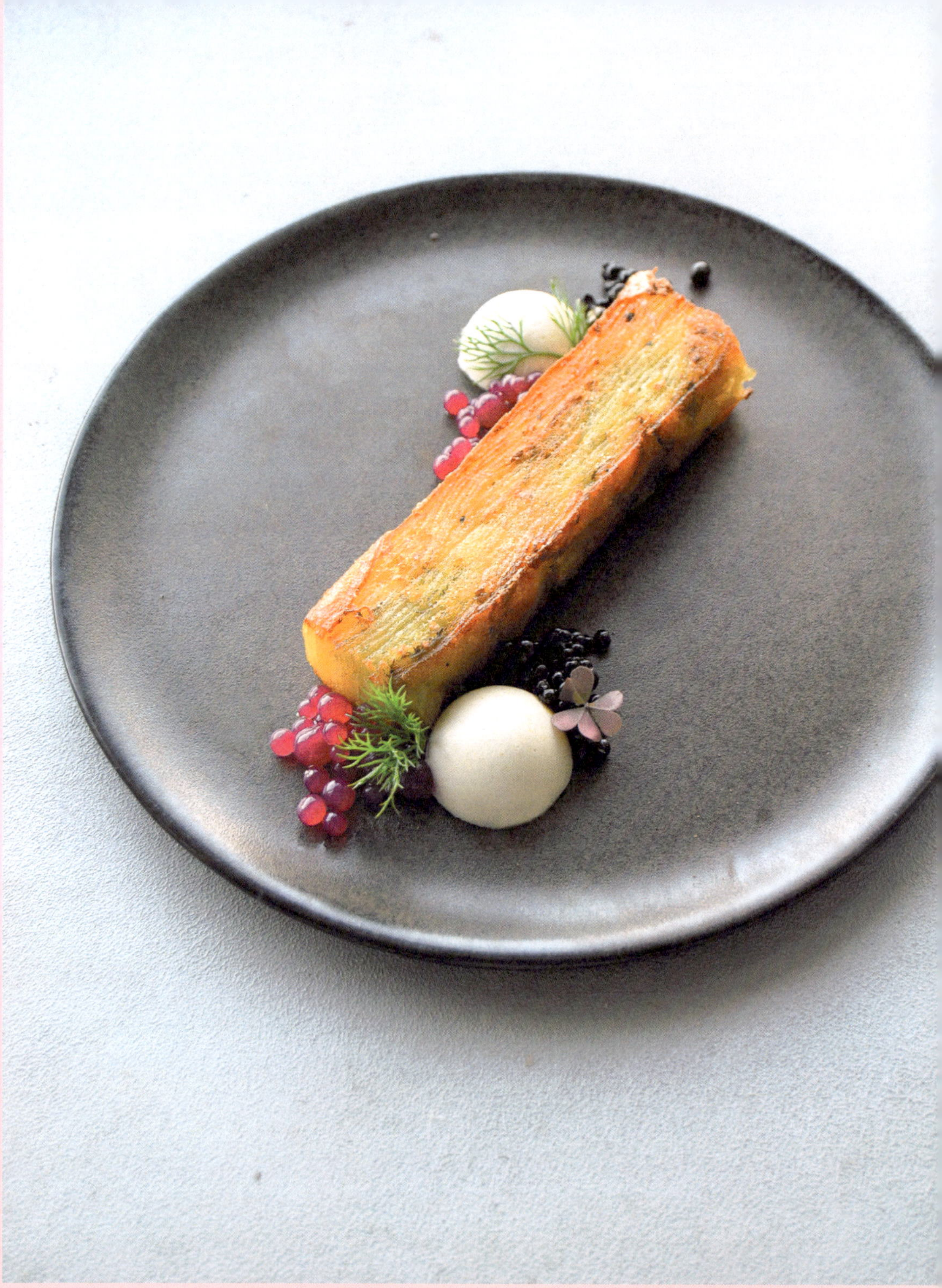

Serves: 4

**Pavé**

1 kg Yukon gold potatoes

200 ml olive oil

Balsamic to brush

**Cashew Cheese Balls**

120 g cashews soaked

150 ml water + more as needed

30 ml lemon juice

2 tbsp olive oil

1 tsp salt

1 tsp mustard

**Coconut Aminos Pearls**

160 ml coconut aminos

4 g agar agar

**Blood Grapefruit Pearls**

160 ml blood grape fruit juice

4 g agar agar

*Thinly layered potatoes, baked to golden perfection, creating a crispy, tender, and elegant side.*

**Pavé**

1. Peel your potatoes and slice on a mandoline as thin as possible. Line a loaf pan with parchment and place down a layer of the potato slices, then brush with olive oil. Repeat this layering until all the potato has been used.
2. Cover the loaf pan with a lid or foil and bake for 1 hour 20 minutes or so, until the potato is tender. Allow to cool.
3. Cut a sheet of parchment to lay on top of the terrine in the loaf pan and top with a heavy weight so that the terrine will compact and become stable for slicing.
4. Refrigerate overnight with the weight on top.
5. Remove the weights from the Potato Pavé, unmould and trim the edges if you prefer.
6. Slice lengthwise into pieces.
7. Place the pieces onto a parchment-lined baking sheet, brush some balsamic and warm gently in the oven for about 20 minutes.
8. Serve with cashew cheese balls, coconut aminos pearls and blood grapefruit pearls.

**Cashew Cheese Balls**

1. Place all ingredients in a food processor, blend until smooth.
2. Transfer to 3cm half sphere molds.

**Coconut Aminos Pearls**

1. Place coconut aminos in a small pan, add agar powder, bring to a simmer. 2. Transfer to a syringe or dressing bottle. Drop the pearls into cold olive oil in a tall, deep jar.

3. Then strain the pearls and transfer them to cold water. Then strain and store in a small jar, will keep for up to a week in the fridge.

**Blood Grapefruit Pearls**

1. Place blood grapefruit juice in a small pan, add agar, bring to a boil. Transfer to a syringe or dressing bottle. Drop the pearls into cold olive oil in a tall, deep jar.
2. Then strain the pearls and transfer them to cold water. Then strain and store in a small jar, will keep for up to 2-3 days in the fridge.

# APPLE TERRINE

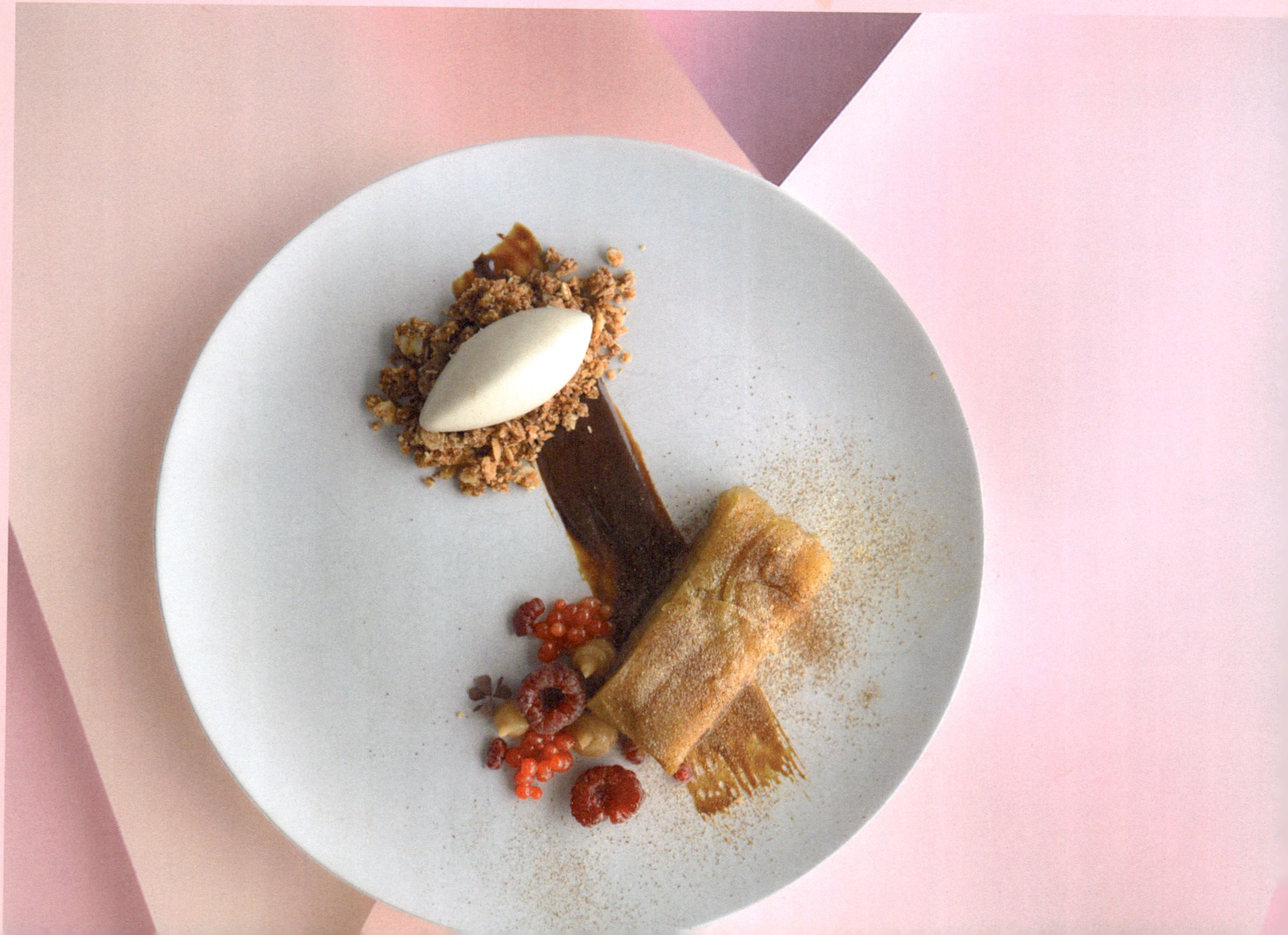

**Apples**

2 kg golden apples mandoline sliced
30 ml maple syrup
30 ml lemon juice
1 tsp vanilla
1 tsp gingerbread spice blend

**Coconut Caramel**

100 g coconut sugar
300 ml full fat coconut milk

**Cashew Coconut Cream**

150 g cashews soaked
100 ml coconut milk
50 ml coconut cream
50 ml maple syrup
30 g coconut oil melted
15 ml cacao butter melted

**Oat Crumble**

120 g rolled oats
75 g coconut oil
25 g almond flour
100 g coconut sugar
1 tsp cinnamon
1/8 tsp cardamom
1/4 tsp pink himalayan salt

**Pearls**

160 ml beetroot juice
15 ml maple syrup
4 g agar agar powder

**For serving**

Oxalis
Fresh Raspberries
Quince Puré (page 49)

**Apples**

1. Thinly slice the apples and place in the lemon juice.
2. Put the lemon juice in a bowl. Add the maple, vanilla and spices to the apples and stir to fully coat.
3. Place a layer of apples in the bottom of the tin. Keep layering until all the apple is used up.
4. Cover the dish with foil and bake in a preheated oven at 180 C for 1 hour and 30 minutes.
5. Remove the foil and cook for a further 30 minutes. Allow to cool with the foil loosely placed on top. Cover the top with foil and place a couple of tins on top to compress the apples. Leave in the refrigerator overnight before turning out and serving.

**Coconut Caramel**

1. Combine all ingredients in a medium saucepan. Bring to a boil. Let it boil for around 3-4 minutes, stirring continuously, then lower to a simmer.
2. Let it simmer—stirring as needed—until it cooks down to about half its volume and thickens.
3. Turn off the heat, stir in the vanilla, and let it sit for about an hour. Cover and refrigerate overnight – it continues to thicken as it sits.

**Cashew Coconut Cream**

1. Place all ingredients in the blender except oils, blend until smooth.
2. Lastly add the melted oils, and blend again.
3. Pour mixture over quenelle molds. Freeze at least 1 hour.

**Oat Crumble**

1. Place all ingredients in a baking pan, toss well together.
2. Bake at 150 C for 25-30 minutes or until golden brown.

**Pearls**

1. Fill a tall glass with olive oil and freeze for 1-2 hour. In a small sauce-pan, mix beetroot juice, maple and agar powder together, bring to boil.
2. Then immediately transfer to a piping bottle. Drop the pearls in cold olive oil glass. Then strain and keep in a small jar in the fridge.
3. Arrange the components on the plate as shown in the picture.

# LIONS MANE & PADRONS

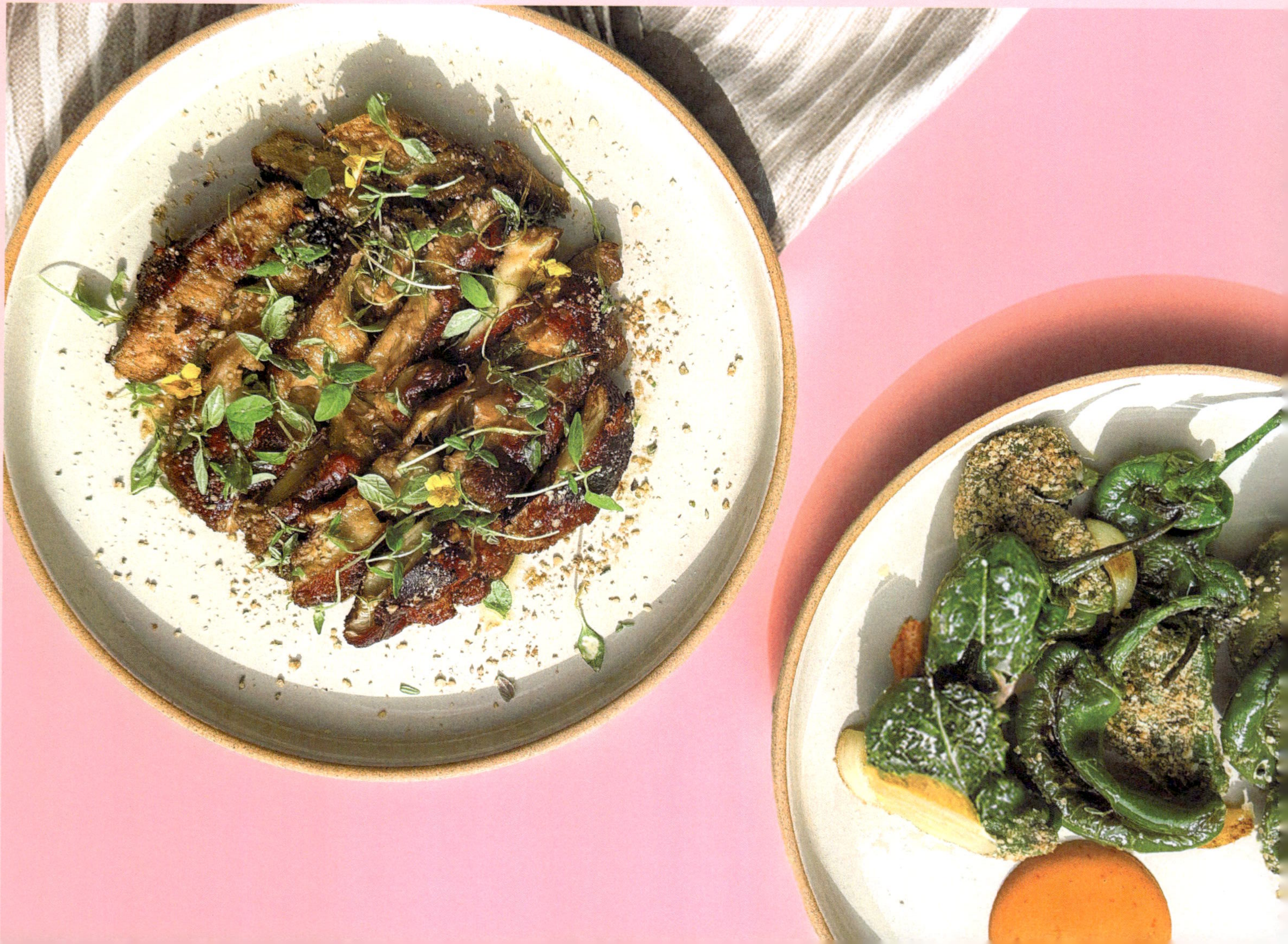

*Meaty lion's mane mushrooms, lightly sautéed to develop a golden, tender texture reminiscent of seafood. Accompanied by Padrón peppers, which offer a delicate smokiness with occasional gentle heat, this dish is finished with a drizzle of spicy, tangy sriracha sauce that adds depth and complexity.*

**Serves: 2**

**Ingredients**

300 g lions mane mushrooms
3 cloves garlic
2-3 sprigs of thyme
2-3 tbsp olive oil
Black pepper and salt

**Padrons**

20 pimiento de padron
2 tbsp olive oil
1 tsp flaked salt
50 g vegan parmesan (page 23)

**For serving**

Lemon
Sriracha (page 17)

**Lion´s Mane**

1. Since the mushrooms are grown without soil, they do not need to be cleaned.
Cut the mushrooms into slices about 1.5 cm.
2. Fry the mushroom pieces like meat in a hot pan with olive oil, garlic and thyme.
3. Season with salt and plenty of black pepper. Turn and fry the mushroom pieces until golden brown on both sides. Press firmly until the mushrooms are browned and pressed to less than half their original thickness, about another 5 minutes.

**Padrons**

1. Fry the small peppers in the oil in a hot frying pan. They should get a lot of color. Stir occasionally.
2. Season with salt flakes. Top with hemp parmesan when serving.
3. Serve with sriracha mayo and lemon wedges.

PLANT BASED UMAMI

# MUSHROOM QUICHE

## WITH JERUSALEM ARTICHOKE PURÉ

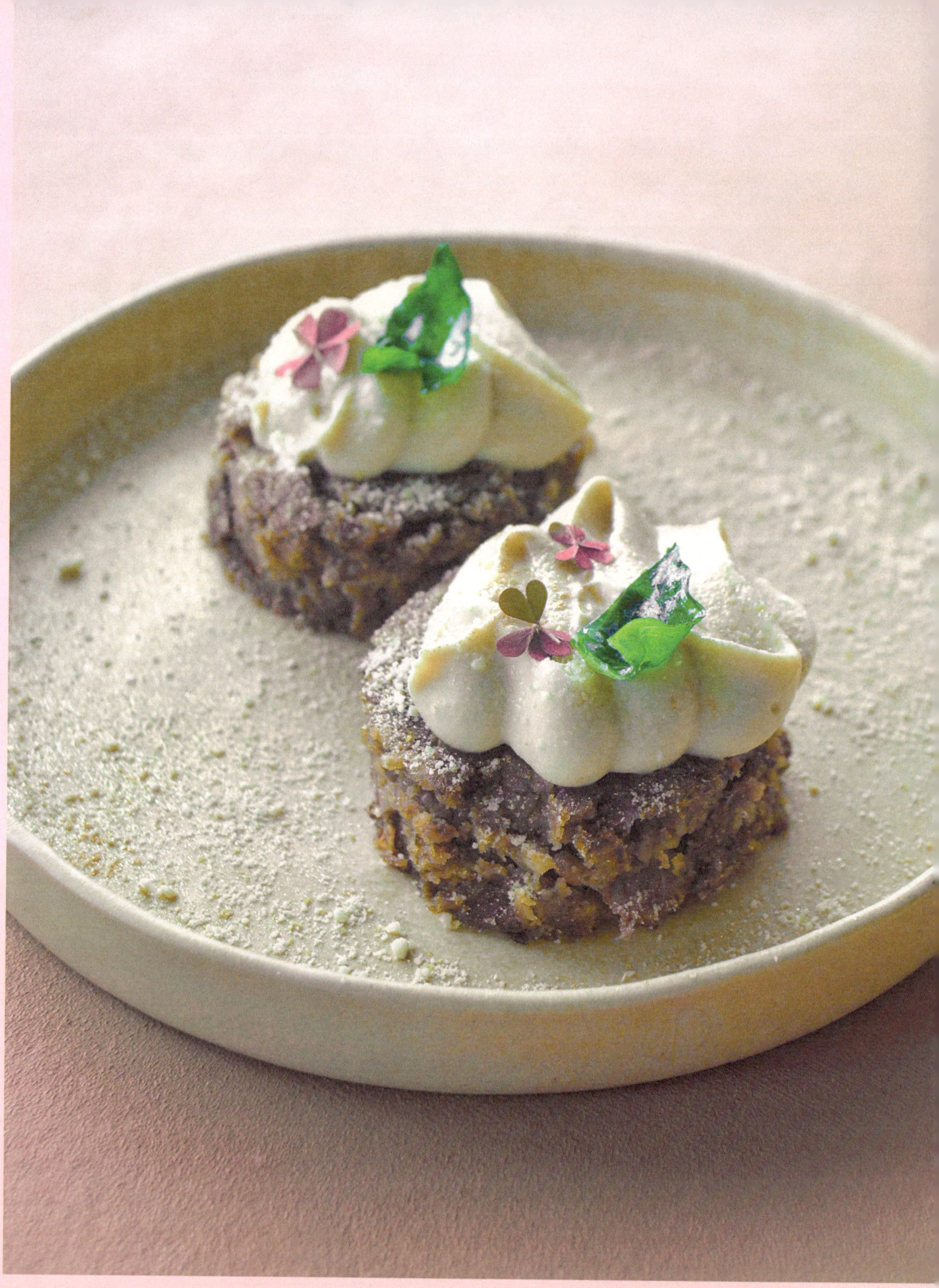

*Earthy mushrooms and crunchy walnuts meet tender quiche, topped with silky artichoke cream and crisp Brussels sprouts.*

**Serves: 5**

**Ingredients**

1 cup walnut flour
1/4 cup chopped walnuts
1 cup rice flour
1/2 cup tapioca flour
1/2 cup oat milk
300 g mushrooms diced
1 onion finely diced
4 garlic cloves minced
1/4 cup chopped olives
2-3 tbsp coconut aminos
2 tbsp olive oil
1 tsp umami mixture (page 23)

**To serve**

1 cup multi-purpose cashew cream (page 18)
1/4 cup jerusalem artichoke purée or 1 tbsp white miso
Parmesan topping (page 23)

**To decorate**

Pan-fried brussels sprout leaves
Red oxalis

1. Place diced onion, mushrooms, olives, garlic, coconut aminos and olive oil in a pan, saute until cooked enough.
2. In a bowl, mix walnut flour, rice flour, tapioca, umami mixture and chopped walnuts together. Then add the sauted mushrooms and onions. Mix together. Add oat milk + more as needed and knead until you get a dough like texture.
3. Transfer dough into a 15 cm round cake tin lined parchment paper. Bake at 200 C for 20-30 minutes until the top gets brown. Let it cool for 20 minutes before unmould. Then using a 4- 5 cm round cake mold, cut your quiche into small circles.
4. In a food processor, mix 1 batch cashew cream with jerusalem artichoke puree or white miso. Let it cool for 2 hours, then transfer to a pipping bag, decorate the quiche rings.
5. Sprinkle some parmesan topping on the top. Decorate with brussels sprouts chips (to make it just, brush with olive oil and bake in the oven until crispy) and oxalis if desired.

# PAPRIKA SOUP WITH ROASTED OLIVES

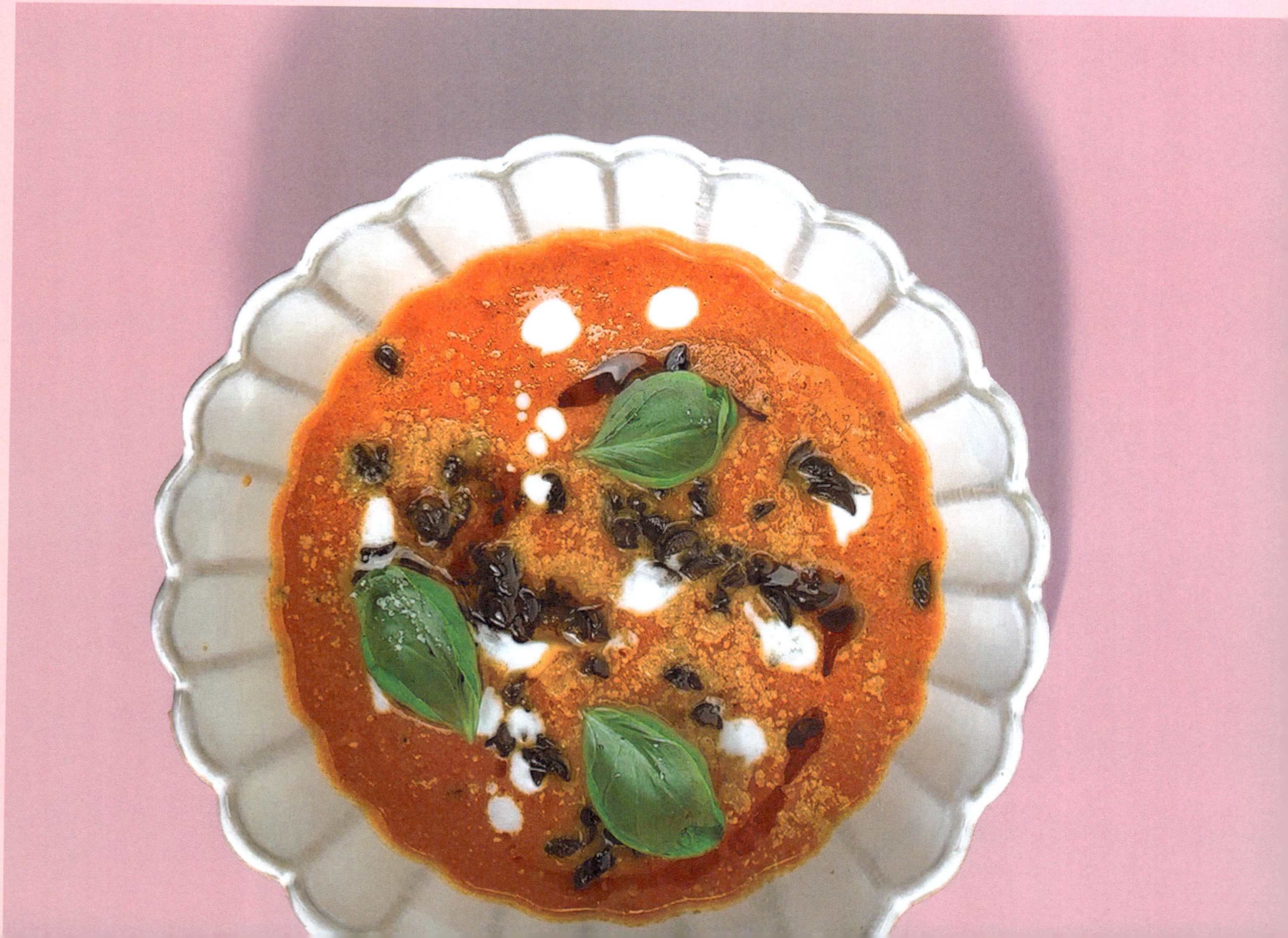

*A vibrant, plant-based soup that delights the senses with its smoky, sweet roasted paprika base, complemented by the briny richness of olives. Silky coconut cream adds a smooth texture, while vegan parmesan brings depth and a subtle umami note with the olives. Smoky, creamy, savory, and slightly tangy—all in a single comforting bowl.*

**Serves: 3**

**Ingredients**

4 red peppers
4 large tomatoes
1 large red onion
6 dl water
2 tbsp olive oil
2 dl coconut cream
Salt and black pepper

**For serving**

70 g olives, pitted and finely chopped
Parmesan topping (page 23)
Basil
Chili oil

1. Preheat the oven to 200 C.
2. Place the red pepper, onion, garlic and tomatoes on a baking sheet with olives, salt, pepper and olive oil.
3. Roast in the oven for about 40 minutes at 200 degrees.
4. Remove from the plate and scoop out the roasted vegetables and mix in a blender until smooth.
5. Season with salt and pepper.
6. Return the soup to the pot and add the coconut cream, cook for about 2-3 minutes until well mixed.
7. Chop your olives, on a non-stick pan, with a little olive oil, fry them. You can also roast them in the oven.
8. Serve with parmesan topping, finely chopped olives, basil, chili oil and a little extra coconut cream.

# JACKFRUIT CUTLETS

## WITH MAYO, CAPERS AND CHILI

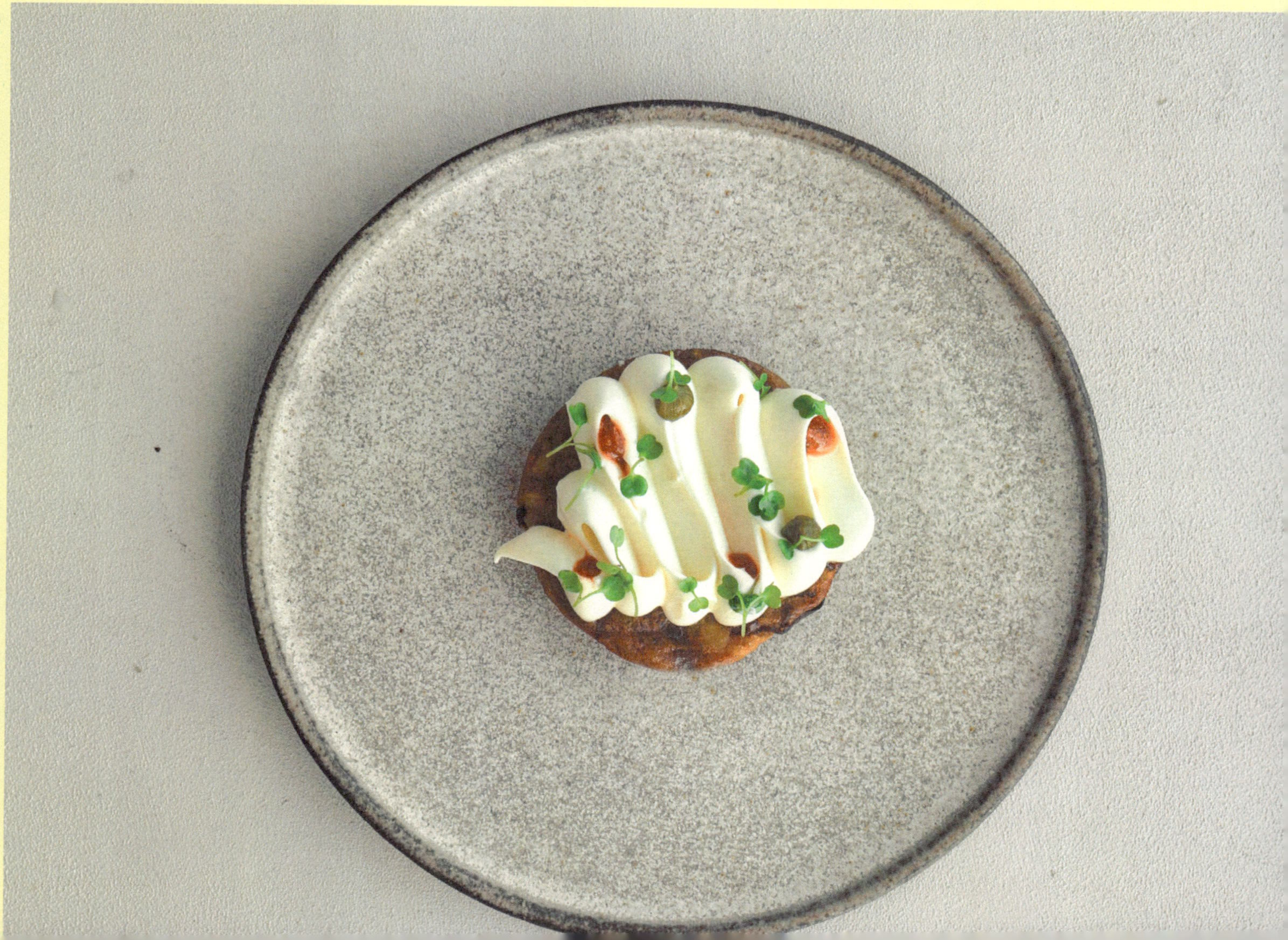

*Tender, shredded jackfruit cutlets are lightly crisped to perfection, offering a meaty, satisfying texture. Finished with creamy mayo, briny capers, and a hint of spicy chili, each bite delivers a harmonious balance of savory, tangy, and mildly fiery flavors.*

**Serves: 4**

**Ingredients**

170 g pulled young jack fruit cooked
120 g boiled potatoes
80 g cooked white beans
1/4 cup finely chopped green olives
2 tbsp tapioca flour
1 tbsp olive oil for brushing
1/4 tsp red chilli powder
2 cloves garlic, chopped
3 tbsp mushroom sauce or coconut aminos
1/2 bunch scallions, chopped
1 tsp pink Himalayan salt

**For serving**

Capers
Chili sauce
Microgreens
Plant-based mayonnaise (page 16)
100 g cooked rice (optional)

1. Boil your potatoes until soft. Once cooked, peel and mash with a fork.
2. Pull the cooked jackfruit with your fingers so that it looks shredded instead of mashed.
3. Combine both jackfruit, olives, cooked beans and mashed potatoes in a bowl, add tapioca flour, salt to taste, chopped garlic, scallions, coconut aminos and red chili powder.
4. Mix well, shape them into round cutlets using a 5-6 cm ring mold with push handles. Then refrigerate for 1 hour before cooking.
5. Brush a little oil on both sides of the cutlets before placing them on the baking sheet lined with baking paper. Bake in the oven at 200 C with fan for 15-20 minutes or until crispy and golden brown.
6. Top with plant-based mayonnaise, capers, chili sauce and microgreens, serve with rice if desired or as a side dish.

PLANT BASED UMAMI

# OAT CAROB THINS

## WITH CHESTNUT & ROSEHIP MARMELADE

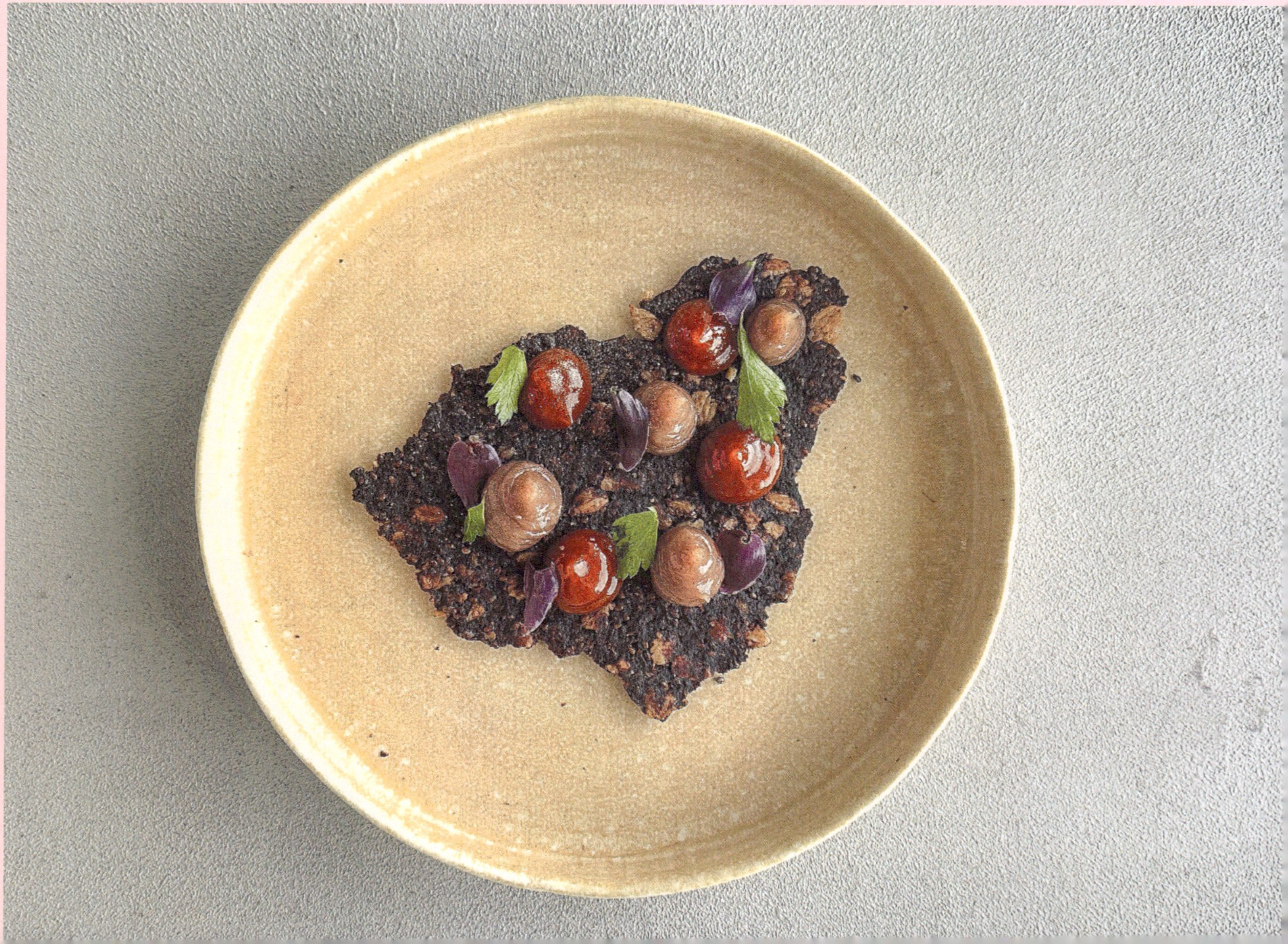

**Serves: 6**

**Oat Biscuits**

65 g oats
50 g flaxseed
30 g sunflower seeds
50 g almond flour
15 g psyllium husk powder
65 g date paste
25 g carob powder
20 g coconut sugar
30 ml olive oil
130 ml warm water
2 g pink Himalayan salt

**Chestnut Jam**

300 g chestnuts
30 g coconut sugar
50 ml water
1/4 tsp pink Himalayan salt

**Rosehip Jam**

300 g rosehips
2 apples cored and peeled
200 g coconut sugar
1 lemon juice

**Oat Biscuits**

1. Place oats, flaxseed, sunflower seeds, almond flour, psyllium husk powder, carob powder, coconut sugar and salt in a bowl. Mix together.
2. Then add date paste, olive oil and hot water. Mix to combine well. Let the dough rest for 5 minutes.
3. Then divide in half. Between two sheets of baking paper, roll out the dough thinly.
4. Repeat the process for the rest of the dough. Bake at 150 C for 35-40 minutes, turning the biscuits at the end of baking and keeping in the oven for another 5-10 minutes if necessary.

**Chestnut Jam**

1. Cut the chestnuts across the top and place in a saucepan. Fill with enough cold water to cover the chestnuts and place over medium heat. Cook for 30-35 minutes. They are ready when they are no longer chalky and difficult to break apart.
2. Peel them as quickly as you can, without burning yourself as it is much easier to remove the skins while they are still quite warm.
3. In a food processor fitted with an S blade, crush the chestnuts and add the sugar. Process until a crumbly consistency is formed.
4. Add the water and process until you have a puree consistency. Set aside.

**Rosehip Jam**

1. Wash the rose hips well and drain, cut off the ends and tails, remove any leaves, otherwise the green tails and leaves can give them a bitter taste. Chop roughly and place in a saucepan and cover with 250ml water.
2. Add the zest of half a lemon.
3. Cook slowly, partially covered, until they are soft. Check the hips by picking one and letting it cool, squeezing it between your fingers if it breaks and has a soft consistency. You can do one of two things; pulse the hips and water in a blender to break them up, strain or just mash with a potato masher and then strain. Coarsely grate the apples.
4. Now put the strained liquid back into the saucepan and add the grated apple with the lemon juice.
5. Now add the sugar. Stir over a low heat until the sugar has dissolved. Increase the heat and continue cooking for about 30 minutes.
6. Place the jam jars in the oven to sterilize. Then let them cool overnight.

# FINGER FOOD

PLANT BASED UMAMI

# FLOURLESS SWEET POTATO CANNELLONI

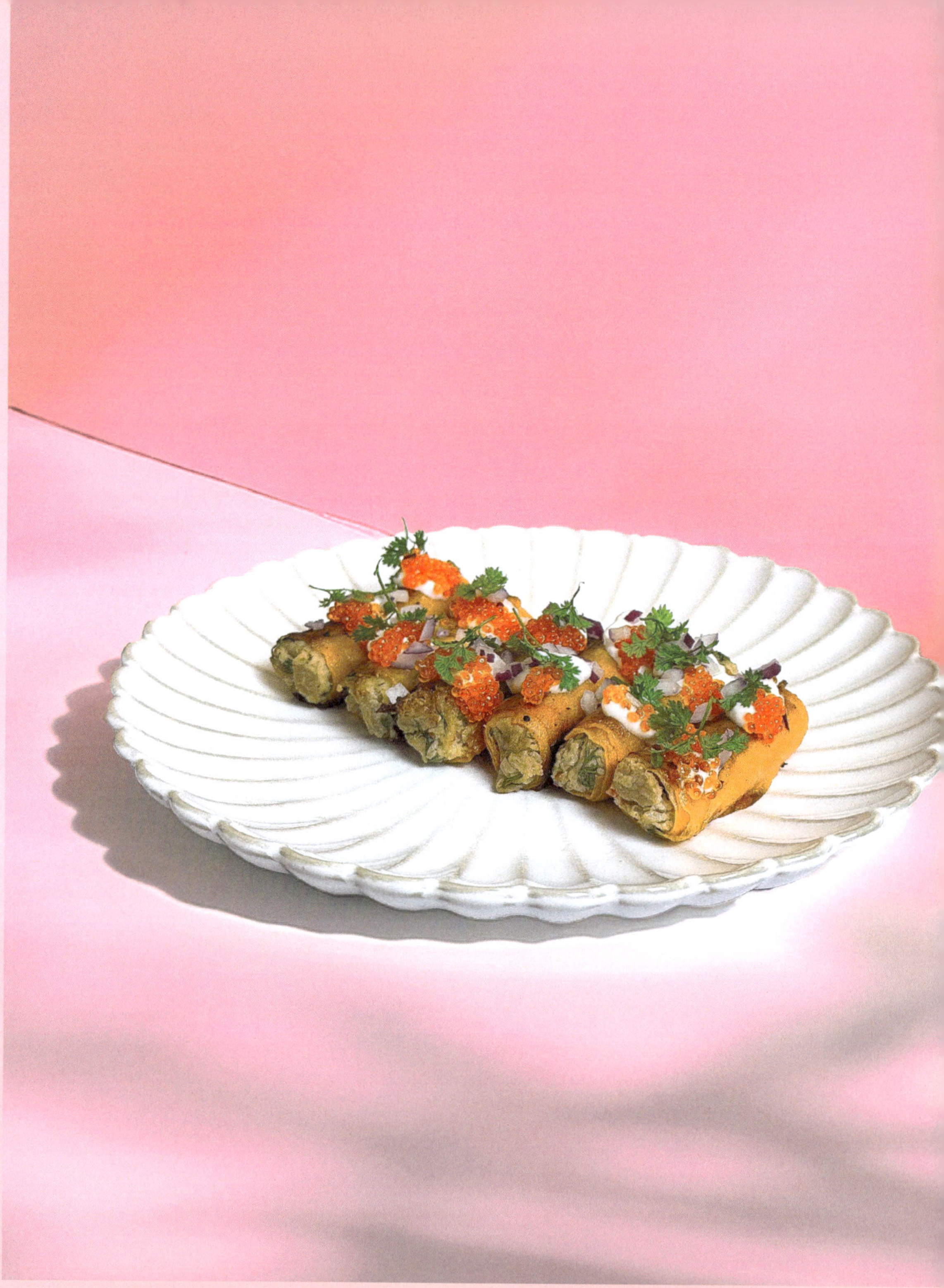

*Thin sheets of roasted sweet potato take the place of traditional pasta, creating a naturally gluten-free, subtly sweet small wrap bites that hold a creamy, briny filling. Inside, the classic Swedish Skagen mix is reimagined with tender jackfruit, delicately seasoned to evoke the taste of the sea while staying entirely plant-based.*

**Serves: 4**

**Ingredients**

250 g sweet potato (sliced into sheets using a chiba tsumataro or vegetable sheet cutter)

**Filling**

350 g young jackfruit
120 g vegan mayonnaise (page 16)
1 tsp seaweed mix (nori, dulse, wakame)
1/4 cup finely chopped red onion
1/2 tbsp dijon mustard
2 tbsp capers
1/4 cup chopped celery stalks
1 tbsp lemon juice
1/2 tsp garlic powder
1 tbsp coconut aminos
1/2 tsp apple cider vinegar
1/2 bunch fresh dill
Salt to taste

**Serving**

Chopped red onion
Chives
Seaweed caviar
Chervil
Plant-based yogurt (page 17)

1. Preheat the oven to 200 degrees.
2. Cut the jackfruit into small pieces, fry in a pan with a little olive oil.
3. Place the jackfruit in a large bowl and mash them with a fork.
4. Add the vegan mayonnaise, finely chopped red onion, seaweed mixture, lemon juice, finely chopped capers, garlic, chopped celery stalk, coconut aminos, Dijon mustard, dill, vinegar and salt and pepper.
5. Place the jackfruit stems at one end of the sweet potato lasagna sheet. Roll up and then place the cannelloni seam side down on a baking sheet lined with parchment paper. Repeat with all the sheets.
6. Just before they go into the oven, brush them with water. Place in the oven and let them bake for 10 minutes. Remove the sheet and brush them with water again. Place back in the oven and let them finish cooking for about 5-7 more minutes.
7. Place 6-7 cannelloni on each plate. Top with yoghurt, chopped red onion, chives, seaweed caviar and chervil.

PLANT BASED UMAMI

# PEACH SALSA

## WITH TEMPEH AND SALAD

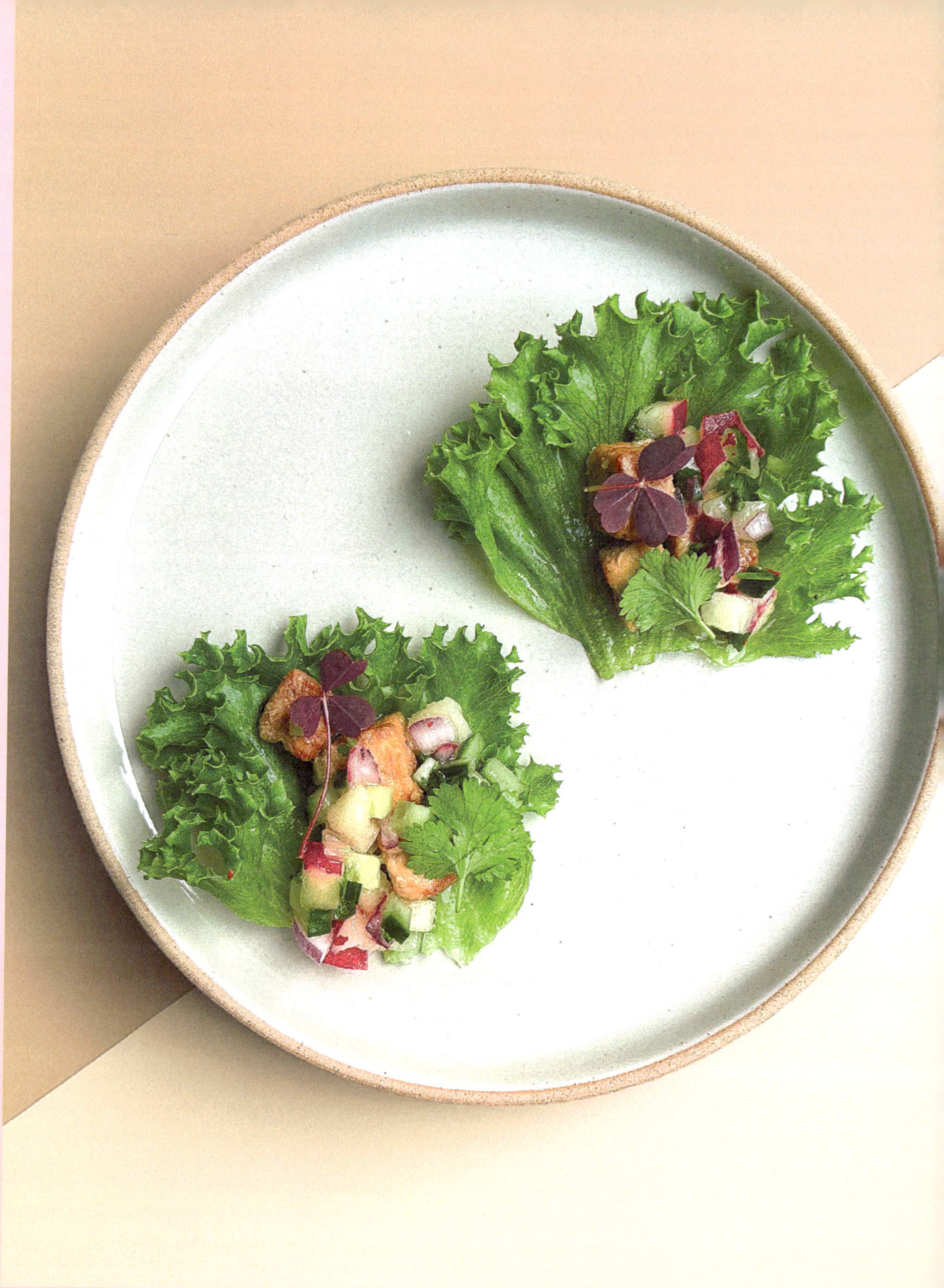

*Peach salsa is unbeatably delicious, easy to make and a must-have addition to tacos or salads! The salsa is made with Japanese peaches, chilies, red onions, freshly squeezed lime juice and coriander, served with umami-rich tempeh.*

**Serves: 2**

**Ingredients**

200 g tempeh diced
2 tbsp olive oil
2 tbsp coconut aminos
1 tbsp maple

**Peach Salsa**

5 Japanese peaches diced
1/3 cucumber, finely diced
1 finely chopped red onion
1 squeezed lime
1 finely chopped chili
2 tbsp olive oil
1/4 bunch coriander
Salt to taste

1. Dice your tempeh, marinate in coconut aminos, maple and olive oil for couple of hours or overnight.
2. Fry the tempeh cubes on medium heat in a non-stick pan on both sides until brown and crispy. It also can be done in the oven.
3. Mix all the salsa ingredients in a large bowl and let it marinate for 20-30 minutes.
4. Serve your crispy salad leaves with peach salsa and tempeh.
5. Add cilantro leaves and oxalis to decorate.

# FILLED PIMIENTOS DE PADRON

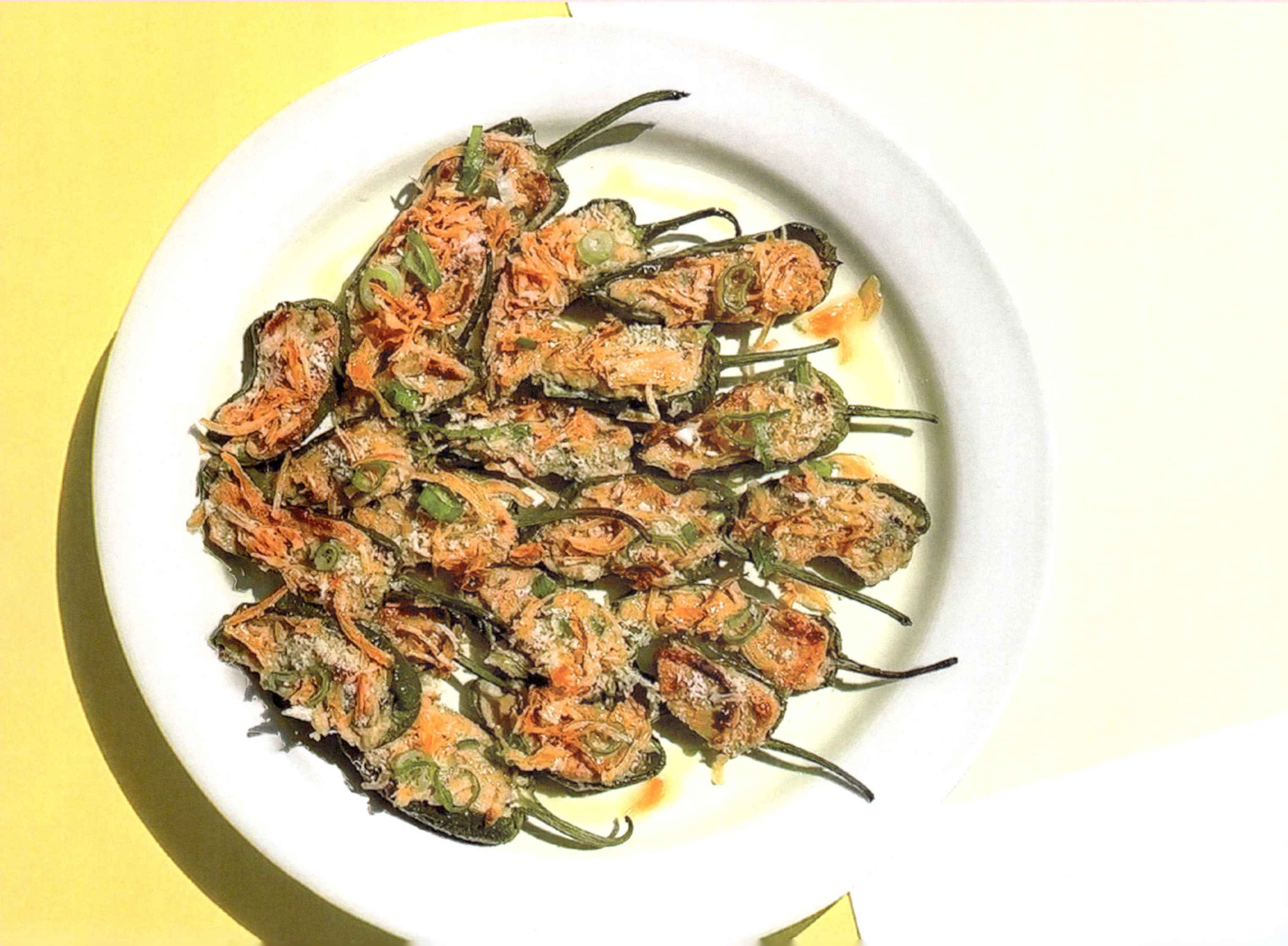

*Pimientos de Padrón are tender, mildly sweet and grassy peppers that, when blistered in olive oil and salted, develop smoky, nutty notes—though every so often one surprises with a burst of heat.We've stuffed them with almond ricotta, a dash of spicy jalapeño, and topped them with crispy onions. They're the perfect finger food.*

**Serves: 4**

**Ingredients**

250 g pimentos de padron

1 tbsp olive oil

**Filling**

225 g almond ricotta (page 18)

1 tsp white wine vinegar

2 tbsp pickled jalapeños, finely chopped

3 scallions, finely chopped

1 tbsp dill, finely chopped

Salt

Black pepper

**For serving**

2 cups gluten-free panko or roasted crispy onions

1. Preheat the oven to 200 degrees.
2. Mix the ingredients for the cheese cream.
3. Rinse and dry the padrons. Cut them lengthwise and remove the seeds.
4. Fill each half with 1 teaspoon of the cheese mixture and sprinkle with panko or roasted onions.
5. Brush with the oil and roast them in the oven, 220° for about 8-10 minutes until they have a nice color and the cheese has melted. Serve immediately.

# MAKI COCONUTRÖRA

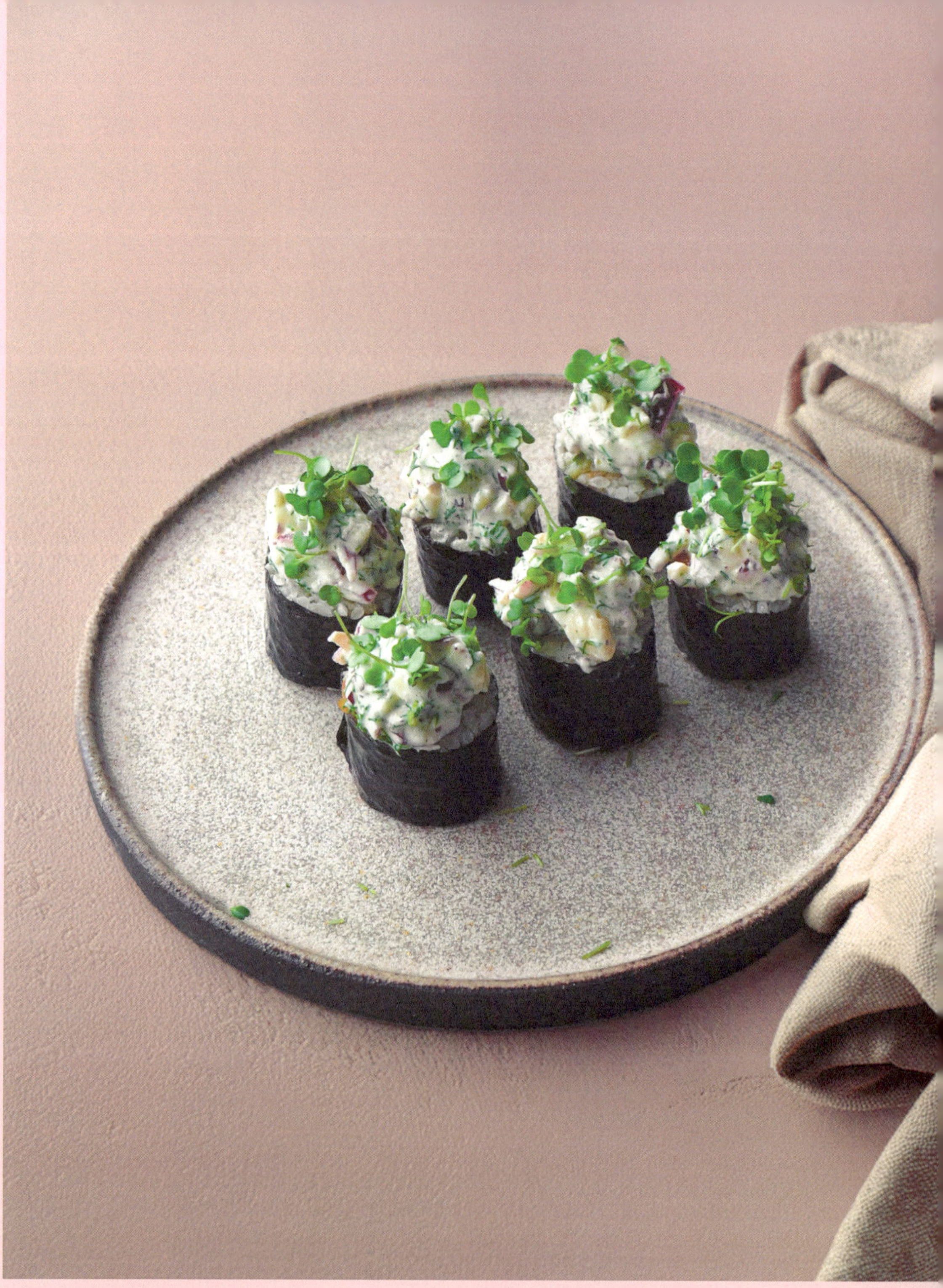

*Delicate maki rolls filled with creamy, savory skagenröra, combining subtle flavors of plant-based seafood alternatives with fresh seasonings. Topped with vibrant micro-greens, each bite offers a refreshing crunch and herbal brightness.*

**Serves: 4**

**Maki**

225 dl sushi rice
300 ml water
2 tbsp vinegar seasoning
4 nori sheets

**Coconutröra**

200g young coconut meat
120g vegan mayonnaise (page 16)
1 tsp seaweed flakes (nori, dulse or wakame flakes)
1 small red onion, finely chopped
1/2 tbsp dijon mustard
2 tbsp capers
1/4 cup chopped celery stalks
1 tbsp lemon juice
1/2 tsp garlic powder
1 tbsp nutritional yeast (optional)
2 tbsp coconut aminos
1/2 tsp apple cider vinegar
1/2 bunch fresh dill
Salt and black pepper

**Toppings**

Broccoli microgreens

**Maki**

1. Soak your sushi rice in water for 20 minutes. Then cook for 15 minutes. Once done, let it cool for at least 10 minutes.
2. Mix cooked sushi rice with vinegar seasoning while still warm using a wooden rice paddle. Let the rice cool.
3. Add a nori sheet to the sushi mat with the short side facing you and the matte side facing up.
4. Add a layer of rice to the nori sheet.
5. Press firmly and roll up the roll. Moisten the rice-free part of the nori sheet with a little water and press to hold the roll together. Do the same with all the rolls, then cut into bite-sized pieces.

**Coconutröra**

1. Cut young coconut meat into small strips.
2. Add young coconut meat pieces, vegan mayonnaise, finely chopped red onion, seaweed mix, lemon juice, finely chopped capers, garlic, chopped celery stalk, nutritional yeast, coconut aminos, Dijon mustard, dill, vinegar, and salt and pepper, toss together.
3. Taste and add more salt and pepper if needed.
4. Top chilled skagen mix on top of your maki rolls.
5. Garnish with optional microgreens.

# MUSHROOM TART BITES

## WITH CASHEW BECHAMÉL

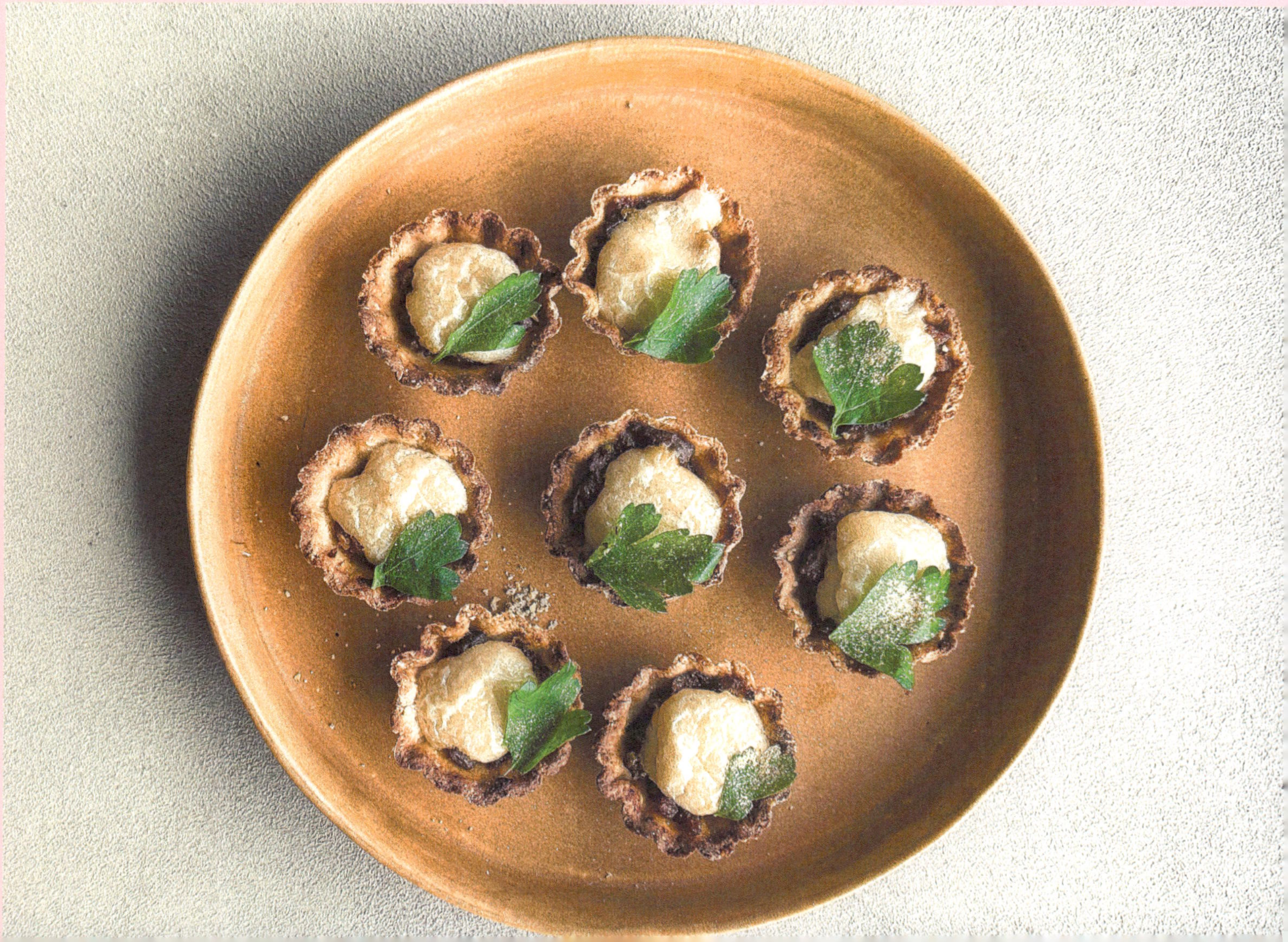

**Serves: 34 x 5cm**

**Tart Dough**

125g almond flour
40 g tapioca flour
35 g rice flour
2 tbsp maple or agave syrup
1/2 tsp salt
3 tbsp water

**Mushroom Filling**

400 g cremini mushrooms diced
1 large carrot slow cooked and diced
1 large onion finely chopped
4 garlic cloves minced
1 carrot diced
1 chili pepper diced
1 tsp dried thyme
1 tsp salt
1 tbsp olive oil
1 tbsp chickpea miso + 2 tbsp water

**Cashew bechamél**

100 g raw cashews soaked
2 tbsp lemon juice
3 garlic cloves minced
2 tbsp nutritional yeast
100 ml almond milk
2 tbsp olive oil
Water as needed
1 tsp salt

1. To make dough, preheat oven to 175 C, and bring 34 pcs, 5cm silicon tart tins.
2. In a mixing bowl whisk together the almond flour, tapioca, rice flour and salt.
3. Add 2 tbsp of water, and use a large spoon to thoroughly combine. Add agave syrup, whisk it into 1 tbsp of water, and add that now. Mix very well. Squeeze a handful of the mixture to see if it holds together yet. It should hold together, otherwise add additional 1/2 tbsp water.
4. Place the dough on a large piece of parchment paper. Use your palm to gently flatten the dough into a disc.
5. With a rolling pin, use firm and steady pressure and slow movements to roll the dough into an even circle. If the dough sticks to the rolling pin, sprinkle tapioca flour on top. Using a 5cm round cutter, cut the dough into small rounds. Knead the dough and repeat the process for the rest of dough until you get 34 rounds.
6. Place the rounds into silicon molds. Without stretching the dough, use your fingers to gently press it into the corners of the silicon molds. Patch any holes or tears with excess dough from the edges.
7. Use a fork to poke vent holes in the bottom of the crust.
8. Bake for 15 minutes. When done, the very center of the crust may feel slightly soft, but it will crisp up as it cools. It's important not to overbake this crust so that it doesn't crack or become hard. Allow to cool and proceed with fillings.
9. In a pan, place all mushroom filling ingredients and cook on medium-high heat until mushrooms and carrots are soften enough and absorbs all water content.
10. Place all cashew bechamél ingredients in a blender, blend on high speed until silky smooth.
11. Fill your tarts with mushroom and top with cashew bechamél.
12. Continue to bake in the oven additional 10 minutes until the sauce thickened and slightly turns golden brown. Serve with fresh parsley if desired.

# JACK-SKAGEN CANAPÉS

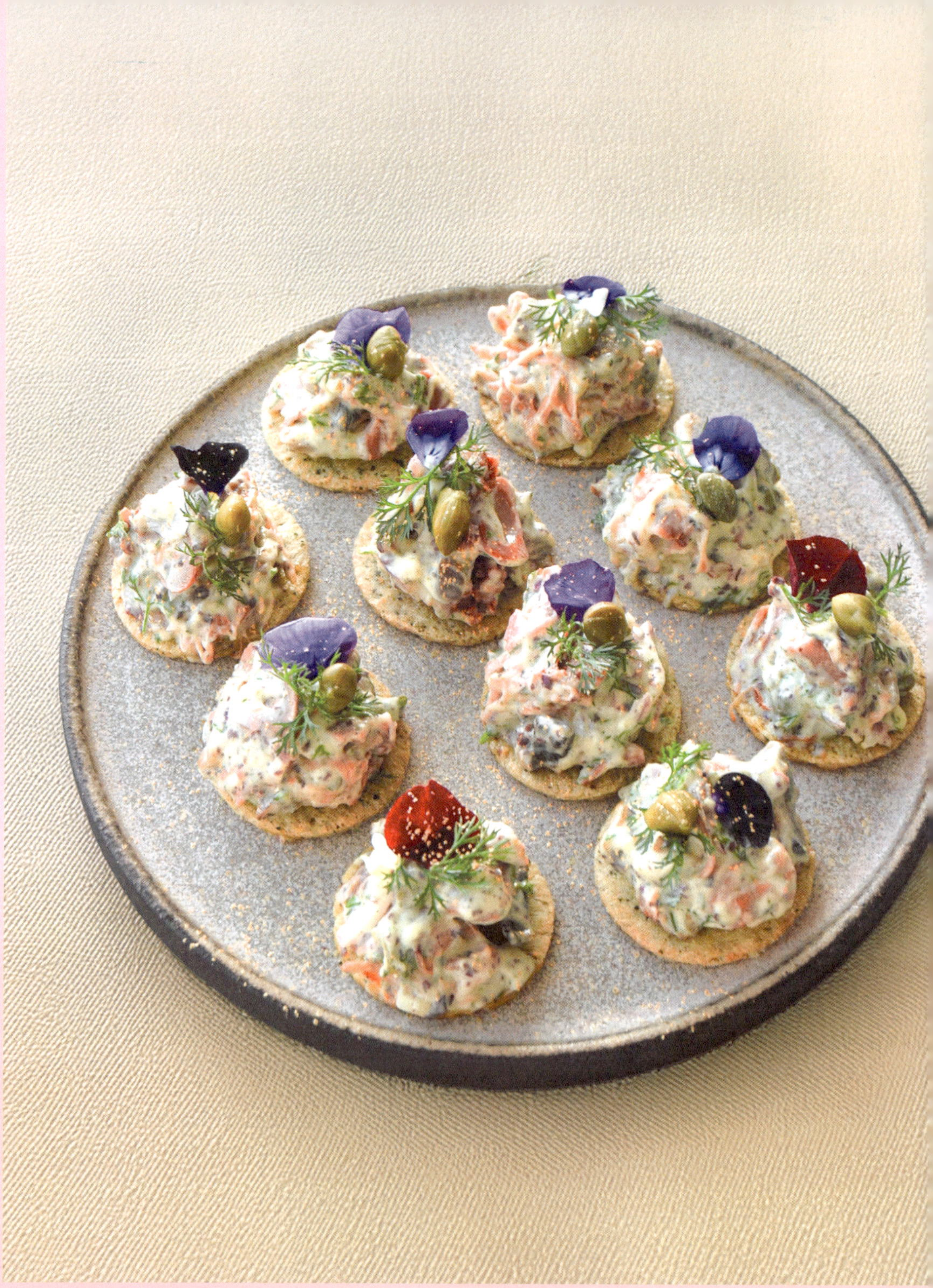

*Elegant bite-sized canapés topped with creamy, savory jackfruit Skagen, offering the flavors of classic seafood-inspired skagen in a plant-based version.*

**Serves: 2**

**Rice Crackers**

1 cup rice flour
1 cup almond flour
1 cup tapioca flour
1/2 cup buckwheat flour
1/4 cup olive oil
1 tsp pink himalayan salt + more as needed
Water as needed to knead
3 tbsp rice vinegar

**Skagenröra**

200 g young jack fruit chopped
120 g vegan mayonnaise
1 tsp seaweed blend (or mix nori,dulse, wakame together)
1/4 cup red onion finely chopped
1/2 tbsp djon mustard
Salt and black pepper to taste
2 tbsp capers
1/4 cup chopped celery stalks or leek
1 tbsp lemon juice
1/2 tsp garlic powder
1 tbsp nutritional yeast
2 tbsp coconut aminos
1/2 tsp apple cider vinegar
1/2 bunch fresh dill

**Toppings**

Capers, fresh dill ,pansies

**1.** To make rice crackers, mix all ingredients with just enough water to blend and knead with your hands.

2. Divide mixture into three equal pieces. Season each piece with different flavors as given above, then knead again until you get a smooth elastic dough.

3. Roll the dough between two parchment papers using a rolling pin. 4. Repeat the process for the rest. Using a cookie cutter, cut in rounds.

5. Bake at 180 C in the oven for 15-20 minutes or until golden brown.

6. Let them cool at least 20 minutes before serving.

7. To make skagenröra, add the jackfruit chunks into a large bowl and mash them with a fork.

8. In a pan with little olive oil and a dash of water, cook them until soften.

9. In a bowl, add vegan mayonnaise, finely chopped red onion, seaweed blend, lemon juice, finely chopped capers, garlic, chopped celery stalks, nutritional yeast, coconut aminos, dijon mustard, dill, vinegar and salt and pepper.

10. Taste and add more salt and pepper if needed. Serve chilled or at room temperature. Top on your canapes.

Storage: Leftovers keep very well in the fridge for 2-3 days.

# KIMCHI MAKI

## WITH BLACK RICE AND AVOCADO

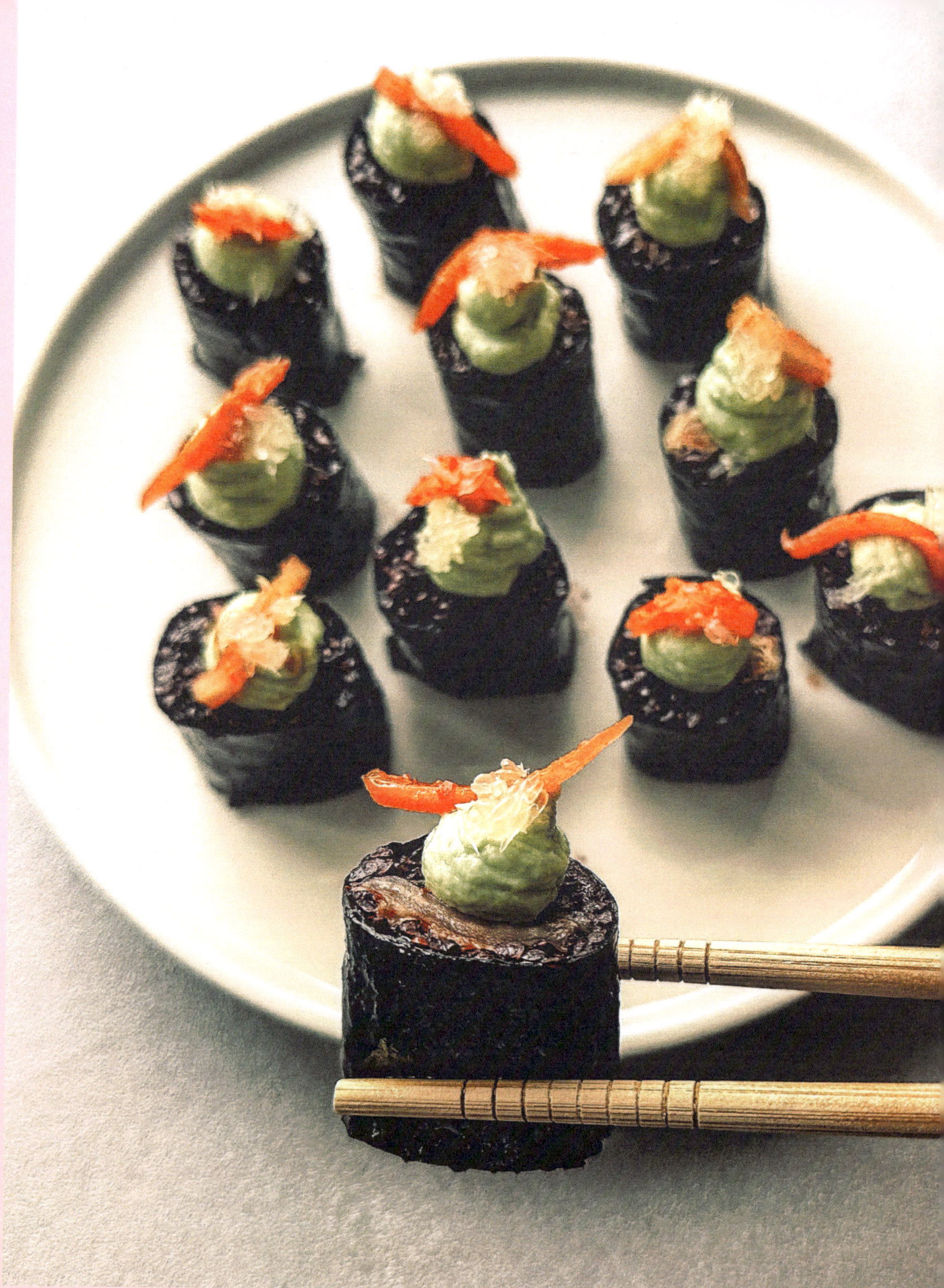

**Serves: 6**

**Ingredients**

250 g black rice
700 ml water (may vary depending on the type of black rice you use, follow the instructions on the package)
6 nori sheets

**Kimchi Filling**

220 g vegan kimchi (page 21)

**Avocado Cream**

2 avocados
1/2 lemon juice
3 cloves garlic, minced
1 tsp salt

**Serving**

Fermented carrot strips from kimchi
4 limequat

1. To cook black rice, add water and rinsed black rice to a saucepan. Bring the water to a boil over medium heat. Add the salt, reduce heat, cover, and cook for about 30 minutes until the rice is tender and all the water has been absorbed.
Turn off the heat and let it sit, covered, for about 5 to 10 minutes, then fluff it with a fork. Don't skip this step because black rice, unlike regular sushi rice, is not naturally sticky.
2. Drain the kimchi from the water to remove as much water as possible, as this will help you roll the kimchi up so it holds together. Set aside a few carrot slices from the kimchi for garnish.
3. Peel the avocado, remove the pit, and place the avocado flesh in a food processor, add the lemon juice, minced garlic, and salt. Blend until creamy. Pour the cream into a piping bag and set aside.
4. Once the rice has cooled, place a sheet of nori, shiny side down, on a sushi mat.
5. Using a rice spoon, spread the rice thinly and evenly over the nori sheet, leaving about 1 inch (2.5 cm) of space at the top. Make sure the rice covers the sides as well. You can also use a maki tool to make the filling easier.
6. Then spread out some kimchi.
7. Lift the underside of the mat with your thumbs and gently press the filling into place with your other fingers. Roll up so that the underside is just above the filling.
8. Press the sushi mat with your fingers to tighten them. Continue rolling and pressing with the sushi mat.
9. To seal the roll, moisten the top edge of the nori sheet with water using your finger.
10. Repeat the sushi rolling process with the remaining ingredients.
11. Cut each sushi roll in half, then cut each half in half again and repeat until you have about 6-8 pieces of sushi from each roll.
12. Top with avocado cream, fermented carrot strips from kimchi and limequat.
Best when consumed in the same day but can be stored up to 3 days.

PLANT BASED UMAMI

# BUTTERFLY URAMAKI

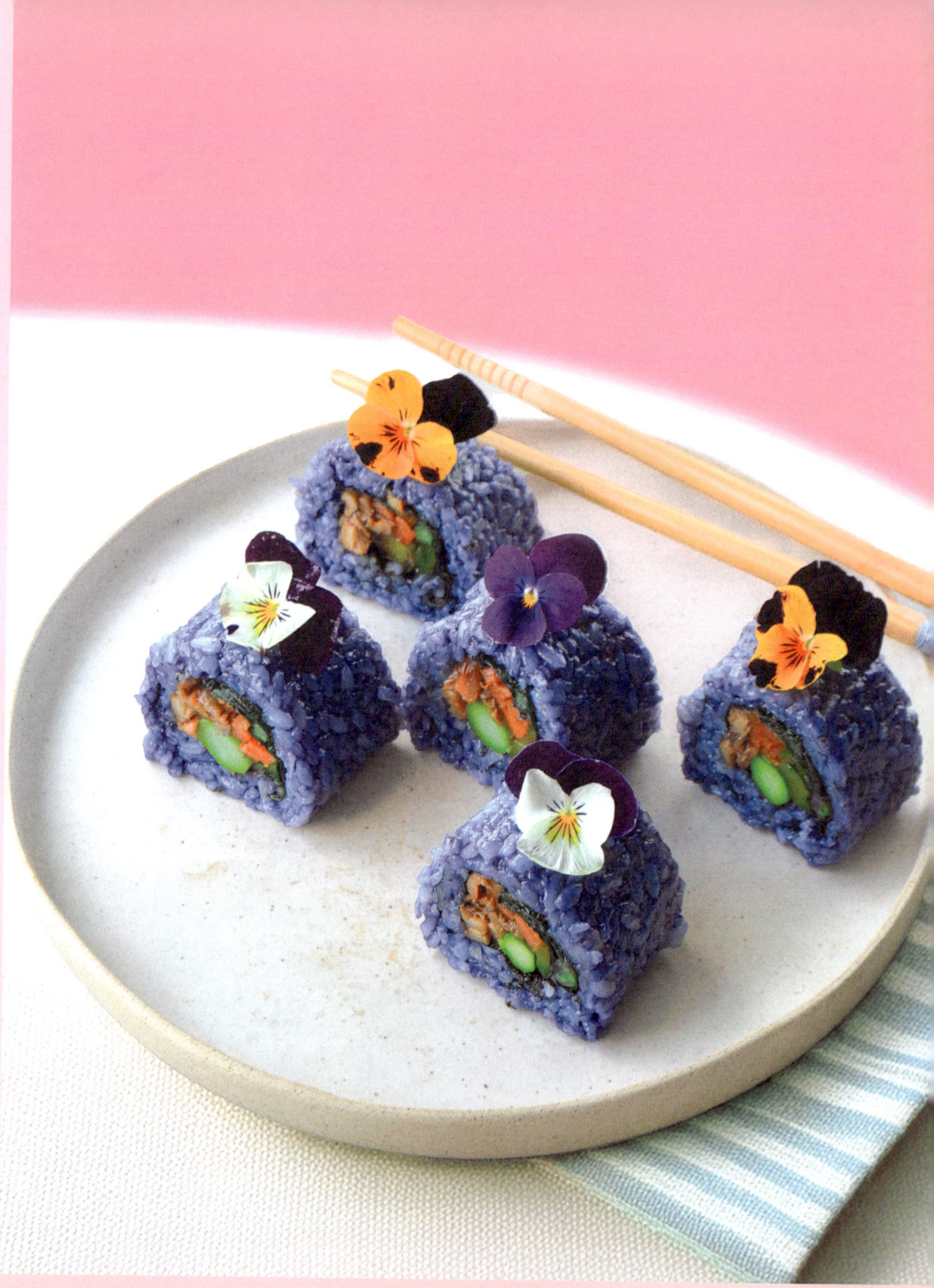

*Vibrant uramaki rolls wrapped in naturally blue butterfly pea flower rice, filled with tender asparagus, sweet carrot, and earthy mushrooms*

**Serves: 4**

**Ingredients**

4 sheets of nori, cut in half
1 cup sushi rice
1+1/4 cup water
2 tbsp rice vinegar
1 tbsp coconut nectar
1 cup long thin cut carrot slices (sauté in the pan with a little bit water)
4 asparagus (sauté in the pan with a little bit olive oil and water)
1 cup sauted mushrooms (sauté in the pan with a little bit coconut aminos and olive oil)
2 red onion caramelized (sauté in the pan with a little bit olive oil and coconut sugar until soften)
1 cup kale sauted (wilt in the pan until slightly soften and crispy)
2 tbsp butterfly pea flower powder-
Pansies to decorate
Sesame oil to brush

1. To make sushi rice, combine 1 cup of sushi rice and 1 + 1/4 cup water in an instant pot on high for 4 minutes.
2. After it naturally releases, add in 2 tbsp rice vinegar, 1 tbsp coconut nectar, agave or maple syrup, and a dash of salt. Keep covered with wet paper towel. Once done, add butterfly pea flower powder and using a fork or rice paddle, gently mix the rice until all turns into blue color.
3. Wrap a sushi mat with a long piece of plastic wrap and fold the edges around to seal it nicely. Lay one half sheet of nori shiny side down on the plastic-wrapped bamboo sushi mat.
4. Set a small bowl with a wet paper towel and a little water next to your mat. Wet your fingers on the paper towel and place about 1/2 cup of sushi rice in an even layer across the nori sheet.
5. Carefully flip the nori over so that the rice side is now facing down.
6. About half an inch from the edge, layer sautéed and caramelized veggies in a line from end to end.
7. Using the sushi mat and both hands, start rolling from the bottom of the roll, tucking the edge of the roll to fully enclose the filling. Once you reach the end, use the mat to rotate the roll inside to make sure you have an even and consistent sushi roll.
8. Then brush your sushi with sesame oil. Using a sharp knife, cut it in half first, then cut each half in thirds.

Place your sushi on a serving dish and enjoy with pickled ginger and wasabi if desired.

# BEETROOT FUTOMAKI

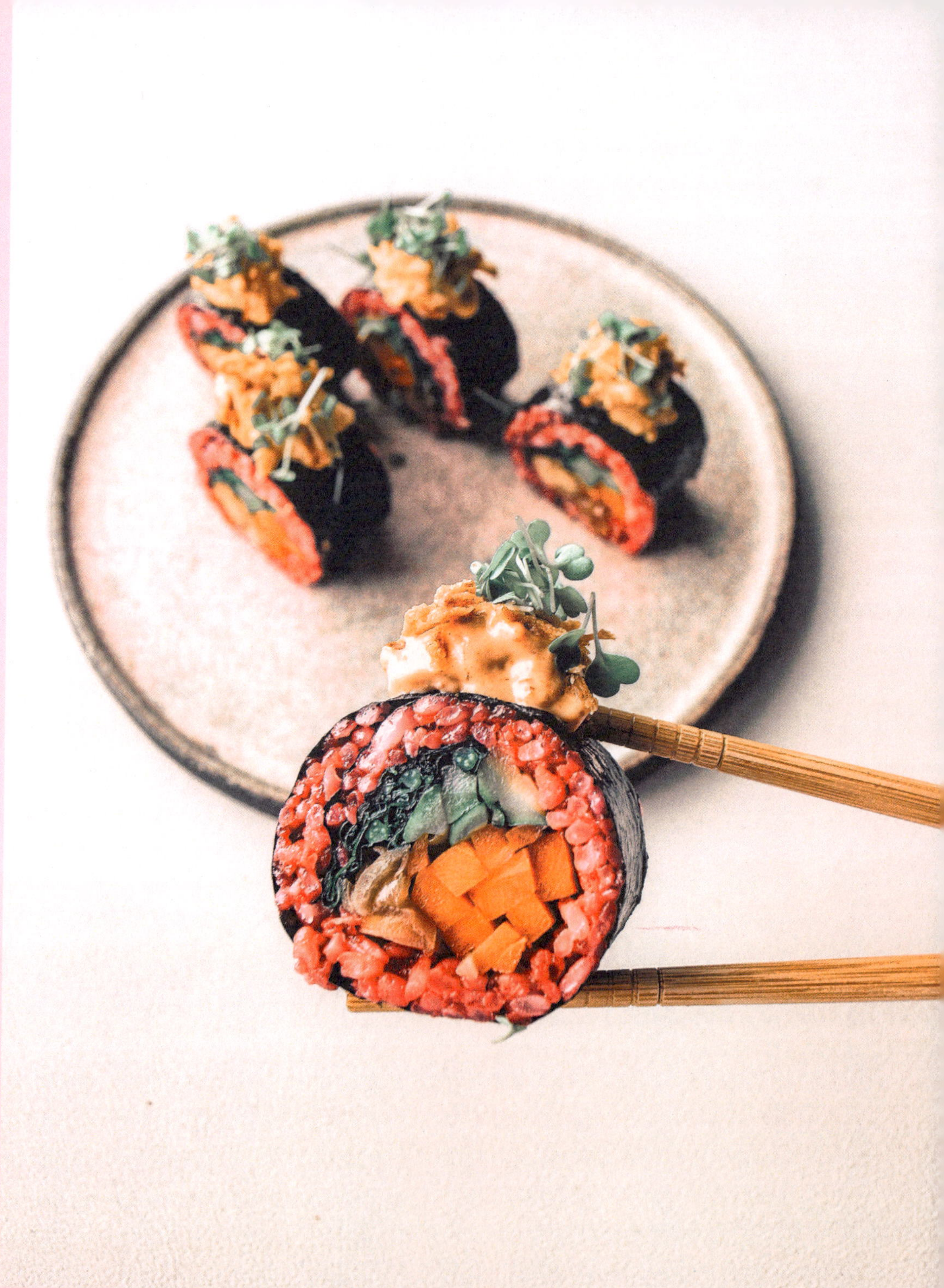

**Serves: 12**

**For the rice**

440 grams sushi rice

480 ml water

60 ml rice vinegar

1 tbsp coconut sugar

1.5–2 tbsp beetroot powder

1/2 tsp salt

5–6 nori sheets

**For the veggies**

4–5 asparagus or 1 zucchini

A bunch of kale or spinach

1 large carrot, sliced

200 g mushrooms or tempeh

**For serving**

Coconut aminos

Sriracha mayonnaise (page 17 - mix sriracha with mayonnaise)

Chili

Fried crispy onions

Microgreens

1. Place the rice in a bowl and add cold water. Mix the rice into the water with your hand, drain and repeat until the water runs clear. Rinse a few more times. Once the rice has rinsed, let the rice drain in a colander or sieve for 1 hour.
2. Once the rice has drained, place the rice in a heavy saucepan, add the water and bring to a boil over medium heat; bring to a boil, reduce heat to low and simmer, cover and cook for 15 minutes. Turn off the heat and let the rice sit with the lid on for another 15 minutes.
3. While the rice is cooking, prepare the vinegar mixture. Combine the rice vinegar, coconut sugar and salt in a small saucepan over medium heat. Heat the mixture until the sugar has dissolved (do not let it boil). Remove from the heat and let cool to room temperature.
4. Once the rice is done, carefully spread the rice out onto a baking sheet. Spread the cooled vinegar mixture evenly over the rice. Then add the beetroot powder. Gently turn the rice occasionally with a spatula or wooden spatula so that the rice cools evenly and turns pink.
5. Press out some rice. Place a sheet of nori on the mat, shiny side down. Dip your hands in water and then press out handfuls of rice on top in a 1cm thick layer, leaving the longest edge free.
6. Add sautéed carrots, zucchini, asparagus, spinach or kale, long strips of tempeh or sautéed mushrooms. To sauté, cut each vegetable into long thin strips (do not use the inner parts of the zucchini, only the outer ones), fry each vegetable separately in a pan with a little coconut aminos and oil until tender.
7. Lift the edge of the mat over the rice and press down slightly to keep everything in a tight roll.
8. Attach the sides like a stamp. When you get to the edge without rice, brush with a little water and continue rolling into a tight roll.
9. Brush the rolls with sesame oil and cut them with a very sharp knife.
10. Top with sriracha, chili, fried onions and microgreens if desired.

# EVERDAY GOURMET

PLANT BASED UMAMI

# WINTER KITCHARI

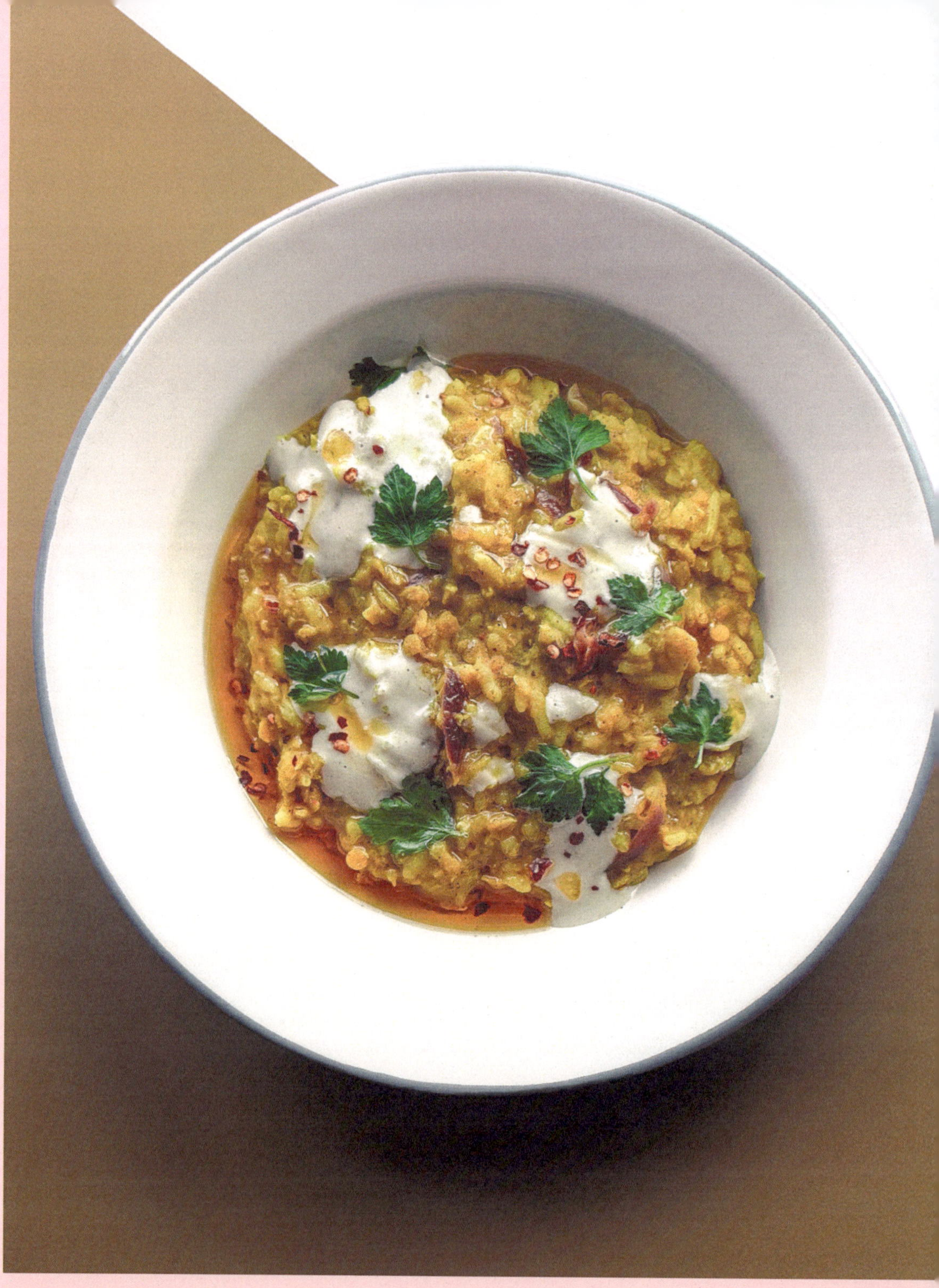

*A comforting, nourishing one-pot dish rooted in Ayurvedic tradition, Winter Kitchari combines lentil, rice, seasonal root vegetables, and warming spices such as turmeric, ginger, and cumin. This plant-based dish is easily digestible, supports immune function, and promotes gentle detoxification, making it perfect for cold winter months*

**Serves: 3**

**Ingredients**

100 g red lentils
100 g basmati rice
1 tsp turmeric
2 cloves garlic, peeled and kept whole
250 ml coconut milk
25 g coconut oil
1 tbsp olive oil
10 fresh curry leaves
1 tsp black mustard seeds
pinch dried red chilli, thinly sliced
1 small red onion, thinly sliced
salt, to taste

**For serving**

Coriander
Chili
Yoghurt (page 17)

1. Wash the lentils and rice several times in clean water to remove the starch.
2. Place them in a large saucepan and add 500 ml water, turmeric and garlic. Bring to the boil, then reduce the heat and simmer for about 15 minutes.
3. Stir in the coconut milk and continue to cook for a further 5 minutes or until the lentils are cooked and the dal has thickened. Season with salt.
4. In a separate small frying pan, add the oil over a low heat.
5. Add the curry leaves, mustard seeds and chilli. Fry gently for 1-2 minutes, then add the onion and continue to fry for a few minutes, stirring constantly until the onion is golden and caramelised.
6. Add this mixture to the lentils and stir together. Remove the garlic cloves before serving.
7. Serve with oat yoghurt, chillies and coriander.

# POTATO WAFFLES

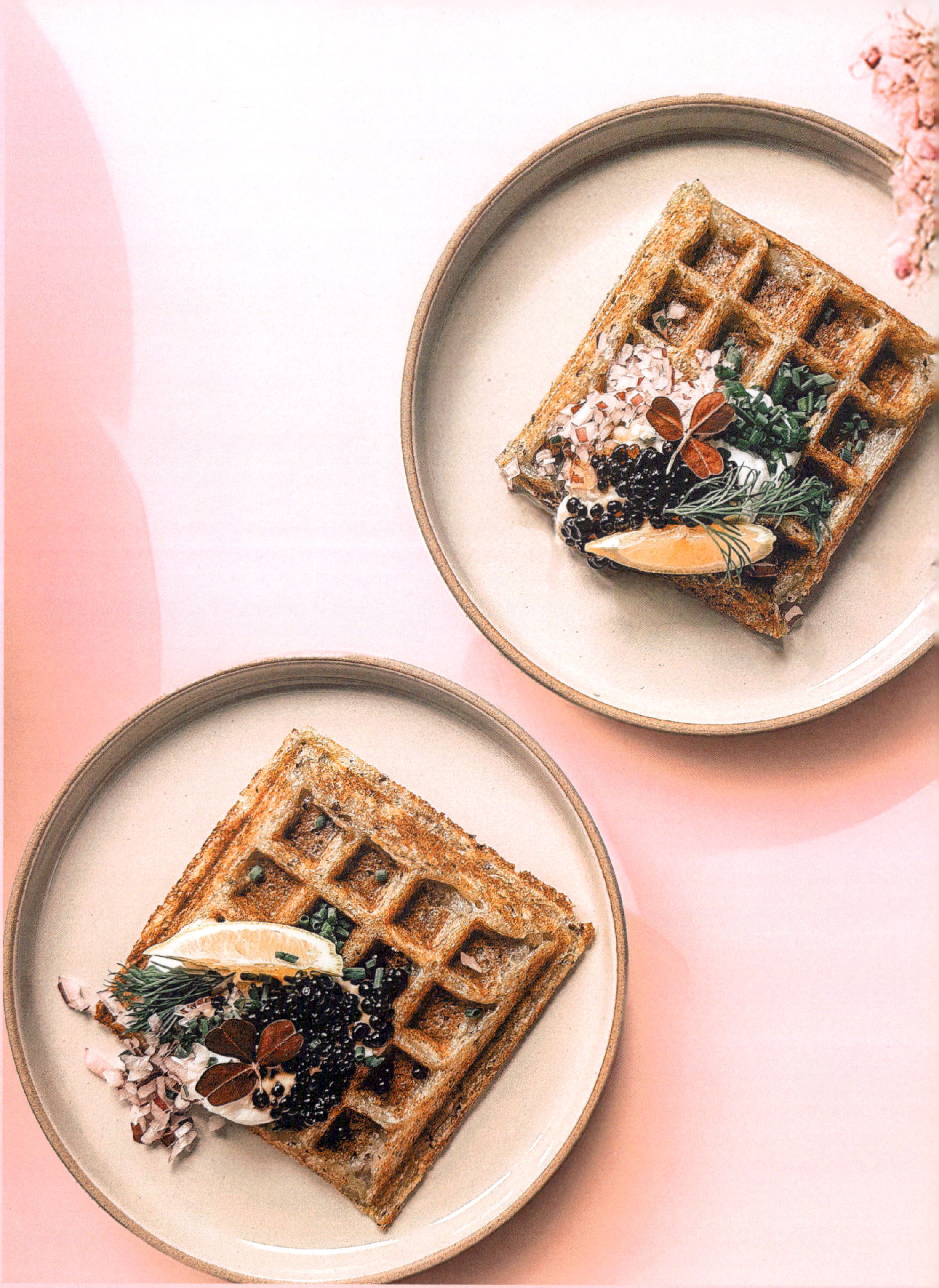

**Serves: 3**

### Potato Waffles

350 g boiled potatoes (4 potatoes)
1 tbsp ground flaxseed
3 tbsp water
1-2 tbsp olive oil
2 tsp garlic powder
2 dl tapioca
3-4 tbsp rice flour + more as needed
1/4 tsp baking powder
1 tsp salt

### Coconut Aminos Pearls

130 ml coconut aminos
2 g agar agar
300 ml cold seed oil or olive oil
300 ml cold water

### For serving

Plant-based crème fraîche or multi-purpose cashew cream (page 18)
Dill
Chives
Red onion
Lemon
Red sorrel

### Potato Waffles

1. Mix ground flax with water in a bowl. Set aside for 5 minutes.
2. In a large bowl, grate the potatoes. Add garlic powder, salt, baking powder, tapioca, rice flour, olive oil and flaxseed mixture.
3. Mix everything together until you get a dough. If it is too sticky, add a little more rice flour.
4. Divide the mixture into 4 small doughs.
5. Heat the waffle maker, when it is too hot, move the dough balls over. Shape with the spatula.
6. Bake it until it is completely crispy.

### Agave Pearls

1. Pour the oil into a tall container and place in the freezer for 30 min-1 hour.
2. When your oil is almost ready, combine the coconut aminos and agar powder in a small saucepan. Bring to a boil, whisking constantly.
3. Once boiling, turn off the heat on the saucepan and let sit for 2-3 minutes.
4. Remove the oil from the freezer.
5. Transfer the agar-coconut aminos mixture into a small syringe without a needle or a dressing bottle.
6. Drop the coconut aminos-agar mixture into it drop by drop. Do this quite quickly because the longer the mixture sits, the more it will start to solidify in your saucepan. Don't worry if some of the first few drops sit at the top. They will start to sink as you add more.
7. Over a large bowl, pour the oil mixture so that it runs through a fine mesh strainer.
8. Set the bowl of oil aside and transfer the coconut aminos pearls to a bowl of cold water.
9. Store the agar caviar in the refrigerator until you are ready to use it, or add it immediately.

### Assembly

1. Place the waffles on the plate.
2. Top with plant-based crème fraîche.
3. Add finely chopped scallions and red onions.
4. Top with agar caviar.
5. Garnish with dill and oxalis, serve with lemon.

PLANT BASED UMAMI

# INGRID SMÖRREBRÖD

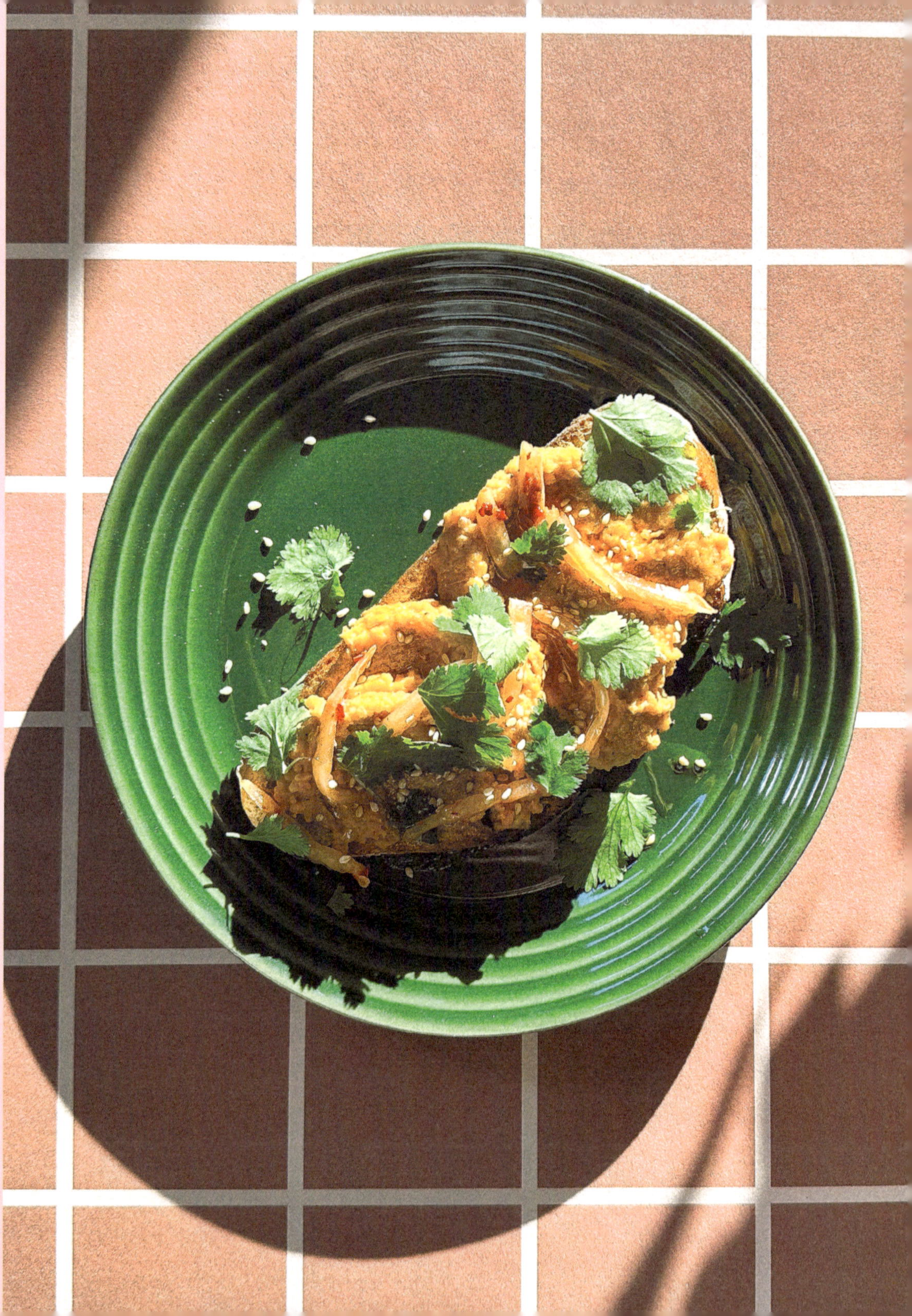

*This dish was born the day I tried a sandwich at RØRT in Cph. It's a spicy carrot and pea mix they call Ingrid. It's not the same but a but similar, my version offers incredible depth and savoryness from the chickpea miso and kimchi. Try it with tahini or hemp butter, both add an earthy flavor to the sweetness of the peas, a perfect balance!*

**Serves: 4**

**Ingredients**

200 g yellow peas
1 onion, thinly sliced
2 garlic cloves, halved
1 carrot, thinly sliced
1 tbsp chickpea miso
1 dl kimchi
2 tbsp kimchi juice
1 lemon juice
3 tbsp tahini or hemp butter
1/4 cup olive oil
1 tsp salt
1 tsp cayenne pepper
1/2 tsp black pepper

**Serving**

Kimchi
Fresh coriander
Sesame
Chili oil

1. Sauté onion, garlic and carrot with a little olive oil in a pan. Add chickpea miso and stir together. Add a little water and cook until the carrots are soft.
2. Cook your yellow peas for about 35-40 minutes until they are soft enough.
3. Put everything in a food processor, blend until smooth.
4. Spread over your favorite bread, preferably Danish rye bread!
5. Top with extra kimchi, coriander, sesame seeds & chili oil.

# UMAMI RISOTTO

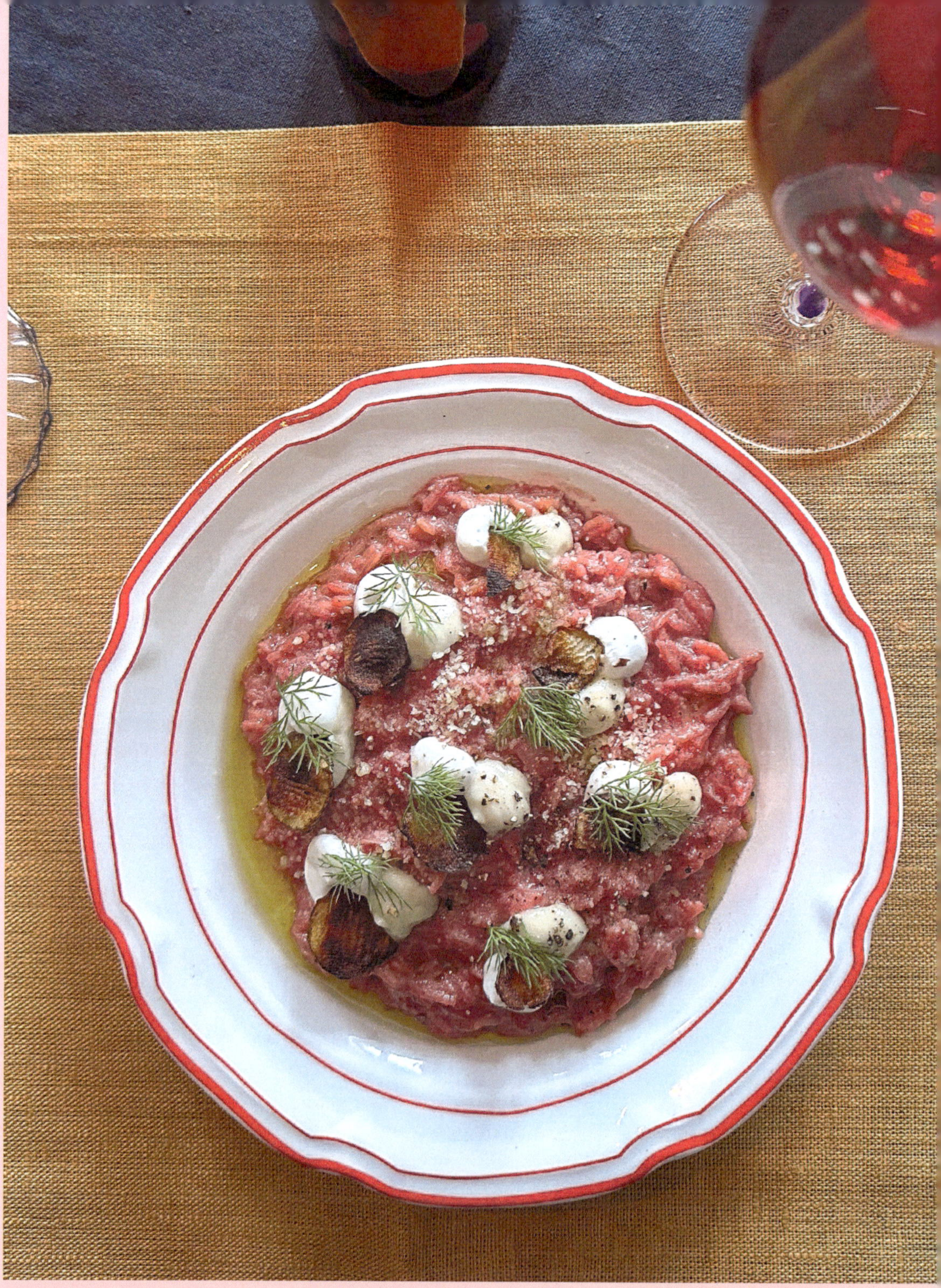

*This Beetroot and Pomegranate Risotto is a vibrant, elegant dish that combines earthy sweetness, delicate acidity, and deep umami richness. The beetroot purée and pomegranate wine create a jewel-toned base with a subtly fruity depth, while the miso–Jerusalem artichoke cream adds silky, savory complexity. Finished with crisp Jerusalem artichoke chips, fresh dill, and a cool dollop of plant-based yogurt, it's a beautifully balanced plate that feels both luxurious and comforting.*

**Serves: 4**

**Ingredients**

2.5 dl risotto rice
1 dl pomegranate wine (or red wine)
150 g beetroot purée (boil and peel beetroots, then blend with a little water)
1 tbsp shiitake powder
1 large onion, finely chopped
50 g grated vegan parmesan
1 tbsp olive oil
2 tbsp coconut aminos or mushroom sauce
Water, as needed
Freshly ground black pepper

**For serving**

Miso–Jerusalem artichoke cream (boil Jerusalem artichokes, peel, and blend with yellow pea miso)
Jerusalem artichoke chips (slice thinly with a mandolin, then dry or lightly fry in olive oil)
Almond or oat yogurt
Fresh dill

1. Heat a little olive oil in a heavy-bottomed pot. Sauté the onion until soft and glossy, but not browned.
2. Add the rice and cook, stirring, until lightly toasted and fragrant, about 5 minutes. Pour in the wine, stir, and let it fully absorb.
3. Add a generous scoop of water along with the beetroot purée and shiitake powder. Let the liquid absorb while stirring, topping up with more water as needed.
4. Continue this process until the rice is al dente, about 15–20 minutes.
5. Add a splash more water to achieve a loose, lightly creamy texture and stir in the parmesan.
6. Mix until the risotto is creamy yet holds its shape—the kind that gently sways on the plate.
7. Serve on warm plates. Top with miso–Jerusalem artichoke cream, almond or oat yogurt, Jerusalem artichoke chips, and dill.
8. Drizzle with a little olive oil, finish with plenty of freshly ground black pepper, parmesan and serve immediately.

PLANT BASED UMAMI

# BUCKWHEAT PASTA

## WITH TOMATO BALSAMIC SAUCE

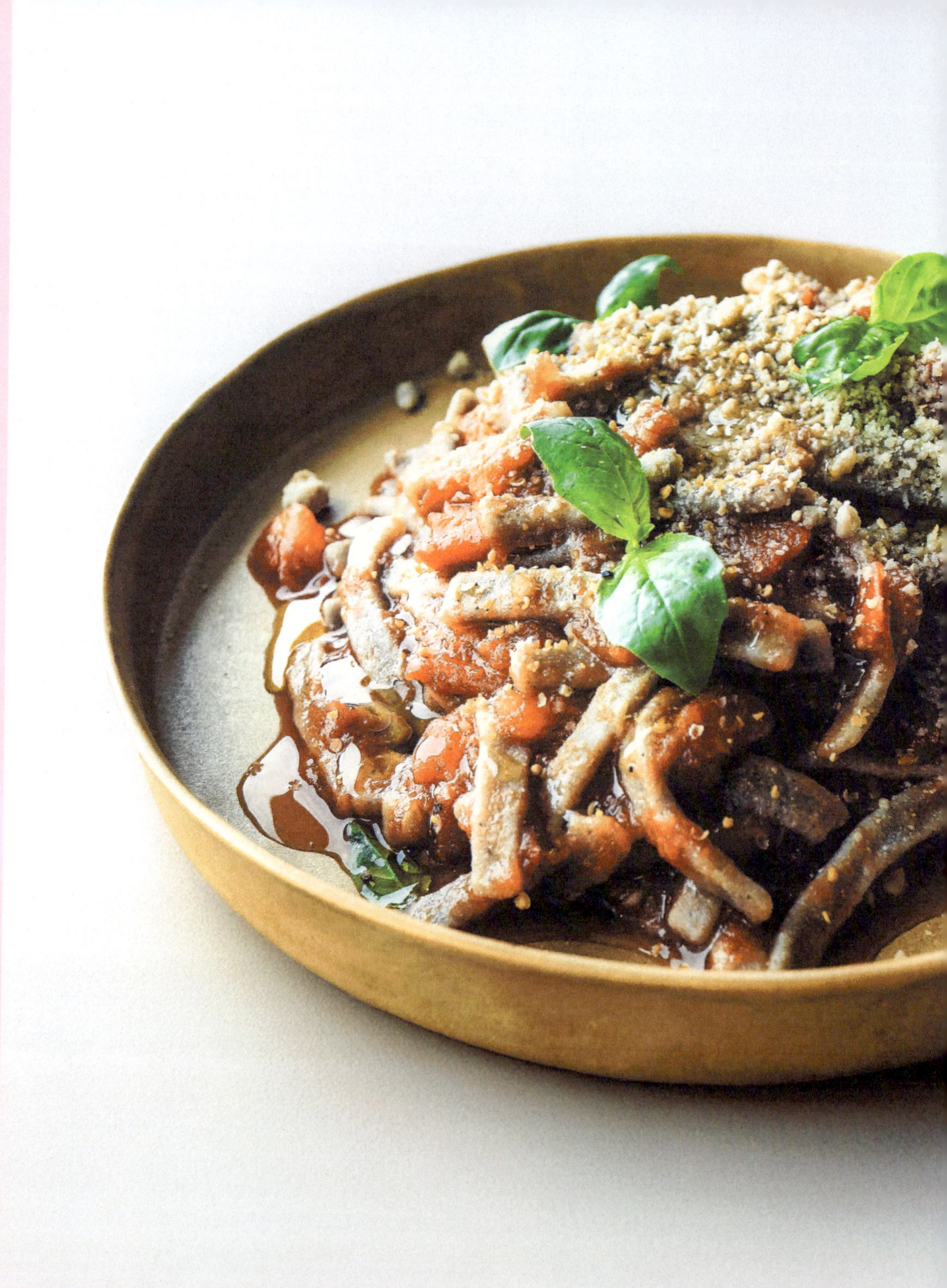

*Our house-crafted buckwheat pasta boasts a perfectly firm, tender texture that holds sauces beautifully. Tossed in a rich, homemade tomato sauce, it delivers a balanced taste profile of earthy, nutty buckwheat, sweet and tangy tomatoes, and aromatic herbs, creating a comforting, satisfying dish.*

**Serves: 2**

1 cup (120 g) buckwheat flour
1/2 cup (65 g) cassava or tapioca flour
90 ml water
1 tbsp psyllium husk powder + 4 tbsp water
1/4 tsp salt (optional)

1. In a bowl, whisk together the buckwheat flour, cassava or tapioca, and salt until well-combined.
2. Add the psyllium, water and start with the first 4 tbsp of water. Mix with a wooden spoon until a nice dough forms. You are looking for slightly moist but not sticky at all.
If your dough is still too dry, add a little more water. At some point you are going to have to ditch the wooden spoon and start using your hands so you can feel the consistency and knead the dough. If it's too sticky add a tablespoon of buckwheat flour until moist but not sticky.
3. Bring a pot of 8 cups of water and a generous pinch of sea salt to a boil.
4. Divide the dough into two smooth balls. Flour your surface with more buckwheat flour and roll out one dough ball as thin as you can. You will notice this dough is beautiful to work with! It should be like elastic and easy to roll out.
5. Using a knife or pizza cutter, create thin strips. Sprinkle with more buckwheat flour to prevent sticking together.
6. Pour into the boiling water in two batches and cook for approximately 2 minutes. Drain and serve immediately.
7. Once cooked, this Buckwheat Pasta has a nutty, dense flavor to it but it doesn't stick to your gut the way most pasta does.

It pairs perfectly with simple tomato sauce or balsamic. Simplicity makes this pasta perfection but really, top it with whatever you want. Do be careful with leaving in the strainer for too long. It will start to stick to the other pasta pieces. Make one batch, drain it from the water with a ladle, set it in the strainer and then place into an individual serving bowl immediately. If you find it sticks still, add a small drizzle of balsamic or tomato sauce and lightly separate.

If you will cook the pasta later, dehydrate until completely dried. Keep in the mason jars. You will need to boil dehydrated pasta for 8-10 minutes.
You can dry them at room temperature by hanging in summer days or dehydrate in a food dehydrator at 46° C for 3-4 hours.

**Balsamic Tomato Sauce**
3 cloves garlic, peeled and sliced
200 g shredded tomatoes
1/2 tbsp tomato paste
1/2 tsp salt
1/2 tsp ground mustard
1 tbsp balsamic
1 tbsp olive oil

In a pot, pour the balsamic and olive oil, add the sliced garlic cloves, cook for 15-20 seconds on medium-high heat until slightly soften. Then add the shredded tomatoes, slow cook for 30-40 minutes. Then add the tomato paste and continue to cook until thicken. Season with salt and freshly ground mustard. Toss with your pasta and serve immediately.

# MAKING TEMPEH FROM SCRATCH

**Time** - 3-4 days
**Serves** - 3-4

**Ingredients**
1 cup legumes of your choice (can be yellow peas, black beans etc)
1 tbsp white vinegar
1 tsp tempeh starter

1. Place the legumes of your choice in a large bowl, cover with clean water soak for 8 hours or overnight.
2. The next day, drain and rinse the legumes. Transfer to a large cooking pot, cover with water (about 2-inch higher than the legumes). Bring to a boil and let simmer for 1 hour. Depending on the size of your legumes it might take up to 1 and 1/2 hour. They must be soft but not mushy. If some foam forms on the surface during cooking, remove it with a spoon to prevent any spillover.
3. Once the legumes are cooked, drain them and leave them in the strainer for 30 minutes. After that, pat them dry using a paper towel to make sure they are mostly dry on the outside. Transfer to a large clean bowl. Add the white vinegar and stir to coat. Add the tempeh starter and mix well using a spoon until uniformly distributed. Using a metal skewer, or chopstick, prick some holes (at about 2-inch intervals) in a clean freezer bag. This step is important to create good air circulation and allow the mold to grow.
4. Transfer the legumes to the freezer bag and form a rectangle of about 5×8 inches with a thickness of about 1-inch. Place the bag of legumes on a baking sheet and put in an oven with the light on for about 14 hours. I set the temperature of my oven to 86°F and let the door very slightly opened because I can't just let the light on.
5.After 14 hours, some white mold (not a lot) should have appeared on the chickpeas. You might also see some condensation inside the plastic bag, this is normal. It's time to remove the baking sheet from the oven and let it ferment for another 24-36H in a dark and warm place. I recommend covering the bag of legumes with a clean towel to make sure it's not under direct sunlight.
6. Your tempeh is ready when it is fully covered with white mold and forms a solid cake, which usually happens at the 48-hour mark. It can be quicker if the temperature in your house is high.

Raw tempeh will keep for up to a week in the refrigerator. If you want to freeze it: steam the tempeh for 25 minutes, let cool completely and wrap in plastic film before freezing.

# TACO SALAD

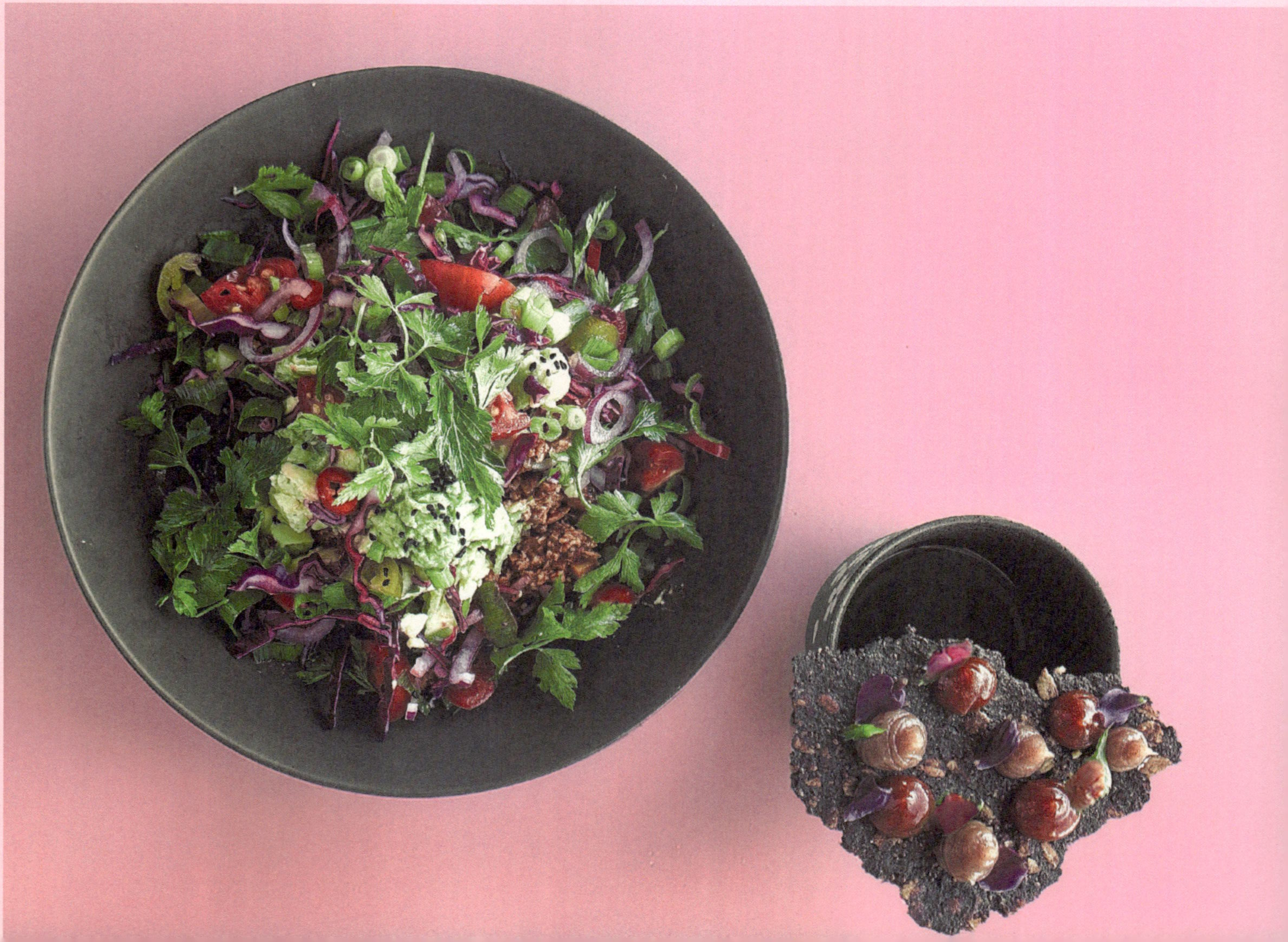

**Serves: 2**

**Ingredients**

1 cup black rice

300 g mushrooms (or jackfruit, pea mince etc)

1 carrot

1 red onion

1 tsp thyme

2 tbsp coconut aminos or mushroom sauce

1 tbsp olive oil

1 tsp sugar kelp powder

1 tbsp tomato paste

4 garlic cloves minced

1/2 tsp salt

**For the salad**

3 spring onions

1 red chili pepper

2 tbsp pickled jalapeno

1 cup shredded red cabbage

1/2 cup fresh cilantro (or parsley)

1 large avocado

1 lemon juice

1 cup tomatoes

1 small red onion or pickled red onion

1/2 tsp salt

1 tbsp black sesame seeds

*I recommend making big batch for busy days. It can be seperarely prepared and stored in the fridge up to 5 days and combined before serving. It can also be served with a stack of warmed tortillas.*
*Add some toasted chopped walnuts, cooked black beans and corn if you like. All goes well together.*

1. If you are going to make it with pea mince, soak your dry pea mince in hot water for a while.
2. Meanwhile, in a pan heat olive oil, add chopped red onion, minced garlic, white parts of spring onion, finely diced carrots and diced 1/2 of chili pepper. Cook until soften, then add the pea mince, toss together and continue to cook until pea mince almost absorbs the water content.
3. Then add tomato paste, coconut aminos, sugar kelp, thyme and salt. Mix together. Cook for additional 1-2 minutes, remove from the heat, set aside.
If you are going to make it with mushrooms or jackfruit, finely dice your mushrooms and cook in the pan along with other ingredients until soften.
4. Rinse and cook your black rice according to package instructions. It should be a bit tender. Once done, set aside to cool down.
5. To prepare salad, wash and dry all ingredients seperately. Deseed and slice your avocado, toss in lemon juice and salt in a bowl. Set aside.
6. Cut your tomatoes in two. Chop your cilantro. Thinly slice red onion and red cabbage along with the rest of chili pepper.
7. Divide your rice between two plates. Add pea mince mixture.
8. Top with avocado, tomatoes, lemon juice, red cabbage, jalapeno, red onion, spring onions, sesame seeds and fresh cilantro.

# LEEK TRIANGLES

## WITH ROSEMARY AND RICE

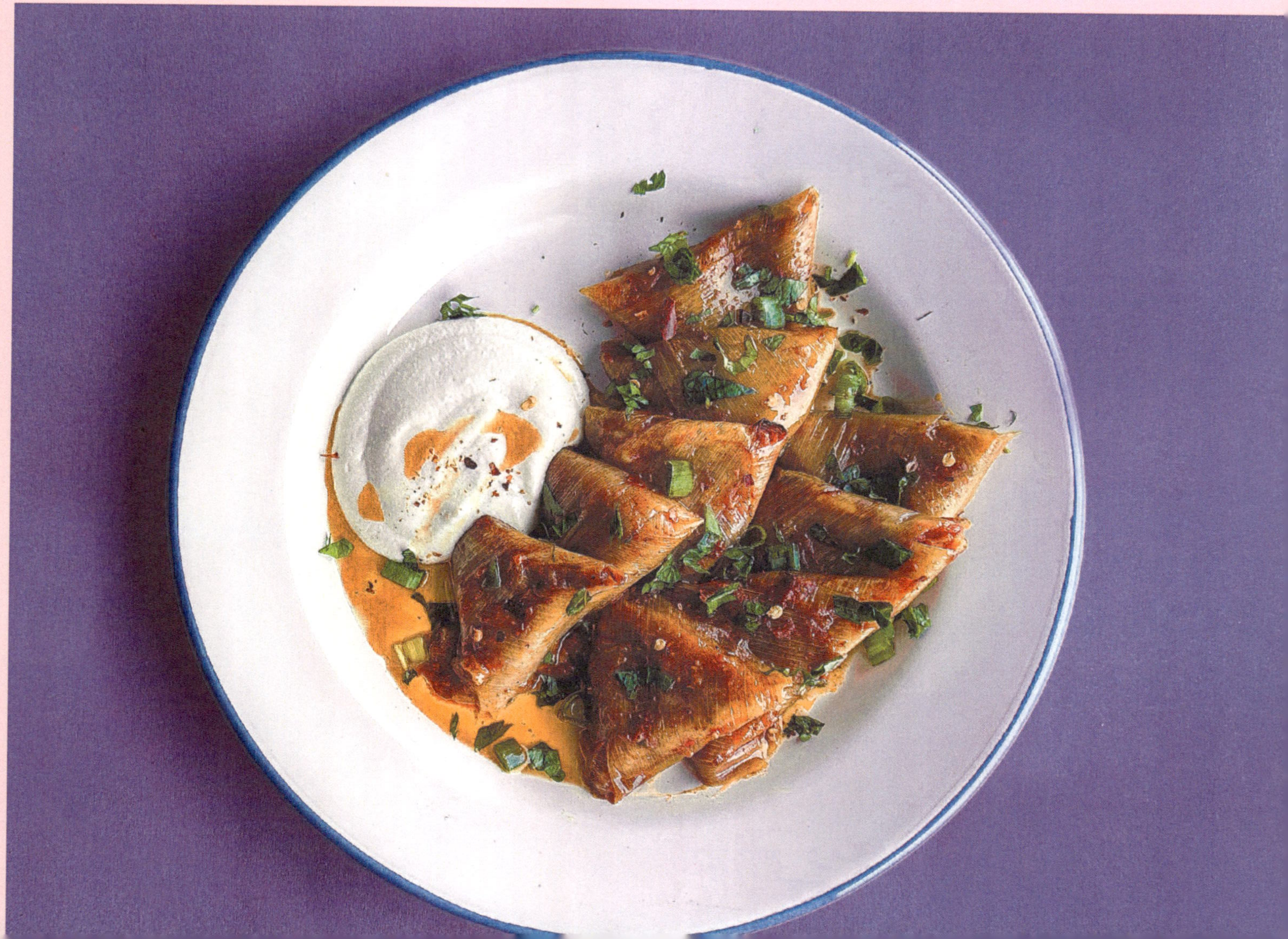

**Serves: 4**

**Ingredients**

1 kg leeks outer large parts
1/2 cup rice
1 1/4 cup water
2 tbsp pea mince
2 tbsp coconut aminos
1/2 carrot diced
1 red pepper diced
1 onion finely chopped
4 garlic cloves minced
1 tbsp seaweed flakes
2 tbsp olive oil
1 tbsp fresh rosemary chopped
1 tsp salt

**For the Sauce**

3 tbsp tomato paste
1 tbsp hot red pepper paste
3 garlic cloves minced
1/3 cup water
3 tbsp olive oil
1 tsp salt
1 tbsp fresh rosemary chopped

**For Serving**

1 cup cashew yoghurt
Fresh parsley leaves and green onion

*Delicate leek triangles encase a savory, umami-packed filling of earthy mushrooms and rich tomato sauce, Served with creamy yogurt and a drizzle of spicy chili oil. Ideal as a sophisticated appetizer or a small plate.*

1. Preheat the oven to 180°C.
2. In a pot, combine all the filling ingredients.
3. Trim the bottom of the leeks, make a lengthwise slit to the center, and separate them into leaf-like layers. Place in a large pot, add 1 lt hot water, let it sit for 10 minutes, then strain and set aside.
4. Wash and rinse your rice. In a pan, add minced garlic, chopped rosemary, onion, diced carrot, peppers and olive oil, cook until golden, then add pea mince and rice mix together.
5. Lastly add salt, coconut aminos, seaweed, tomato paste and water, cover the lid, cook until the mixture absorbs all water content. Your mixture will be semi-cooked as you will continue to baking process in the oven.
6. Place a spoonful of the filling at one end of each leek, fold it into a triangular shape, and continue folding along the length of the leek until it resembles a pastry.
7. Arrange the triangles in a baking dish.
8. Mix all the sauce ingredients and pour them over the triangles. Cover with damp parchment paper and aluminum foil, then bake for an hour.
9. Remove the cover (if the liquids have evaporated, add 1/2 cup of water) and bake uncovered for an additional 15 minutes.
10. You can also arrange the leeks in a flat pot, add an extra cup of water to the sauce, and simmer on low heat until they become tender.

# CREAMY PENNE

## WITH FENNEL AND PAPRIKA SAUCE

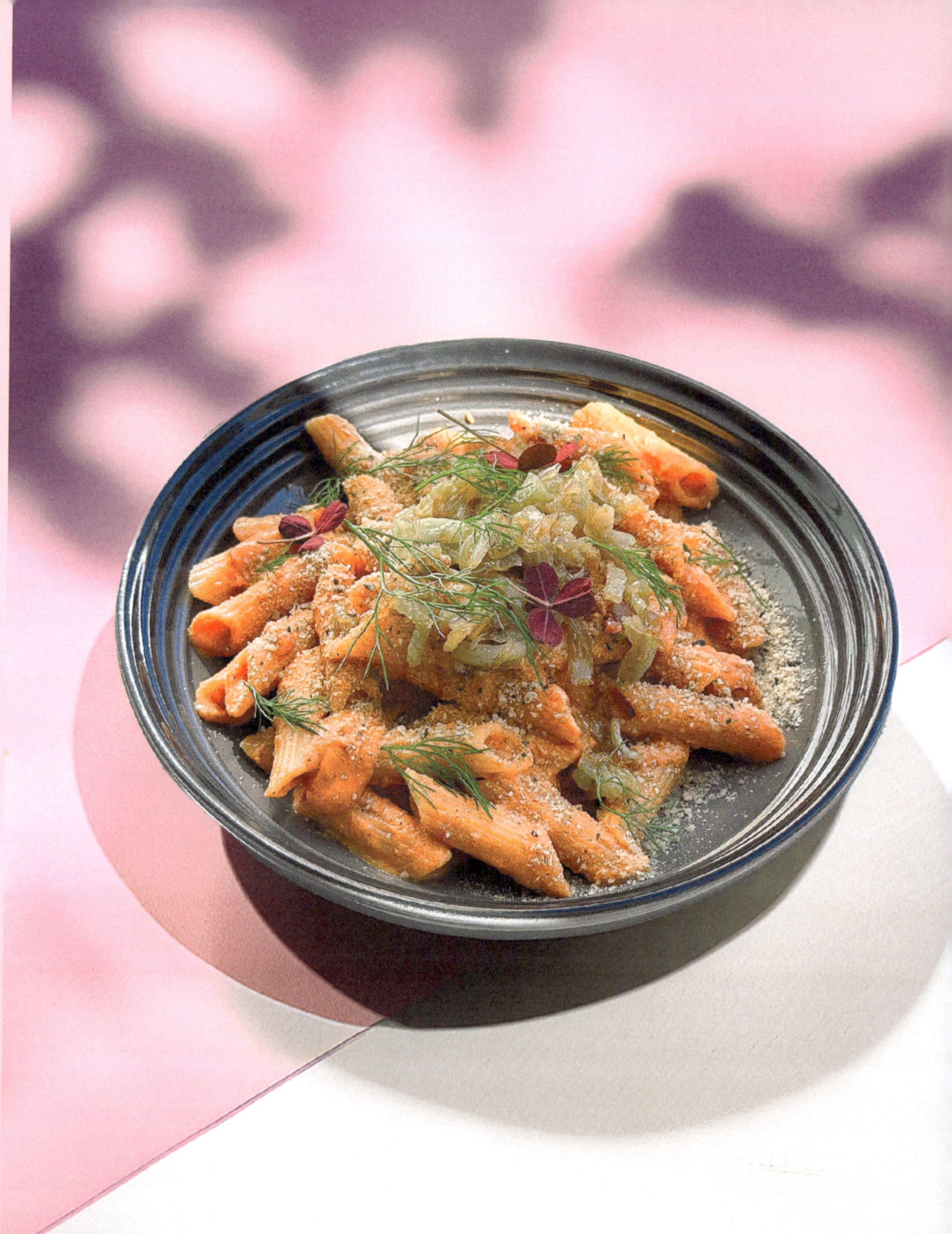

*Tender penne pasta is coated in a creamy, velvety silken tofu sauce, perfectly complementing the sweet, smoky notes of roasted bell pepper and the subtle aniseed aroma of fennel. Perfect for a satisfying lunch or dinner.*

**Serves: 4**

**Ingredients**

500 g gluten-free pasta
400 g silken tofu
250 g roasted bell pepper
150 g roasted tomatoes
100 g roasted fennel
1 dl pasta water
5 roasted garlic cloves
1 tbsp grated ginger
2 tbsp maple syrup
2 tbsp olive oil
5 tbsp tomato paste
3 tbsp nutritional yeast
2 tsp pink Himalayan salt

**For serving**

100 g thinly sliced fennel
100 g thinly sliced red onion
2 thinly sliced garlic cloves
1/2 tsp pink Himalayan salt
1 tbsp olive oil
Parmesan topping (page 23)
Fennel fronds for garnish (fennel fronds can be used as an herb to add fennel's licorice notes to raw and cooked dishes)
Red oxalis for garnish

1. Cook the pasta according to the package directions. Save 1 cup of the pasta water for the sauce.
2. Add all ingredients except the pasta and blend until creamy and smooth.
3. Pour the sauce into a saucepan and heat until bubbling, stirring occasionally. Taste and adjust seasoning.
4. Add the pasta and mix with the sauce.
5. Add the toppings to a frying pan and fry over medium heat until crispy. Top the pasta and sprinkle with a little hemp. Garnish with fennel leaves and oxalis. Enjoy your meal!

# POTATOMMUS

## HUMMUS THE SWEDISH WAY

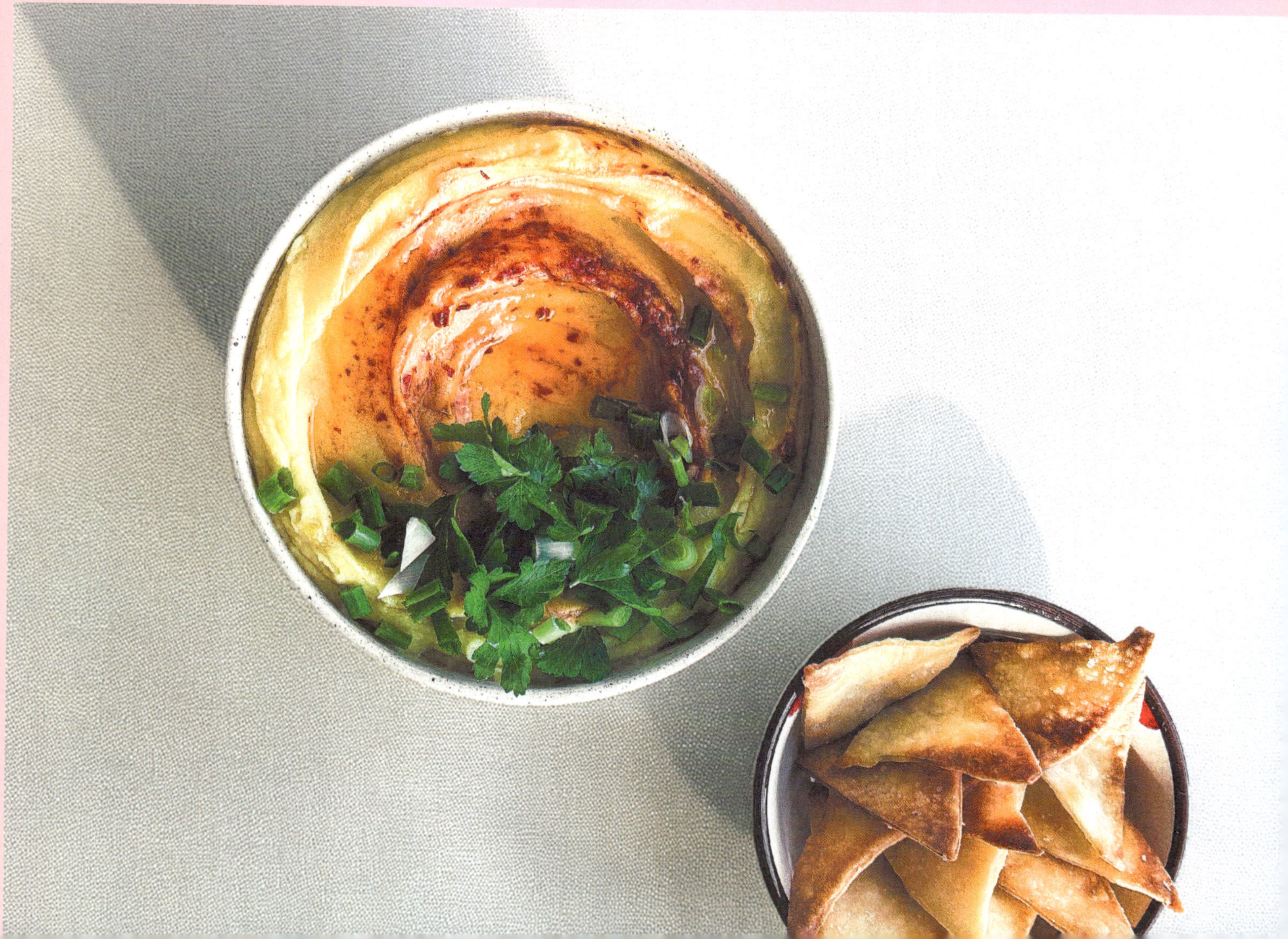

*If you're looking for a light alternative to traditional hummus, this potatommus is great way as the flavour and texture is so similar to regular hummus. This legume-free hummus comes together in just half an hour and is made with Yukon Gold potatoes the swedish way. Alongside a platter of vibrant crudités or tortilla chips, this super-smooth potatommus is sure to be a hit at your next brunch.*

**Serves: 2-3**

**Ingredients**

500 g yukon gold potatoes
2 tbsp extra virgin olive oil
1/2 lemon juice
2 garlic cloves minced
3 tbsp tahini
1 tsp pink himalayan salt

**For Serving**

Tortilla chips
1 tbsp hot red pepper paste
1 tbsp extra virgin olive oil + more as needed
A handful fresh parsley
A handful spring onions

1. Pour water into a saucepan to a depth of about 2 inches, add a few pinches of salt, and set over medium-high heat.
Meanwhile, peel and chop the potatoes.
2. One the water is boiling, cook potatoes for 8-10 minutes, or until tender when pierced with a fork. Drain the potatoes, rinse them with cold water, and put them in the bowl of a food processor.
3. Add salt and the garlic and pulse a few times. Then add the tahini, lemon juice and process until very smooth. With the processor running, add the olive oil in a steady stream and continue to blend until well combined.
4. Transfer to a bowl. Using a small spoon, spread the hot pepper paste on the potatommus.
5. Drizzle with olive oil and sprinkle with parsley and green onion.
6. Serve at room temperature with fresh vegetables or tortilla chips.

# JACKFRUIT BURGER

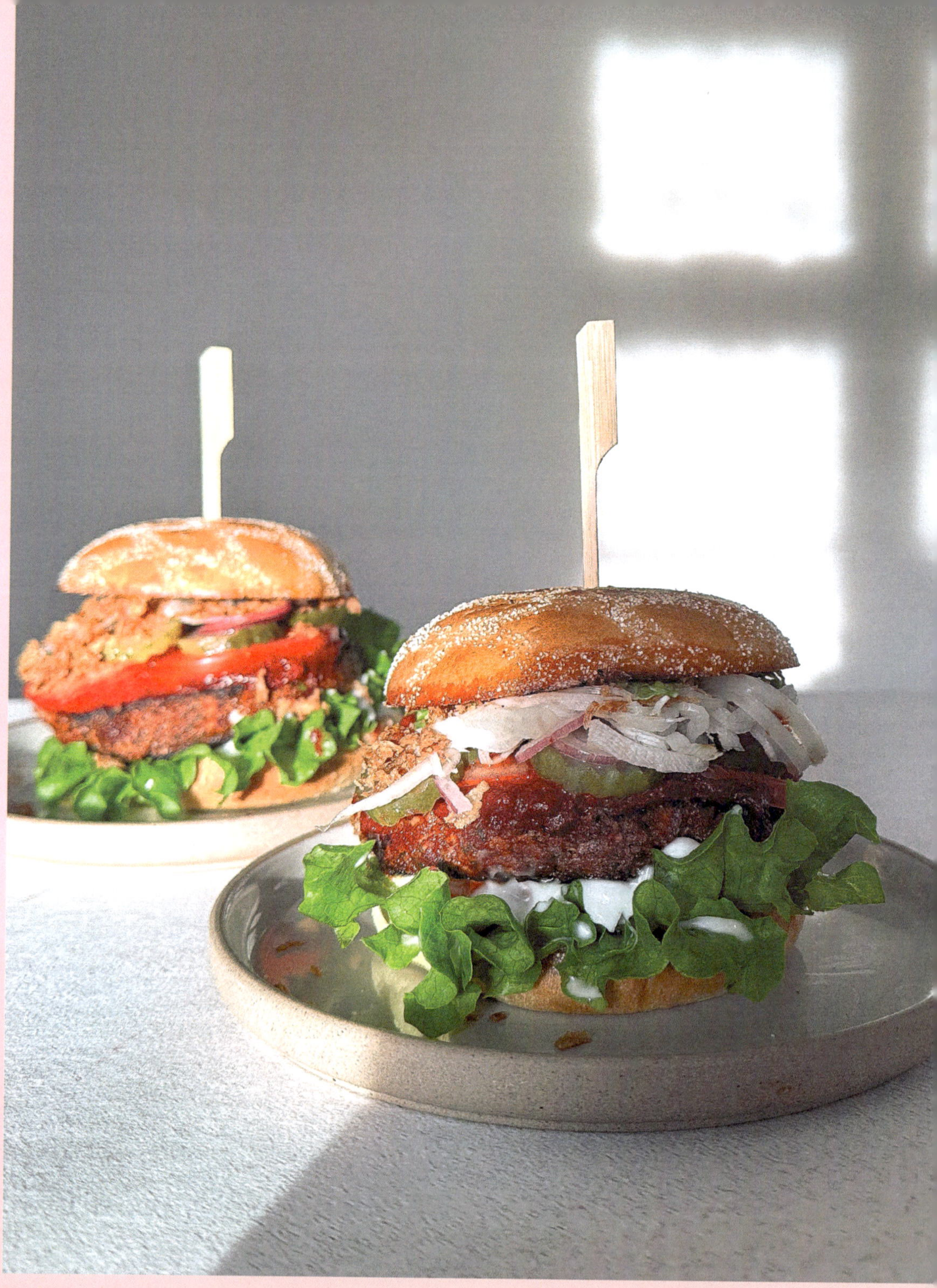

*This jackfruit burger mixes tender jackfruit, lentils, onions, garlic, and a bunch of umami-rich ingredients like miso, nutritional yeast, and tomato paste to create a hearty, savory patty. Brushed with barbecue sauce as it cooks, it develops a lightly caramelized, smoky crust that makes each bite extra satisfying. Stacked on a soft bun with your favorite fresh toppings, it becomes a juicy, flavorful plant-based burger that feels comforting and full of depth.*

**Serves: 4**

**For the Jackfruit Burger Mixture**

100 g oat flour
70 g dry roasted walnut flour
35 g tapioca flour
100 g cooked green lentils
460 g young jackfruit minced
1 tbsp olive oil
1 small yellow onion, finely chopped
4 garlic cloves minced
1/4 cup (12 g) nutritional yeast
5 tbsp tomato paste
2 tbsp agave syrup
3 tbsp miso
1 tsp smoked paprika
1-2 tsp salt
1/4 tsp black pepper
1/2 tsp dried oregano
1/4 cup finely chopped parsley
1/4 cup barbecue sauce, for brushing

**To Assemble:**

Burger buns of your choice.
Toppings of choice: lettuce, tomato, red onion or crispy onions, pickles, ketchup, mayonnaise, cabbage slaw or pickled fennel, etc.

1. To prepare the jackfruit: Rinse, dry and add into your food processor, blend until finely shredded.
2. Blend the dry ingredients: If using oat flour, walnuts, tapioca pulse oats in a food processor until finely ground.
3. Make the patty mixture: Add the jackfruit, nutritional yeast, onion, tomato paste, miso, spices, walnut flour, oat flour and agave to the food processor. Pulse until a moist, cohesive mixture forms.You can alternatively mix everything in a large bowl and knead for a while until it comes together.
4. Chill the mixture: Transfer the jackfruit mixture to a bowl, cover, and refrigerate for 30 minutes to firm up.
5. Shape and cook the patties: Heat a large pan over medium heat and lightly coat it with olive oil. Form the mixture into four thick patties (about 1/3 cup each—expect them to be quite moist).
6. Cook for 3–4 minutes per side, until golden brown and crisp on the edges. Brush lightly with barbecue sauce if desired. Assemble the burgers: Add the patties to buns with your favorite toppings and enjoy!

# PAD THAI

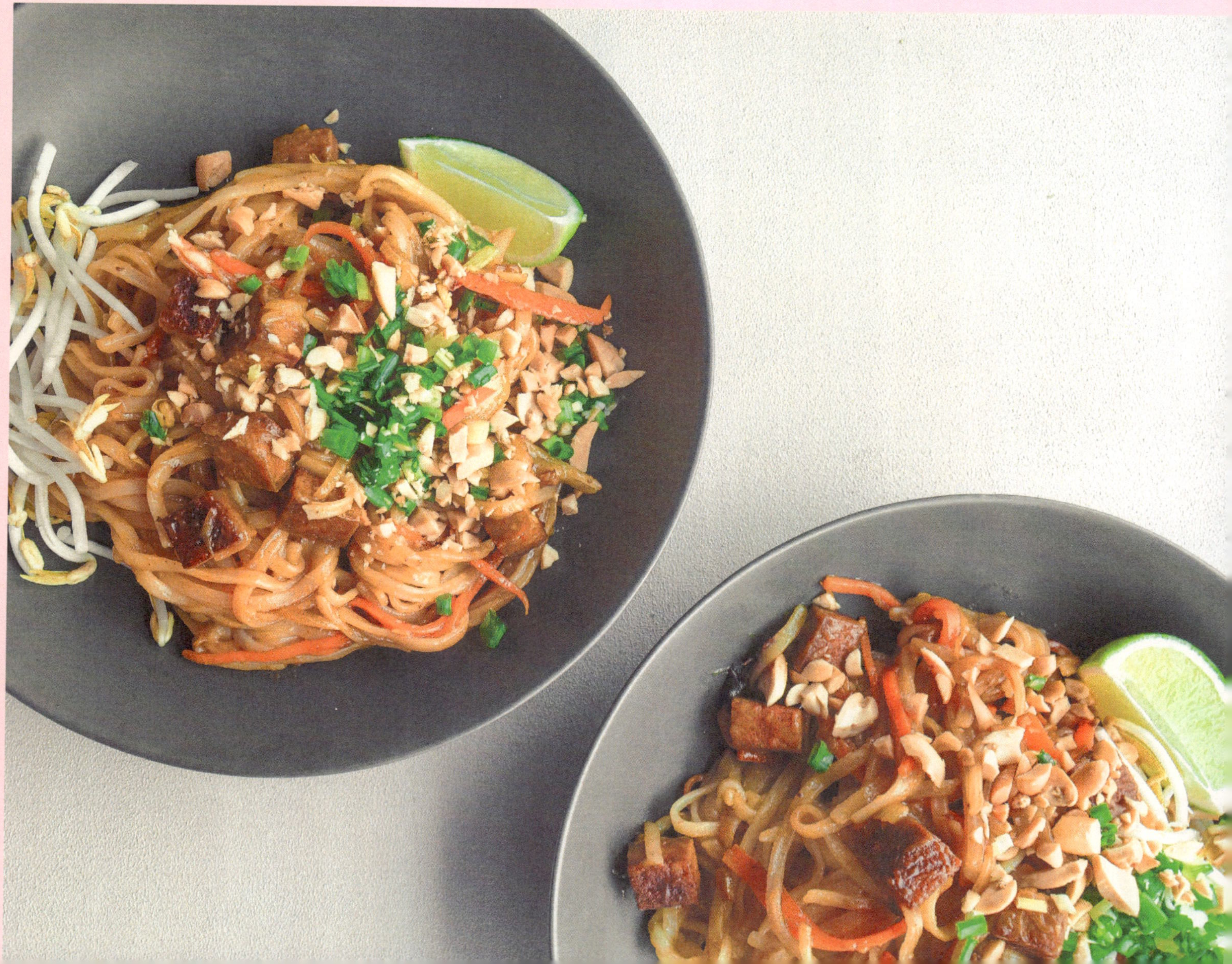

*Pad Thai is one of Thailand's classic dishes and a big favorite here in Sweden. I, who love pad thai so much that I can eat it several days in a row without getting tired, understand completely. Now you can easily make a vegan version at home! It is mild in flavor and garnished with coriander, lime and chopped peanuts to taste.*

**Serves: 2**

**Ingredients**

200 g rice noodles
1/4 small chopped cabbage
1 large chopped onion
200 g mushrooms or plant-based protein of choice (pea protein)
1 tsp salt
4 tbsp olive oil
2 tbsp coconut aminos
Fresh coriander for serving
Sorrel for decoration

**Pad sauce**

4 cm grated ginger
1 tbsp tamarind paste
3 tbsp lemon juice
1 tsp chili pepper
4 cloves garlic, finely chopped
1 tsp mushroom sauce or coconut aminos
1 tbsp sesame oil
2 scallions, thinly sliced
2 tsp coconut sugar

1. Cook your rice noodles in boiling salted water until tender. Follow the instructions on the package for the exact time or taste after 3-4 minutes.
2. Fry the chopped onion, garlic and mushrooms (or plant-based meat alternative) with olive oil in a wok.
3. When the mushrooms are almost cooked, add the chopped cabbage and continue cooking for 3-4 minutes.
4. Add a little more olive oil or coconut aminos if needed during the cooking process to keep the ingredients juicy.
5. When your rice noodles are cooked, remove from the heat, strain and add to the wok. Mix everything together.
6. Then pour the dressing over the noodles. Stir well until everything is well coated with the dressing.
7. Serve your pad thai with coarsely chopped peanuts, coriander and lime to squeeze over.

**Pad thai sauce**

Making your own pad thai sauce is easy. All you need to do is mix the following ingredients together in a bowl. It can also be made in advance and stored in the refrigerator for up to a week.

# SKAGEN PASTA SALAD

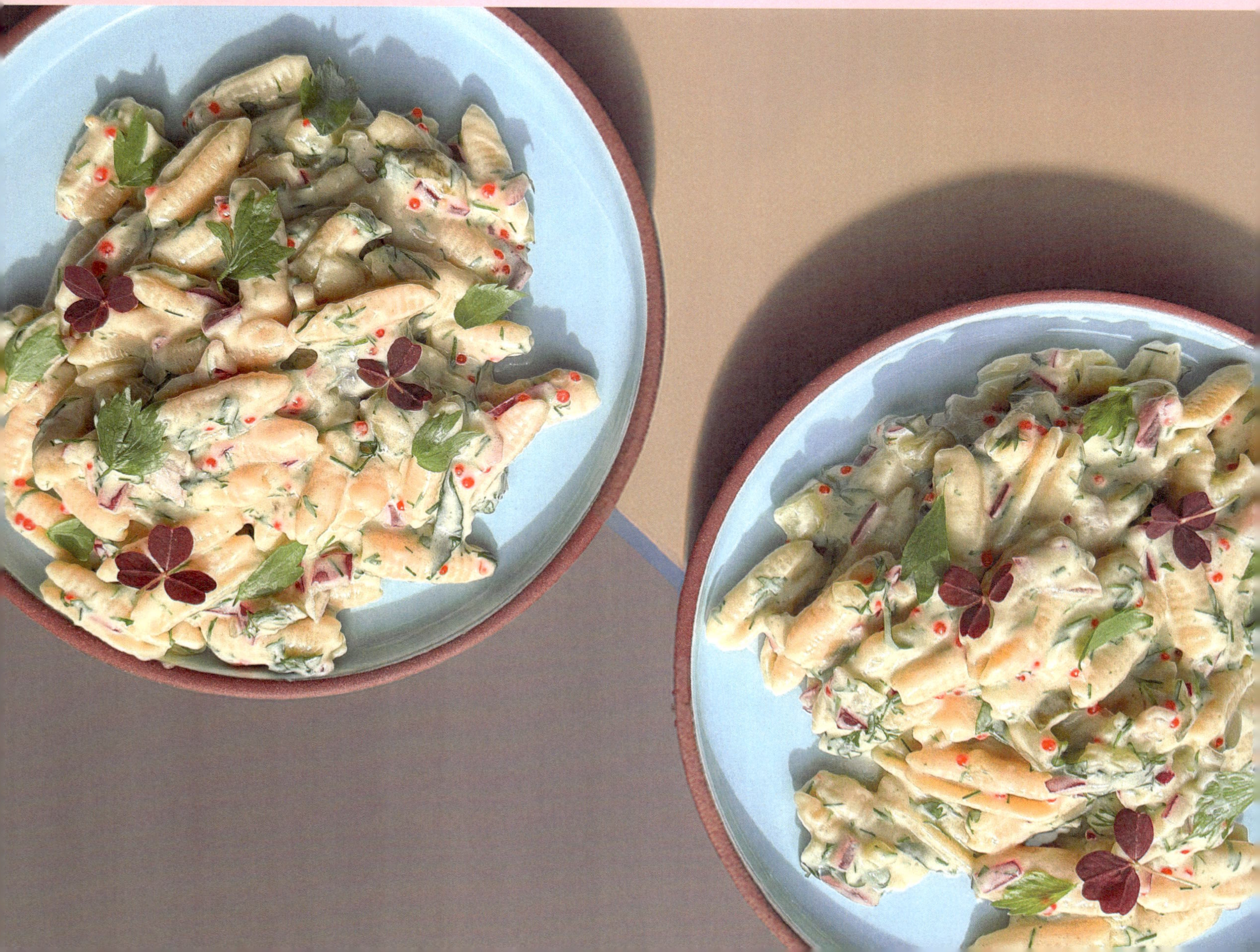

*The creamy, tangy Skagen sauce paired with chilled pasta creates a dish that is cool and satisfying without feeling heavy. Fresh herbs, crisp vegetables, and delicate plant-based seafood flavors make each bite bright, aromatic, and vibrant, ideal for hot days when you want a delicious, easy-to-enjoy meal that still feels indulgent.*

**Serves: 2**

**Ingredients**

200 g cooked pasta of your choice
300 g oat yoghurt (page 17)
1 tbsp dijon mustard
2 tbsp seaweed caviar
1 lime juice
1 tbsp olive oil
2 tbsp coconut aminos
1/2 diced red onion
3 chopped garlic cloves
1/4 bunch fresh lovage chopped
1/4 bunch fresh dill chopped
1/4 bunch finely chopped chives
Red oxalis to decorate

1. Mix all ingredients except pasta in a large bowl.
2. Cook your pasta according to the instructions on the package. Drain under cold running water.
3. Mix the pasta with your Skagen sauce.
4. Decorate with oxalis and lovage leaves.

# JUICY THAI NOODLE SALAD

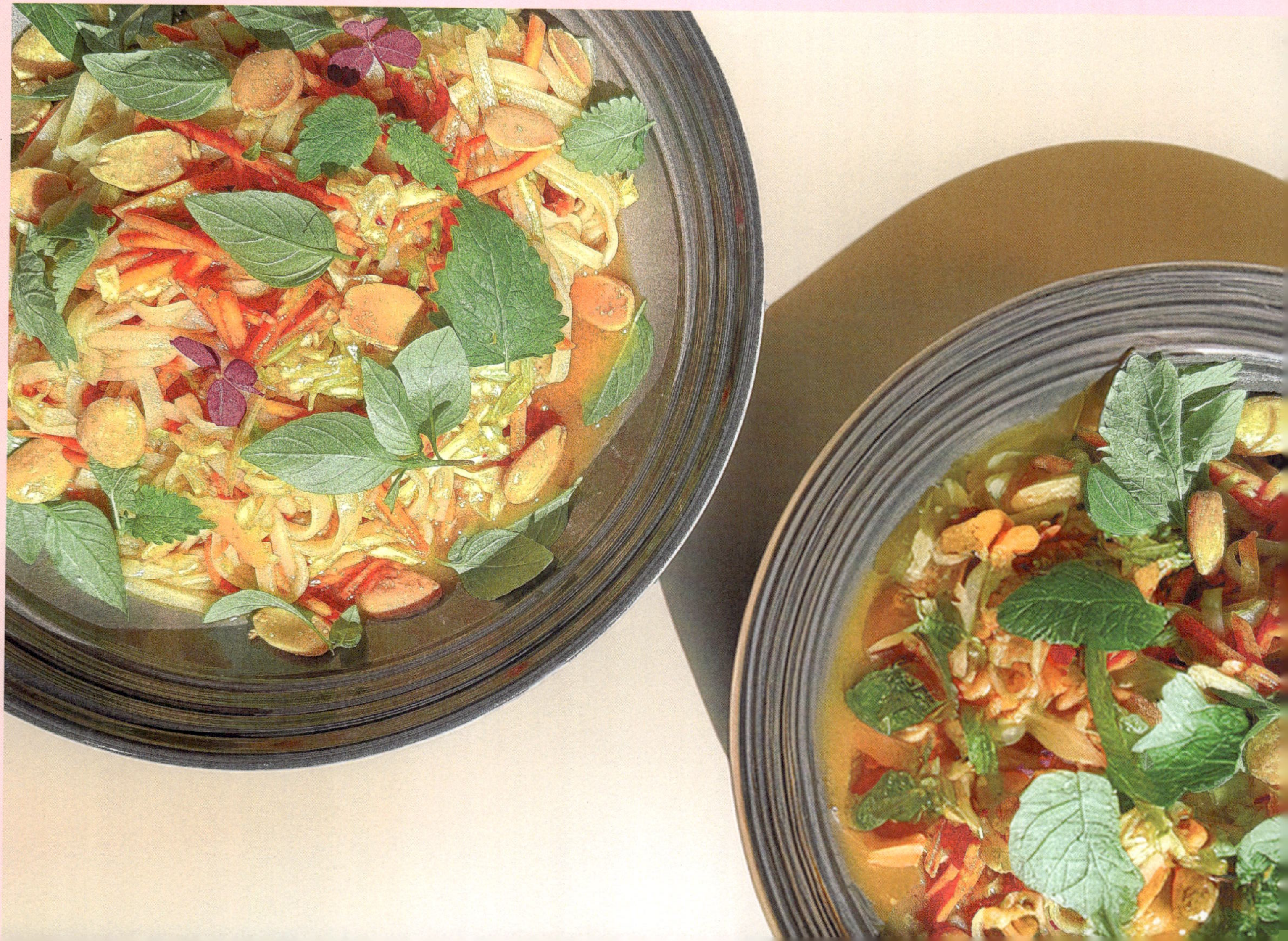

*Rice noodles tossed with crisp vegetables, fresh herbs, and a zesty, tangy dressing inspired by Thai flavors. Each bite bursts with juicy textures, bright citrus notes, and a perfect balance of sweet, salty, and umami flavor.*

**Serves: 2**

**Ingredients**

170 g rice noodles
200 g a mixture of thinly shredded cabbage and julienned carrots

**Dressing**

3 lime juice
1 tbsp extra virgin olive oil
3 tbsp coconut aminos
1.5 tbsp coconut nectar or maple syrup
1 tbsp apple cider vinegar
1/2 tsp pink Himalayan salt

**For serving**

1 dl fresh lemon balm leaves
1/4 bunch Thai basil
1 dl salted blanched almonds
2 chopped garlic cloves
1 tbsp grated fresh ginger
1/2 tsp hot chili flakes

1. Cook the noodles according to the package directions until al dante and set aside.
2. Mix all the dressing ingredients in a bowl.
3. Place the carrot and cabbage in a bowl.
4. Pour the dressing over them. Toss together. Let stand for 7-8 minutes until slightly softened.
5. Add the cooked rice noodles and mix together. Let stand for 5 minutes until the rice noodles absorb all the juicy contents.
6. Serve with almonds and herbs.

# AUBERGINE BELUGA SALAD

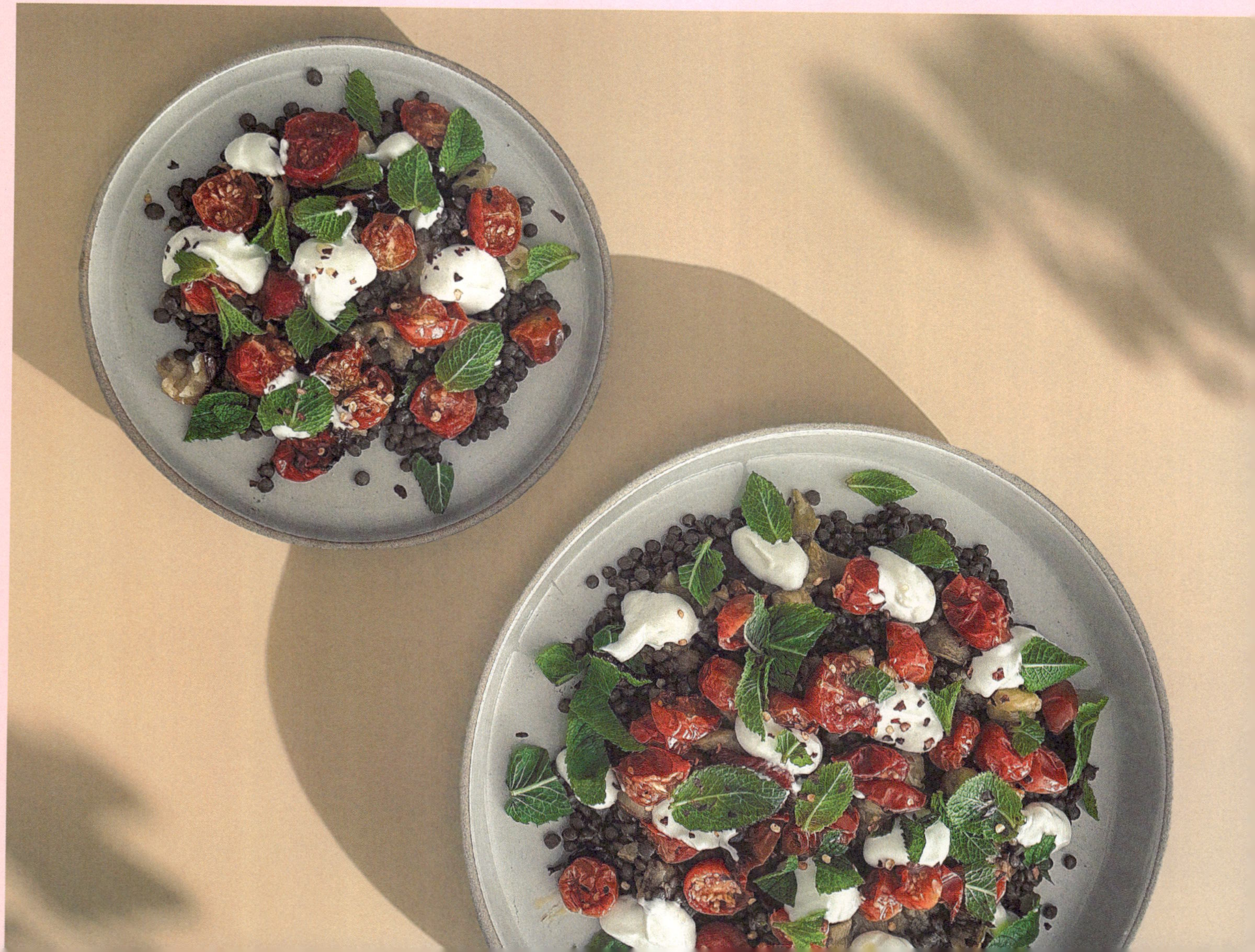

*Earthy beluga lentils provide a hearty base, complemented by smoky roasted aubergine and sweet, caramelized roasted tomatoes. Silky yogurt adds a cooling creaminess, while fresh mint brings a bright, aromatic lift.*

**Serves: 3**

**Ingredients**

4 aubergines
300 g cherry tomatoes
160 g beluga or puy lentils or 350g cooked packaged puy lentils
2 tbsp olive oil
2 tbsp lemon juice
2 small cloves of garlic, chopped
1/4 bunch of chopped mint
1 tbsp chilli
150 g oat yoghurt (page 17)
Salt and pepper

1. Preheat the oven to 220C.
2. To cook the aubergines, place them on a baking tray and roast for 1 hour, turning halfway through, until the flesh is completely soft and slightly smoky.
3. Remove from the oven and, when cool enough to handle, scoop the flesh out into a colander.
4. Set aside, in the sink or over a bowl, for 30 minutes to allow any liquid to drain. The skin can be discarded. Then dice.
5. Place the cherry tomatoes on a baking tray and roast for 12 minutes, until slightly blackened, split and soft. Remove from the oven and set aside.
6. Fill a medium saucepan with plenty of water and place over a high heat. When boiling, add the lentils, reduce the heat to medium and cook for 20 minutes, until tender but still retaining a bite. Drain and set aside to dry out a bit.
7. Place lentils in a large bowl and add the eggplant flesh, tomatoes, oil, lemon juice, garlic, and 3/4 teaspoon salt and a generous grind of pepper.
8. Mix well, then pour into a large shallow serving bowl. Top with yogurt, chili, and fresh mint.
9. Drizzle with a little extra olive oil if desired.

# SAVORY PUFF PASTRY

## WITH MUSHROOM, AVOCADO & PICKLED ONION

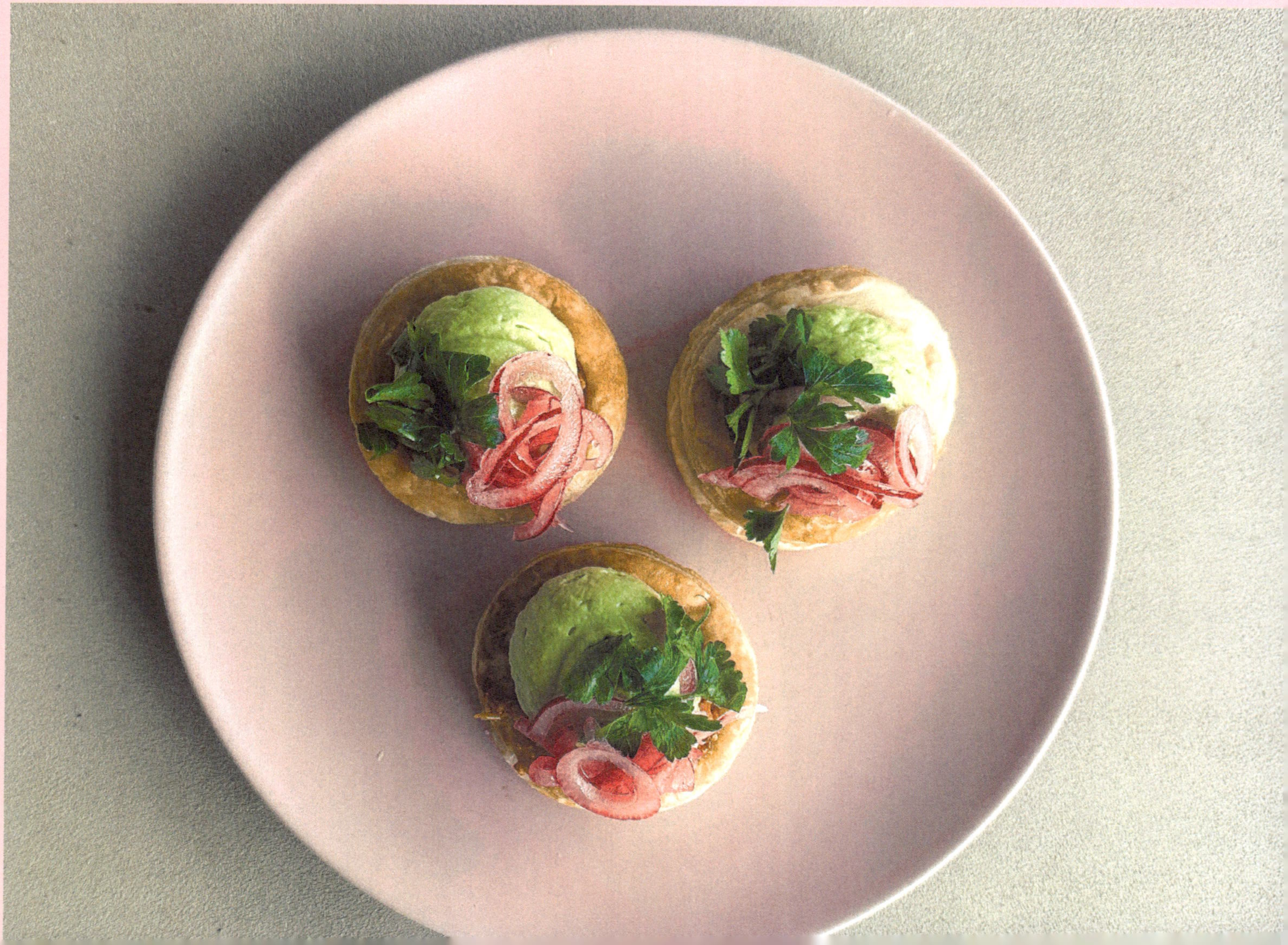

*Flaky, golden puff pastry cradles a savory mushroom mince, layered with creamy avocado mayo and tangy pickled red onion.*

**Serves: 6**

**Ingredients**

500 g puff pastry

200 g mushrooms

1/2 carrot diced

1 onion finely chopped

4 garlic cloves minced

1 red bell pepper diced

2 tbsp olive oil

**Avocado cream**

1 large avocado

2 tbsp lemon juice

1 tbsp water

3 garlic cloves minced

**For serving**

1 cup fresh parsley

1 cup pickled red onion

**Egg wash**

2 tbsp coconut oil

1 tbsp pea milk

1 tsp agave syrup

1. Preheat oven to 210° C.
2. Mix vegan egg wash mixture in a bowl.
3. Using puff pastry dough as cold ad possible. Unfold the pastry sheets and brush the top of the dough with the egg wash. Cut 9 rounds from the puff pastry sheet/sheets using a 2-inch round cutter. Using a 1-½ inch round cutter, cut through the precut 2-inch rounds leaving it together.
4. Place the cut round on top of the uncut 2-inch round. (Note: You can freeze the raw assembled rounds, store in a freezer bag and bake at a later time.)
5. To prepare filling, in a pan, add olive oil and mix finely chopped mushrooms, onion, garlic, pepper, carrot and broccoli stalks. Cook until gets brown, then add a dash of water and continue to cook until the mixture absorbs all water content and tender.
6. ill the puff pastry with your filling.
7. Bake for 15 to 20 minutes until golden brown.
8. In a small blender or food processor, mix avocado, garlic and lemon juice together until smooth. Transfer to a pipping bag. Pipe on the top of filling.
9. Decorate with pickled red onion and fresh parsley.

PLANT BASED UMAMI

# SOM TAM

## THAI GREEN PAPAYA SALAD

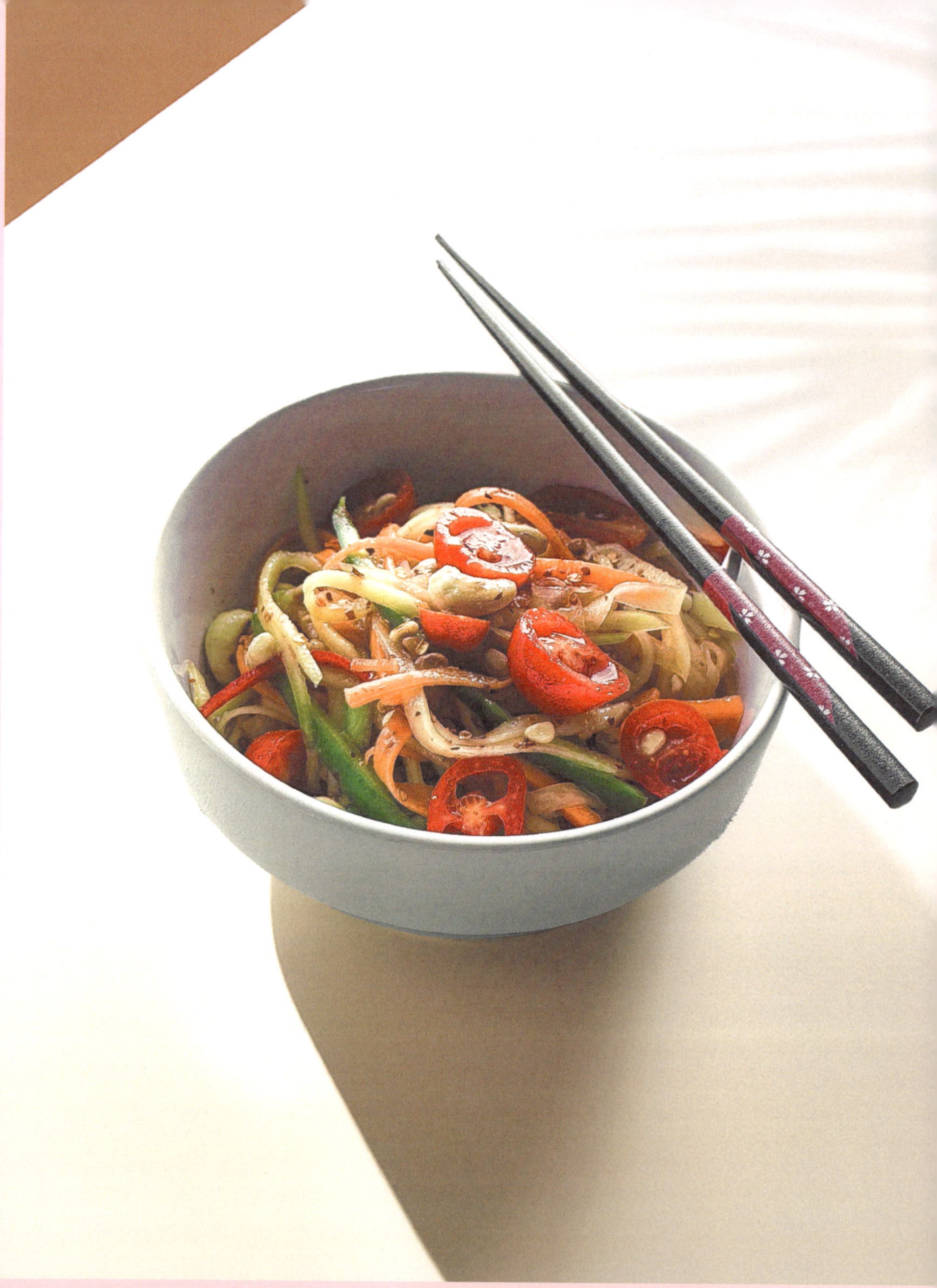

*Som Tam combines crisp shredded green papaya, juicy cherry tomatoes, crunchy long beans, and toasted peanuts. Tossed in a zesty, tangy dressing of lime, chili, and a touch of coconut sugar, each bite bursts with sweet, sour, salty, and spicy flavors.*

**Serves: 2**

**Ingredients**

5 bird's eye chilies
5 minced garlic cloves
2 tbsp coconut blossom sugar
2 long green beans, cut into 1 inch pieces
8 cherry tomatoes, halved
1/2 (400 g) large green papaya, peeled and shredded or julienned
1/2 cup roasted cashews or peanuts
2 tbsp roasted pine nuts
1 julienned carrot

**Dressing**

1 dl lime juice
1 tbsp coconut aminos
1 tsp dulse flakes
5 tamarinds, pitted

1. Toast the cashews over medium heat in a small, dry frying pan until golden brown. Remove from the pan and set aside.
2. Roughly crush the chillies and garlic with a pestle and mortar.
3. Add the coconut sugar, beans and tomatoes. Mix lightly to combine, then squeeze in the lime juice and coconut aminos sauce.
4. Mix lightly again, then add the green papaya and carrot.
5. Stir to combine. The flavours should be a perfect balance of sweet and salty, with a sharp, tangy and spicy note.
6. Pour the salad into a serving bowl and sprinkle with the seaweed and toasted cashews.

# WOK NOODLES

PLANT BASED UMAMI

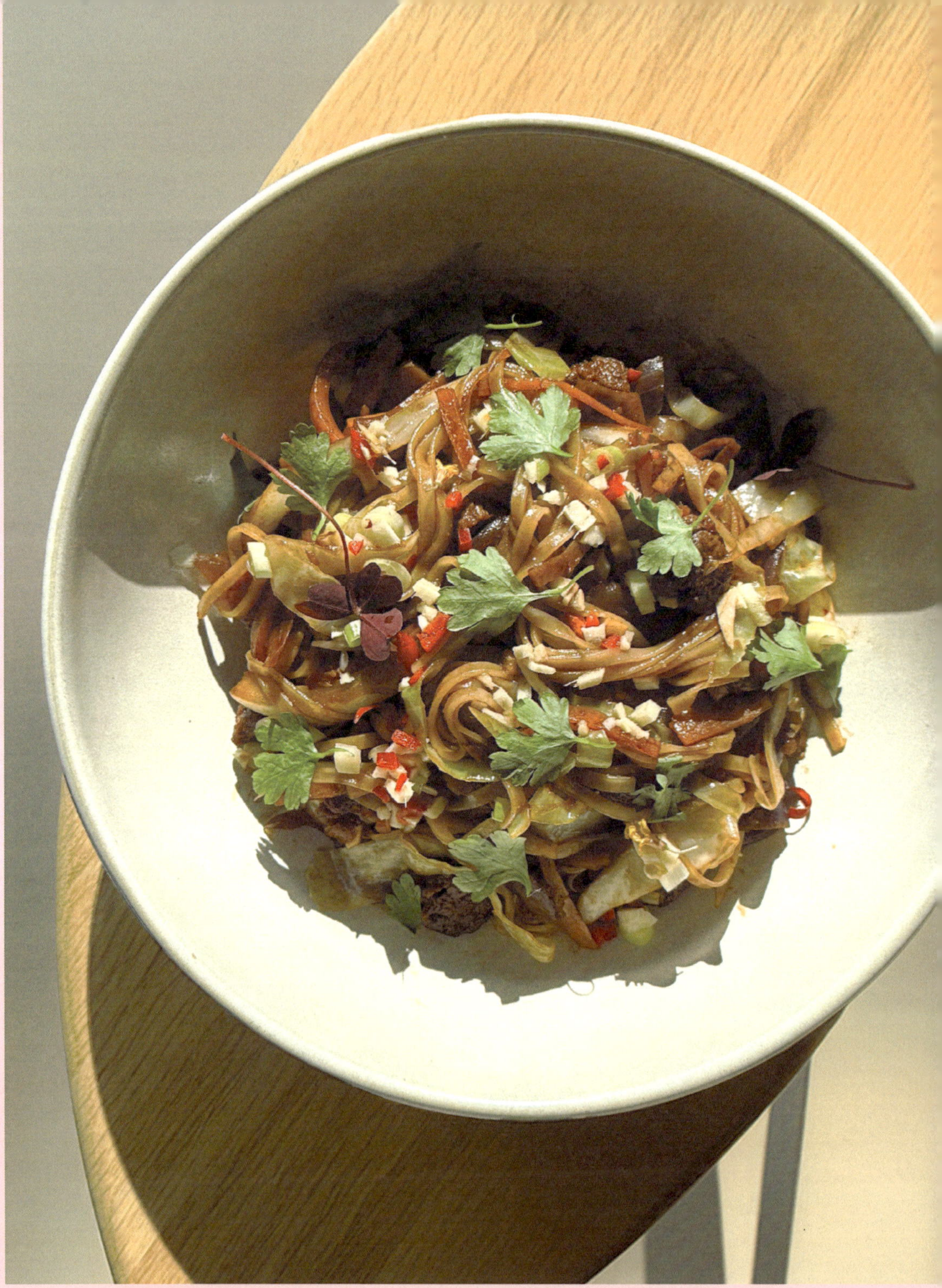

**Serves: 2**

**Ingredients**

200 g young jackfruit diced
200 g rice noodles
1 carrot julienne
4 garlic cloves finely chopped
1 onion finely chopped
3 scallions finely chopped
1 cup white or green cabbage finely shredded
1 tbsp olive oil
1/4 cup water

**For the sauce**

1 tablespoon tapioca
5 tablespoons cold water
1 tsp seaweed powder
5-6 tbsp coconut aminos
1 tbsp mirin or apple cider vinegar
1 tbsp agave
2 tbsp sesame oil

**Optional toppings**

Roasted cashews
Coriander, chili, ginger

1. To make the sauce: Simply mix up the ingredients in a jam jar, or similar, and then throw the sauce straight into the wok for the last 2-3 minutes of cooking time to cook through and thicken up. Set aside.
2. Prepare your jackfruit; cut into small pieces. Pour 2 tbsp of Sauce over the jackfruit, mix to coat, set aside to marinate for 10 minutes.
3. Prepare the noodles according to the packet instructions, then drain.
4. Heat oil in wok or large fry pan over high heat.
5. Add garlic and stir fry for 10 seconds or until it starts to turn golden.
6. Add jackfruit and stir fry until the surface gets a tinge of browning about 2-3 minutes on medium-high heat.
7. Add the cabbage, carrot, and the white pieces of shallots (i.e. from the base of the stalk). Stir fry for 1-2 minutes until the cabbage is mostly wilted.
8. Add the noodles and the rest of the sauce. Stir fry for 2-3 minute, tossing constantly.
9. Remove from heat and serve with roasted cashews, coriander, chili and ginger desired (optional).

PLANT BASED UMAMI

# CHARCOAL TACOS

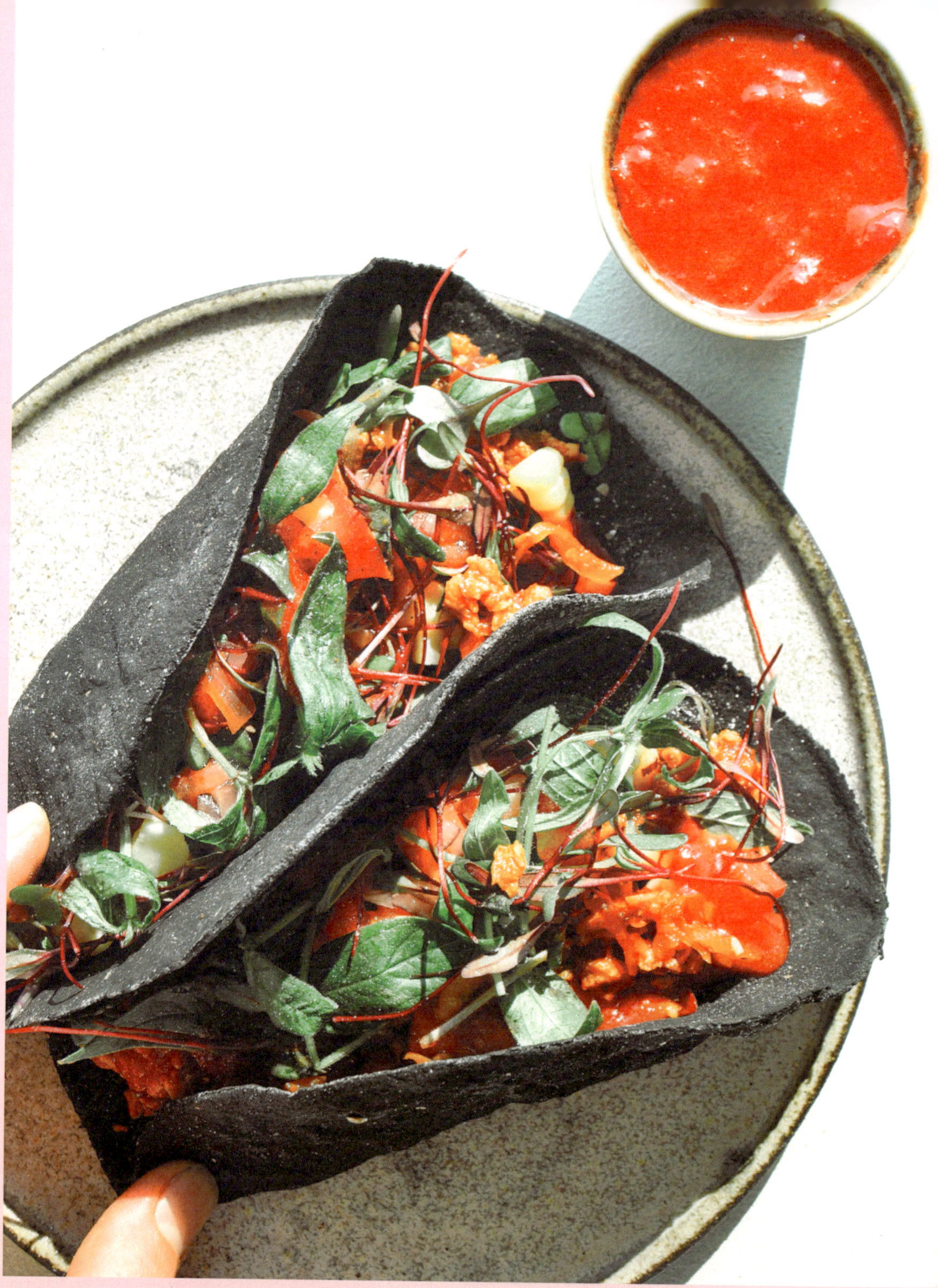

*A visually striking, naturally black taco made from hearty buckwheat flour and activated charcoal. Its robust, nutty flavor and slightly crisp, chewy texture make it a perfect base for plant-based fillings, from fresh vegetables to savory spreads.*

**Serves: 2**

**Ingredients**

120 g (1 cup) buckwheat flour
65 g (1/2 cup) cassava or tapioca flour
1 tbsp psyllium powder + 3 tbsp water
1/4 tsp salt
1/2 tsp activated charcoal
90 ml water

**Filling**

Roasted mushrooms (or tempeh, pea protein, jackfruit)
Hot chili sauce
Thai basil
Beetroot sprouts

1. Mix psyllium with 3 tablespoons of water in a large bowl and stir well.
2. Then add buckwheat flour, tapioca, salt and the rest of the water. Mix well until you get a dough shape.
3. Remove the dough from the bowl and knead it with your hands. Sprinkle a little buckwheat flour on the kitchen counter.
4. Roll out the dough as thin as possible, but avoid breaking it.
5. Use a 7-8 cm round cookie cutter and cut out the dough into small tortillas.
6. Heat a non-stick frying pan over medium heat. Place a tortilla in the pan.
7. Cook on both sides for 1-2 minutes, keeping a close eye on it to avoid burning the tortilla.
8. Repeat the process for the rest.
9. Fill with desired ingredients.

# QUINOA WITH CARROT CREAM

## AND PARSLEY GREMOLATA

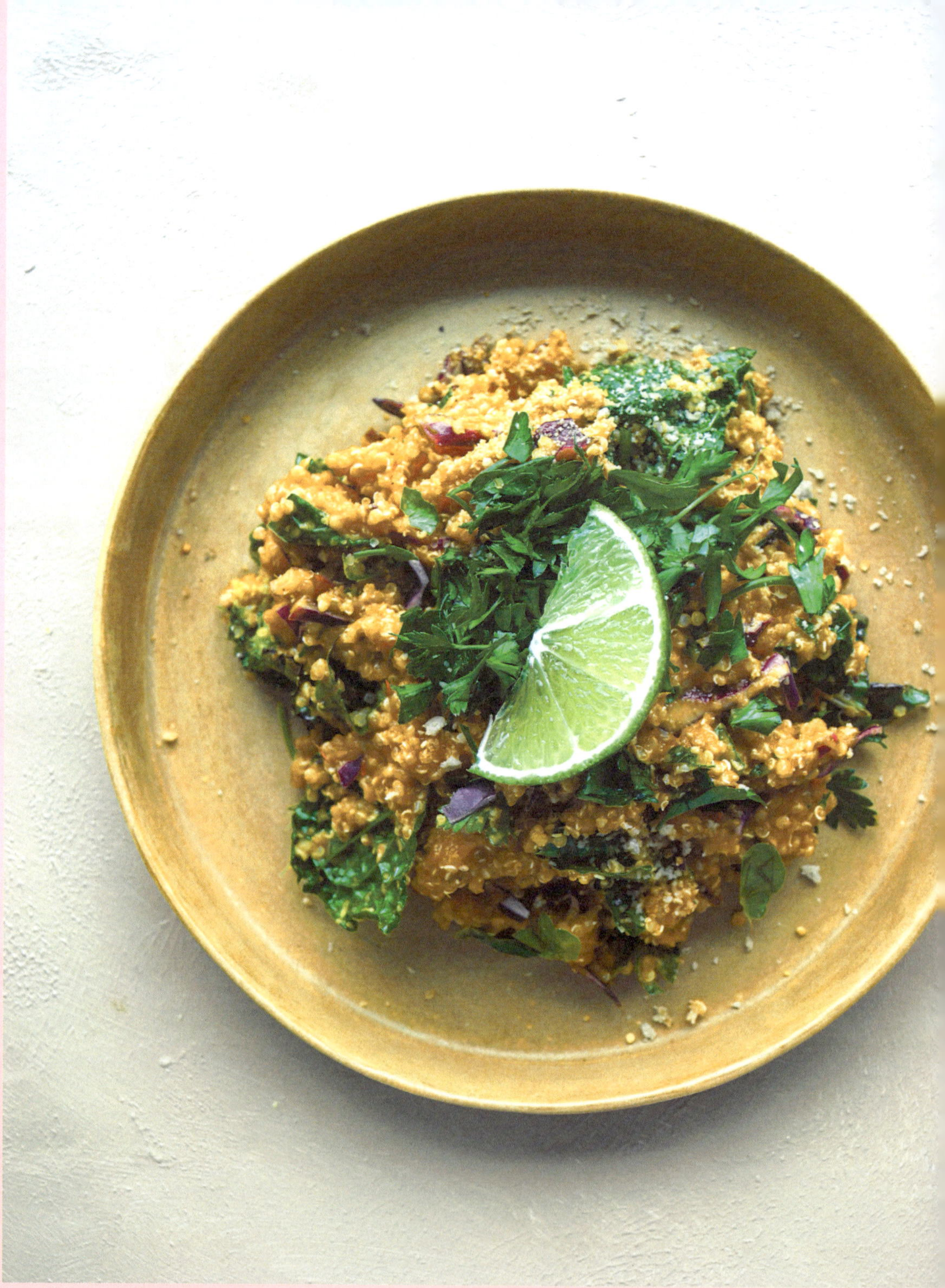

*A warm and delicious dish with crunchy bitter kale, fresh parsley and lemon. Make a big batch and store in the fridge for up to 5 days. It's even better cold, perfect for busy days.*

**Serves: 3**

**Ingredients**

150 g quinoa
240 ml filtered water
1/2 tsp sea salt
1/4 tsp ground black pepper
100 g dinosaur kale
100 g finely chopped red cabbage
Lime wedges to serve

**Carrot Cream**

400 g carrots (or pumpkin)
1 red bell pepper
1 medium red onion
3 garlic cloves
1/2 tsp sea salt
2-4 tbsp water as needed for creamy consistency
1 tsp red pepper flakes

**Parsley Gremolata**

1/2 bunch parsley
Juice of whole lemon
2 garlic cloves
A pinch of salt

1. Pour the water, place a stainless steel steamer basket in the instant pot.
2. Add the carrots in the basket. Pressure cook at high pressure for 2-3 minutes, then quick release.
3. Chop your red bell pepper, onion and garlic. In a pot add 2 tbsp water, place the onion and garlic. Cook at medium heat for 3-4 minutes or until onions are soften enough.
4. Place soften onions and garlic into a high speed blender along with the cooked carrots. Add salt, red pepper flakes and 2 tbsp water. Then blend on high speed until you get a nice smooth carrot cream.
5. Place your quinoa in a small pot, wash and strain. Cover 1 cup filtered water and cook at medium heat for about 15 minutes or until the quinoa absorbs all the water. Once cooked season with salt and black pepper, set aside.
6. Wash and cut your kale leaves into small pieces. Preheat a non-stick skillet over medium heat. Once the pan is ready add the kale and cook for a few seconds then add the water to sautee. Cook until the kale starts to wilt and turns bright green.
7. To make parsley gremolata, remove the stems from the parsley. Chop the parsley with a chef's knife until it is nearly finely chopped. Grate the garlic clove over the parsley. Add fresh lemon juice over the parsley. Toss together.
8. In a bowl, mix all the ingredients together, coat your quinoa with the carrot cream well. Add the parsley gremolata and cabbage. Serve with lime wedges.

# QUINOA CRÊPES

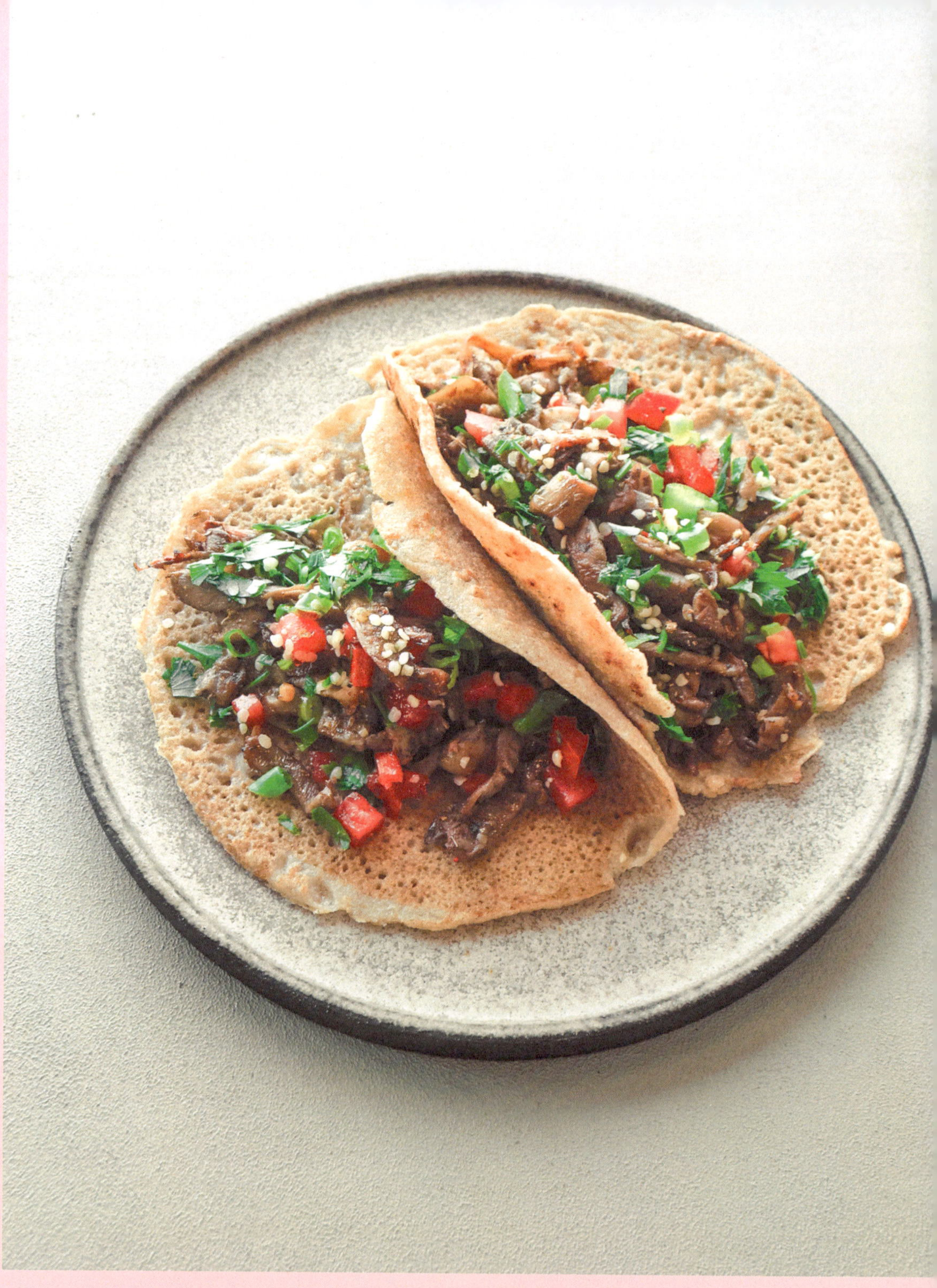

*Quinoa crêpes are made simply with quinoa and water, resulting in a light, nutty, and slightly earthy base that's naturally gluten-free. Filled with a savory mushroom mixture, they are packed with umami-rich flavors that elevate this simple plant-based dish into something deeply satisfying.*

**Serves:** 5 st x 20 cm crêpes

**Crêpes**

90 g uncooked white quinoa
130 g water
1/4 tsp salt

**Pulled Mushrooms**

300 g oyster mushrooms
2 tbsp olive oil
75 ml ketjap manis
3 tbsp coconut aminos
1½ tbsp sriracha sauce
2 tsp mirin
1 tsp lime juice
1 tsp agave
1 tsp tapioca starch + 2 teaspoons water
1 tsp sesame seeds, toasted and 1/2 green onion for garnish

**Crêpes**

1. Soak the quinoa in a bowl for at least 3-4 hours to remove its phytic acid and bitter taste.
2. Once soaked, rinse and strain, transfer to your blender along with the water and salt.
3. Blend for 40 seconds in a high-speed blender or until the batter is smooth. The batter will not be too thick, just runny like a crepe batter.
4. Transfer the batter to a bowl and let sit for 10-12 minutes to thicken.
5. Heat a non-stick pan over medium heat and spray a little olive oil all over the pan.
6. Pour 1/4 cup of the batter into the center of the pan, using the back of a spoon.
7. Cook for 2 minutes on one side, then flip and cook on the other side.
8. Repeat the process for the rest. Make sure to spray the pan with olive oil for each crêpes crêpe.

Storage: up to 2 days in an airtight container.

**Pulled Mushrooms**

1. Preheat oven to 180°C.
2. Line a baking sheet with parchment paper.
3. Pull the oyster mushrooms apart into thick strands. Spread over the baking sheet with oil and 1/2 teaspoon salt.
4. Bake for 20 minutes.
5. For the sauce, heat the coconut aminos, Sriracha sauce, mirin, lime juice and agave in a wok. Make a paste of the tapioca starch and water.
6. Add and simmer until the sugar has dissolved and the sauce thickens.
7. Add the roasted oyster mushrooms to the sauce. Garnish with scallions and sesame seeds.

PLANT BASED UMAMI

# SPAGHETTI SQUASH

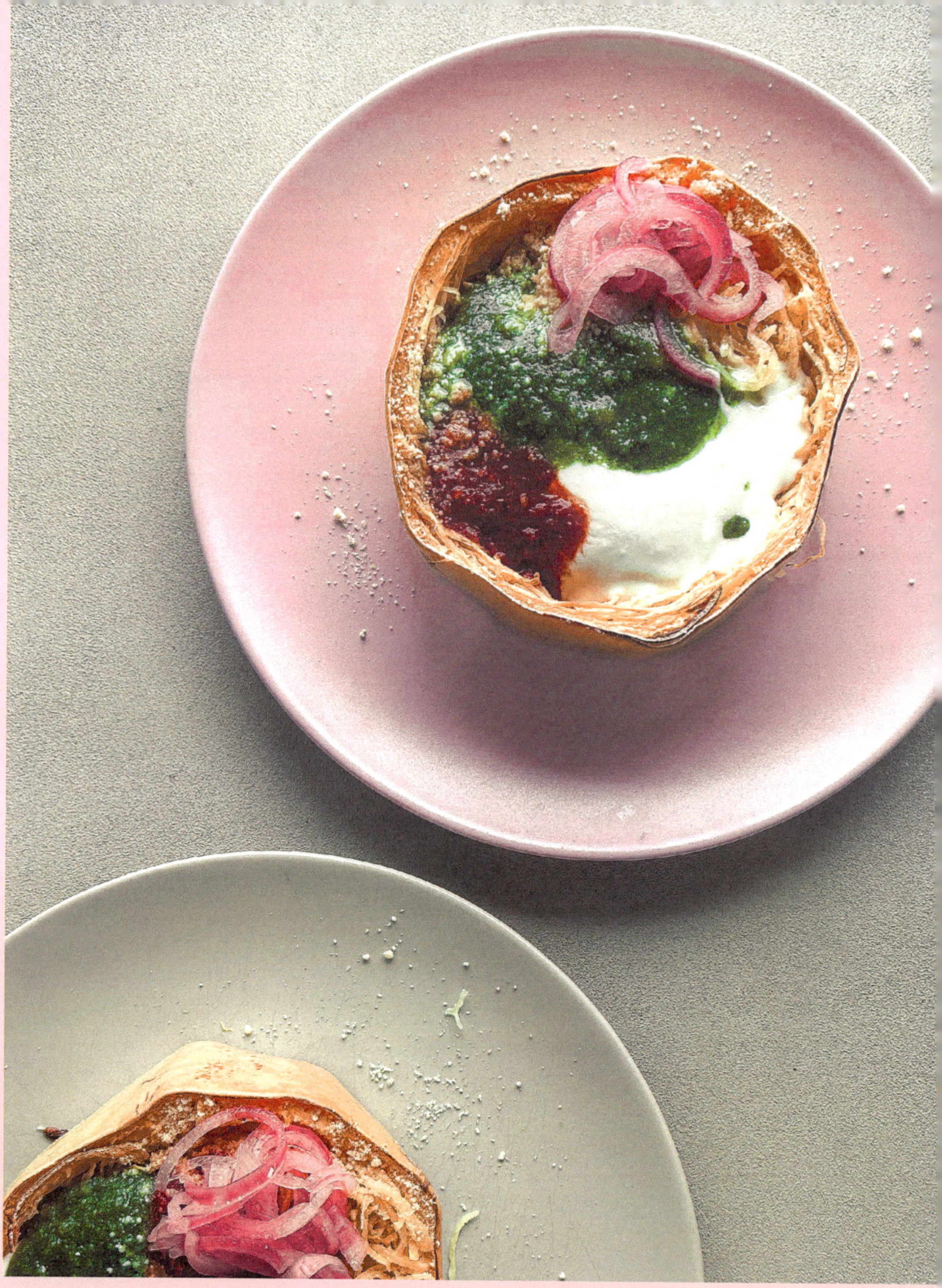

*Tip for making the perfect spaghetti squash: Cut them into rings! When you cut the squash into rings, as opposed to just slicing it down the middle, you work with the strands, not against them, since the spaghetti squash strands run horizontally, in a circle, inside of the squash. When you follow this method you will never get soggy squash anymore, just make sure you don't cook longer than needed.*

**Serves: 4**

**Ingredients**

3 kg spaghetti squash
2 tbsp olive oil
1 tsp salt
Black pepper to taste

**To serve**

1 cup cashew bechamel
1 cup marinara sauce
1 cup pickled red onion
1/2 cup basil pesto

1. Preheat the oven to 210°C.
2. Slice the spaghetti squash into 1 1/2 inch thick rings and scoop out the seeds and ribbing. Make sure that you have an extra-sharp knife to cut through the tough squash. Drizzle the inside of the squash with olive oil and sprinkle with salt and pepper.
3. Do not waste the seeds, they are super delicious! Clean the seeds under the running water. Dry and spread on a tray. While you are cooking your spaghetti squash you can also roast the seeds in the oven for 10-15 minutes.
4. Place the spaghetti squash cut side down on the baking sheet and use a fork to poke holes. Roast for 40-50 minutes or until lightly browned on the outside, fork tender, but still a litte bit firm. The time will vary depending on the size of your squash. I also find that the timing can vary from squash to squash. So it is best to observe after 40 minutes and check with a help of fork if it is soft enough or not. But if you are making it for the first time, keep in mind that it shouldn't be super soft otherwise will loose its consistency.
5. Once time is up, remove from the oven and flip the squash so that it's cut side up. When cool to the touch, use a fork to scrape and fluff the strands from the sides of the squash.
6. Pour the sauces you want, I made marinara, cashew bechamel and basil pesto sauce, sprinkled some hemp parmesan and topped with pickled red onion.

PLANT BASED UMAMI

# BIBIMBAP

## WITH MAYO, CAPERS AND CHILI

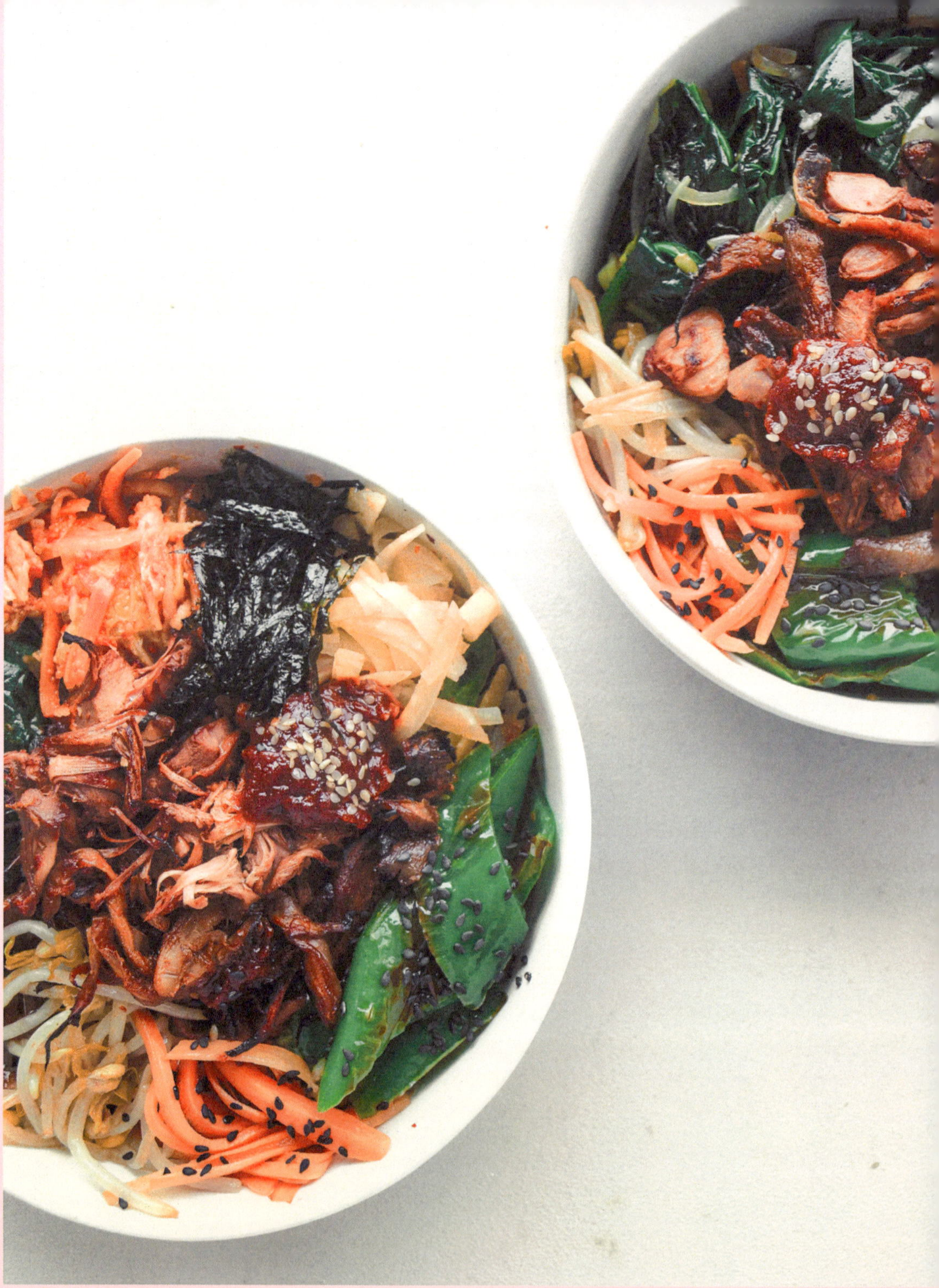

*A plant-based take on a classic Korean mixed rice dish. It's full of flavors and textures, naturally gluten-free, and super delicious! The textures of the crispy rice and the crunchy veggies and the delicious, funky fermented kimchi. Full of umami!*

**Serves: 2**

**Ingredients**

1 cup brown rice or mixed rice
200 g oyster mushrooms
200 g pulled young jackfruit
2 tbsp olive oil
1-2 tbsp coconut aminos
1 tbsp gochujang + more for serving
1/4 cup pickled daikon (see below)
1/4 cup kimchi (page 21)
5-6 shishito peppers
1/4 cup bean sprouts
100 g spinach
1 shallot
3 minced garlic cloves
1 julienned carrot
2 toasted nori sheets

**Pickled daikon**

70g daikon julienne sliced
50ml rice vinegar
50ml water
1 tsp pink Himalayan salt + more as needed
1 + 1/2 tbsp coconut sugar
1/2 tsp gochugaru (Korean red pepper powder)

1. Preheat oven to 200°C with the fan. Roughly chop the mushrooms. Place on a baking tray lined with baking paper.
2. Drain excess water from the canned jackfruit, repeat the process for the jackfruit as well.
3. Drizzle over 1 tbsp of the oil, 1 tbsp coconut aminos and Korean pepper paste. Toss to coat the mushrooms and jackfruit evenly, then bake for 20 minutes, or until the mushrooms and jackfruit are slightly crispy and browned around the edges.
4. To make the pickled daikon, julienne the daikon and place in a jar. Bring the rice vinegar, water, coconut sugar and salt to a boil. Pour the hot pickling liquid over the daikon. Pickles can be eaten straight away, but they are worth making a day in advance as their flavour develops over time. Store in an airtight jar in the fridge. They can be stored for up to 4-5 weeks.
5. Heat 1 tsp oil in a medium non-stick pan. Toss in shishito peppers and fry, pressing down with a lid on the pan from time to time, until nicely browned on all sides. Season with salt and set aside.
6. Toss in spinach and chopped onion and a splash of water. Cook over low heat, stirring occasionally, until spinach is wilted and most of the excess water has evaporated. . Add some finely chopped garlic and stir well. Season with salt and pepper. Set aside.
7. Toss in sliced julienne carrots, 1 tsp olive oil and a pinch of salt, fry over medium heat for 1-2 minutes. Set aside. Repeat the process for bean sprouts or serve raw if desired.
8. Using a sharp knife, slice toasted nori sheets into thin slices. Set aside.
9. Divide all vegetables, kimchi, pickled daikon, thinly sliced nori sheets, oven-baked pulled mushrooms, and jackfruit between two bowls. Sprinkle with black sesame seeds and top with additional gochujang, about 1 teaspoon. Enjoy!

# JAPCHAE

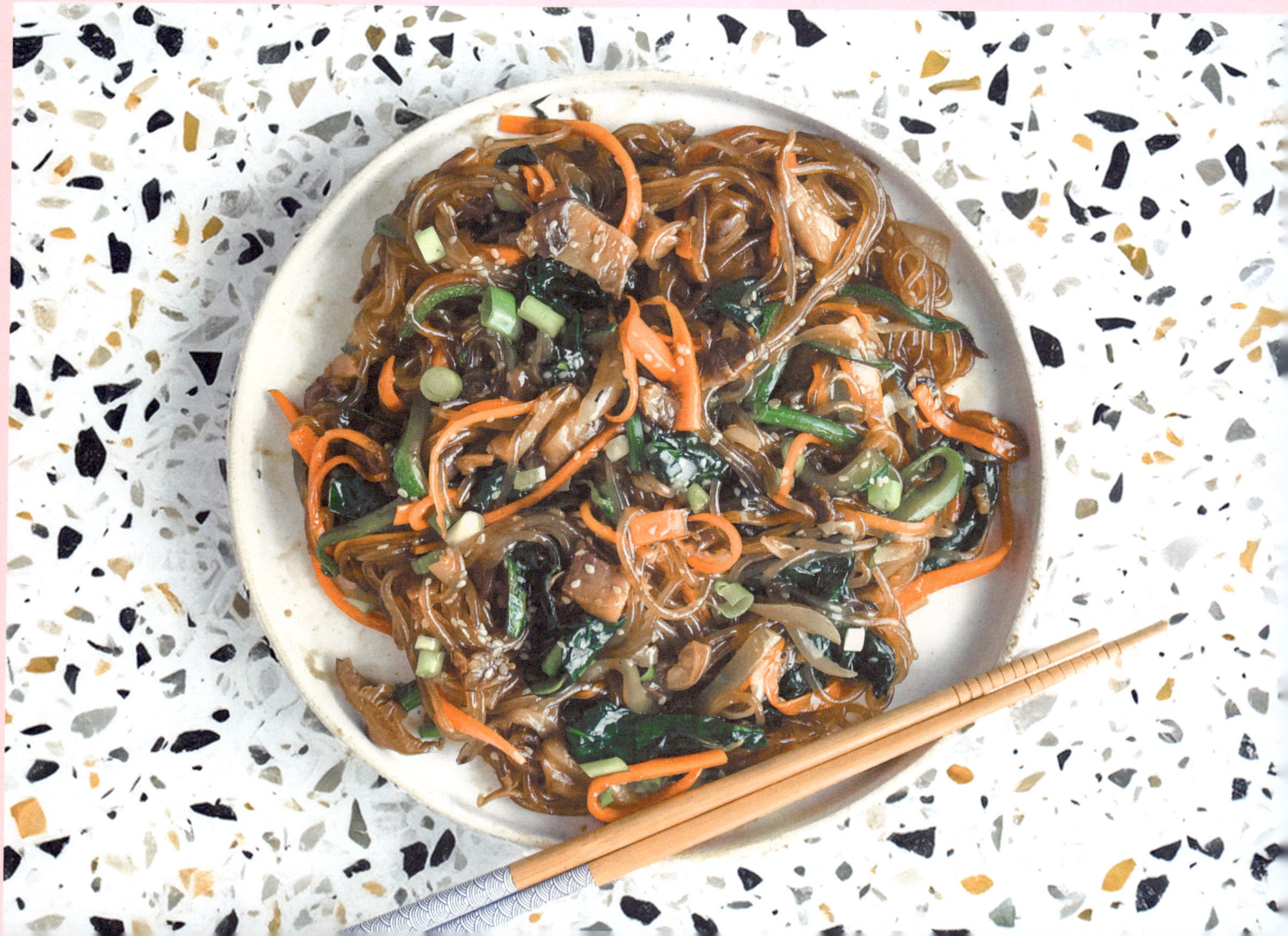

*Japchae is a super popular Korean noodle dish that you will find in every Korean restaurant. It is popular for a good reason, Japchae uses glass noodles made from sweet potatoes and are naturally gluten free. They have a unique springy texture that works perfectly with the crunchy texture of all the vegetables and mushrooms.*

**Serves: 2**

**Ingredients**

100 g sweet potato noodles
200 g shiitake or mushrooms of choice
2 scallion stalks chopped
1/2 medium zucchini julienne sliced
1/2 medium carrot julienne sliced
A handful of spinach
1 small onion chopped
2 cloves garlic chopped
Sesame seeds to serve

**For the sauce**

3 tbsp coconut aminos
1 tbsp coconut sugar
1 tbsp sesame oil
A pinch of pink Himalayan salt

1. Slice the zucchini, mushrooms and carrots into matchstick pieces. Make sure they are the same size for a nice eating experience.
2. Fry the mushrooms in a large wok over medium heat with a little sesame oil until lightly browned on each side. Transfer to a bowl and set aside.
3. In the same wok, repeat the process for the zucchini, when lightly browned, transfer to a bowl.
4. In the same wok, repeat the process for the carrots, adding just a splash of water during the cooking process. When they are slightly soft but still crunchy, transfer to a bowl.
5. Finally, fry the onion and garlic in the wok with a little oil until golden.
6. Then clean the spinach and squeeze out any excess water. Add to the pan and cook for just 1 minute to wilt it with the onion and garlic.
7. Bring a pot of water to a boil and cook your sweet potato noodles according to package directions, about 3-4 minutes.
8. Toss the noodles until all the sauce has been absorbed over medium heat for just 1-2 minutes.
9. Serve with chopped scallion stalks and sesame seeds.

# CHILI CON PEA

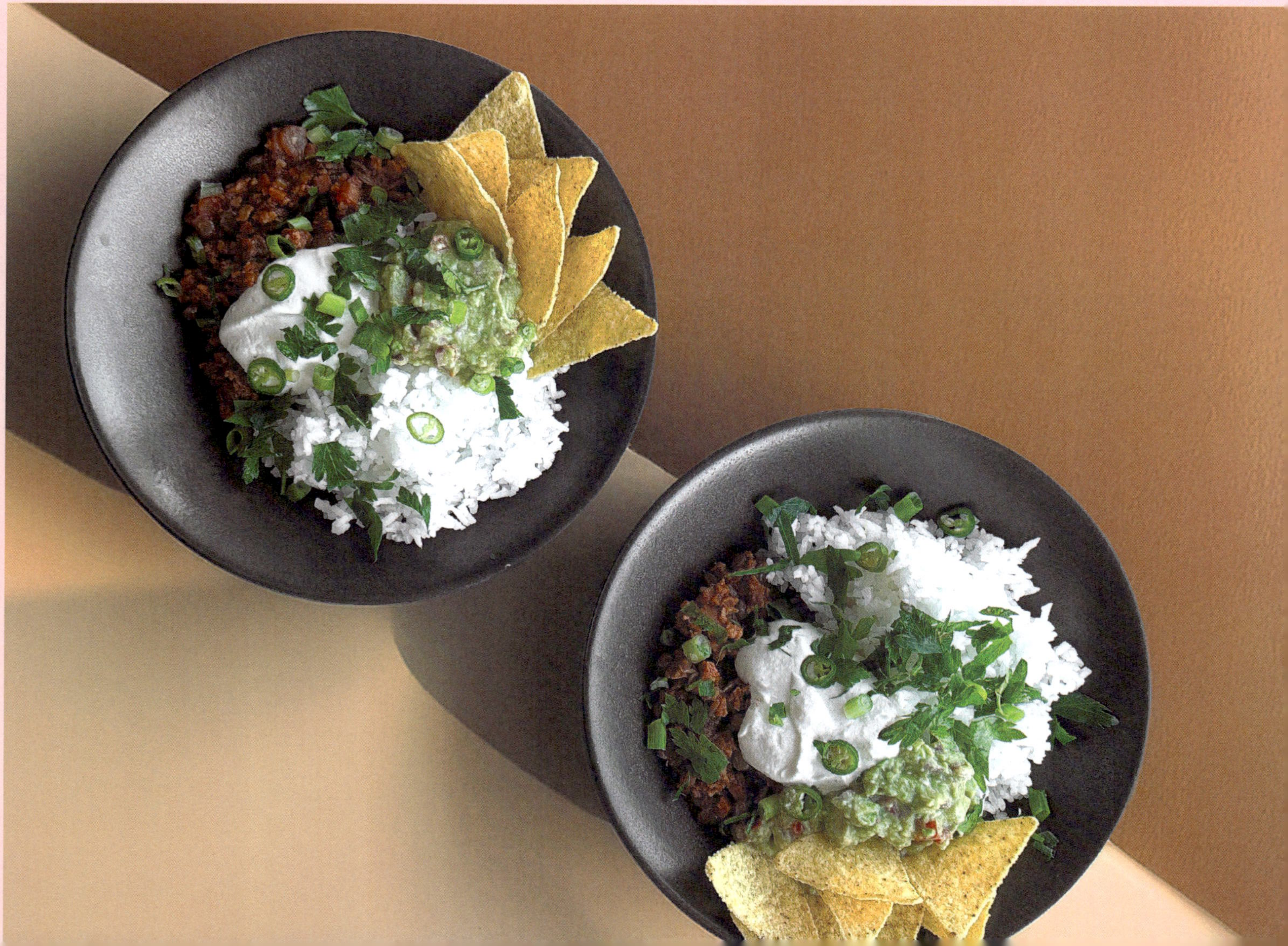

**Serves: 2**

**Ingredients**

70 g pea mince
40 g puy lentils
2 tbsp olive oil
1/2 carrot
1 onion
4 garlic cloves
1 fresh chili
1 tsp oregano
1 tsp red pepper
1 tsp ground coriander
1 tsp cacao (optional)
1 tbsp tomato paste
1 tbsp mushroom sauce or coconut aminos
1/2 tsp salt

**To serve**

1 cup guacamole (see below)
1 cup cashew yoghurt (see below)
1 cup cooked rice
A bunch of fresh coriander (or parsley)
1 cup nachos

**For guacamole**

1 avocado
1/2 lime juice
1 tomato cubed
1 jalapeno diced
1/2 tsp salt
2 garlic cloves minced

**For cashew yoghurt**

90 g cashews soaked
60 g coconut cream
30 ml lemon juice
Water as needed
1 tsp salt

*A rich, hearty meat free vegan chilli recipe packed with flavour. The perfect comfort food to keep you warm during winter nights. This chilli con carne has all the taste and kick of a classic chilli con carne, but with fewer calories and less saturated fat. What's not to love?*

1. To make guacamole, slice the avocados in half, remove the pit, and scoop into a mixing bowl.
2. Mash the avocado with a fork and make it as chunky or smooth as you'd like. Add the remaining ingredients and stir together.
3. Give it a taste test and add a pinch more salt or lime juice if needed. Set aside.
4. To make quick cashew yoghurt, place soaked and rinsed cashews along with all cashew yoghurt ingredients in a blender, blend on high speed, let it sit in the fridge at least 2 hours before using.
5. Pre-heat the oil in a large frying pan and cook the onion for 5-6 minutes or until beginning to soften. Add the red pepper and continue to cook for a further 5 minutes.
6. Add the chillies, garlic and spices and cook for a further 2 minutes stirring continuously.
7. Stir in the tomato puree and mushroom sauce and bring to a gentle simmer for 8 minutes stirring occasionally.
9. Stir in the pea mince and cooked puy lentils and cacao if using. Cook over a gentle heat for a further 10 minutes and season to taste.
10. Stir in the chopped coriander (or parsley if you don't like coriander) and serve with rice, guacamole, cashew yoghurt, jacket potatoes or with nachos for a delicious dinner.

# TEMPEH TORTILLA SALAD

## WITH TOGARASHI FRAICHE AND TOMATO SALSA

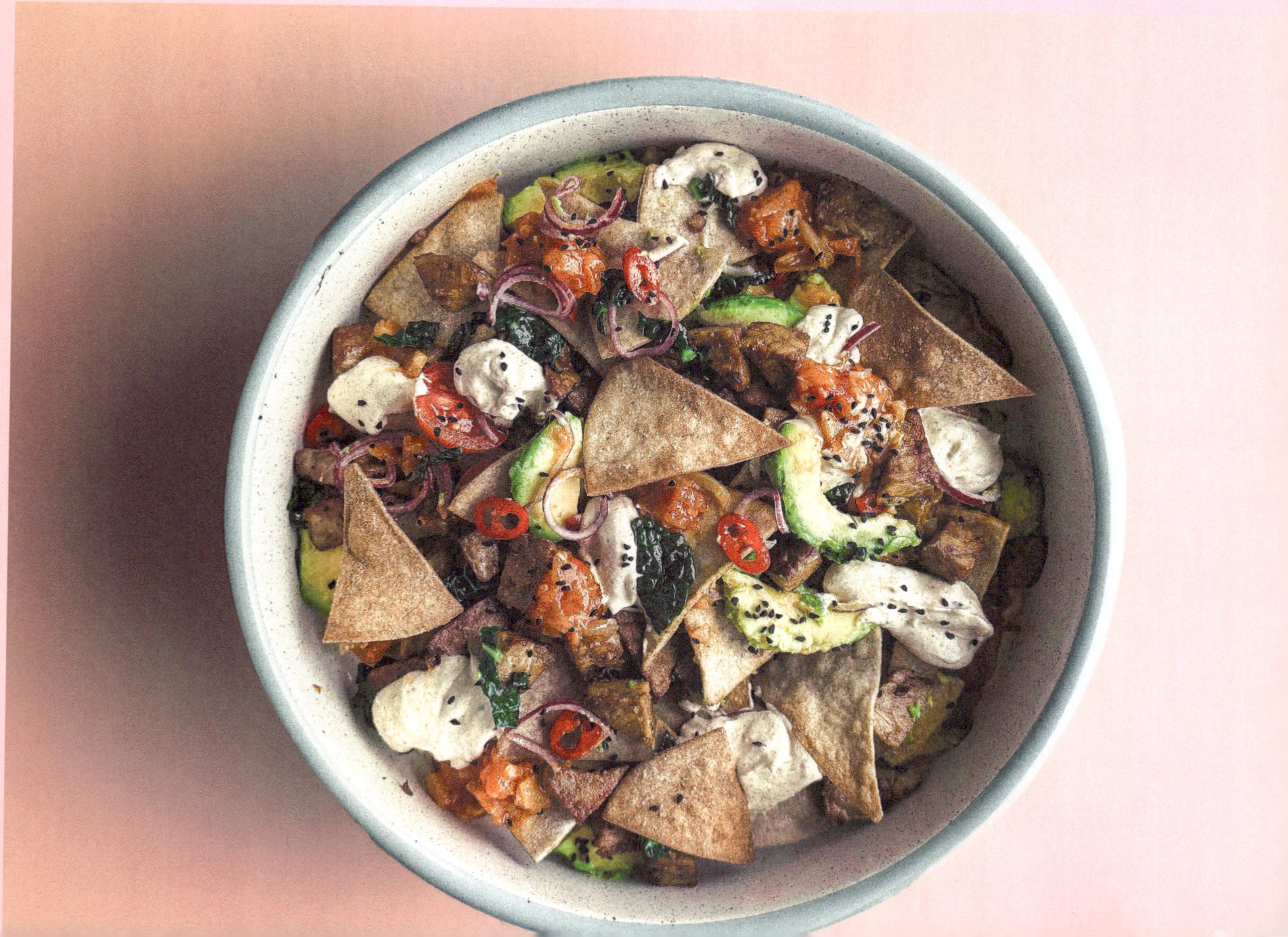

**Serves: 2-3**

### Ingredients

4 buckwheat tortilla, cut into triangles
Olive oil as needed
1 small red onion, finely chopped
200 g tempeh roughly cut into pieces
75 g salad leaves or kale chopped
1 large avocado, sliced
A handful of cherry tomatoes halved
1 cup plant based fraiche
1 cup tomato salsa
1/4 cup fresh parsley or coriander
Sesame seeds to sprinkle

### Buckwheat Tacos

120 g buckwheat flour
65 g tapioca flour
1 tbsp olive oil
1 tbsp psyllium powder + 45 ml water
1/4 tsp salt
90 ml water

### Tomato Salsa

400 g tomatoes
1 red chili
1 large onion
3 garlic cloves minced
1/2 tsp salt

### Fraiche

1 batch cashew cream
2 tsp togarashi spice

*A perfect Spring salad, fresh and crunchy, but still filling and satisfying. I made buckwheat tortilla from scratch, then layered with avocado, cherry tomatoes, and mixed salad leaves. This was topped with spiced tempeh chunks and a rich roasted tomato salsa. Finally I finished the salad with big dollops of fraiche flavoured with chili, which lends the perfect cooling freshness with a slight togarashi.*

1. Toss the tomatoes,red onion and chilli in a little oil, season and roast in the oven at 200 C. for 25 – 30 minutes, until beginning to caramelise. Allow to cool a little then add to a blender/ food processor with the coriander and lime juice and pulse into a salsa.
2. Brush both sides of the tortilla with oil, season and arrange in a single layer on a baking tray. Bake in the oven for 8 – 10 minutes until golden.
3. Fry the finely chopped onion with a little oil, until softened. Add the chipotle chili and cook for a minute before adding the black beans. Season and fry for a couple of minutes to heat through.
4. Finally arrange in layers the baked Tortilla triangles, the salad leaves, sliced avocado and black beans, repeating if necessary. Top with big dollops of Planti fraiche, the tomato salsa and chopped coriander. Put any remaining Planti fraiche and salsa in small bowls and serve on the side.
5. To make tortillas, in a large mixing bowl, mix all ingredients instead water and oil, lastly add the water along with oil and mix together. Then knead with your hands, dust some buckwheat flour on the surface. Roll out the dough as thin as possible. Then cut using a 15 cm round cutter, divide the round into 8 triangles. Cook in the oven at 200 C for 4-5 minutes or until crispy enough.

# ROASTED BEET PESTO

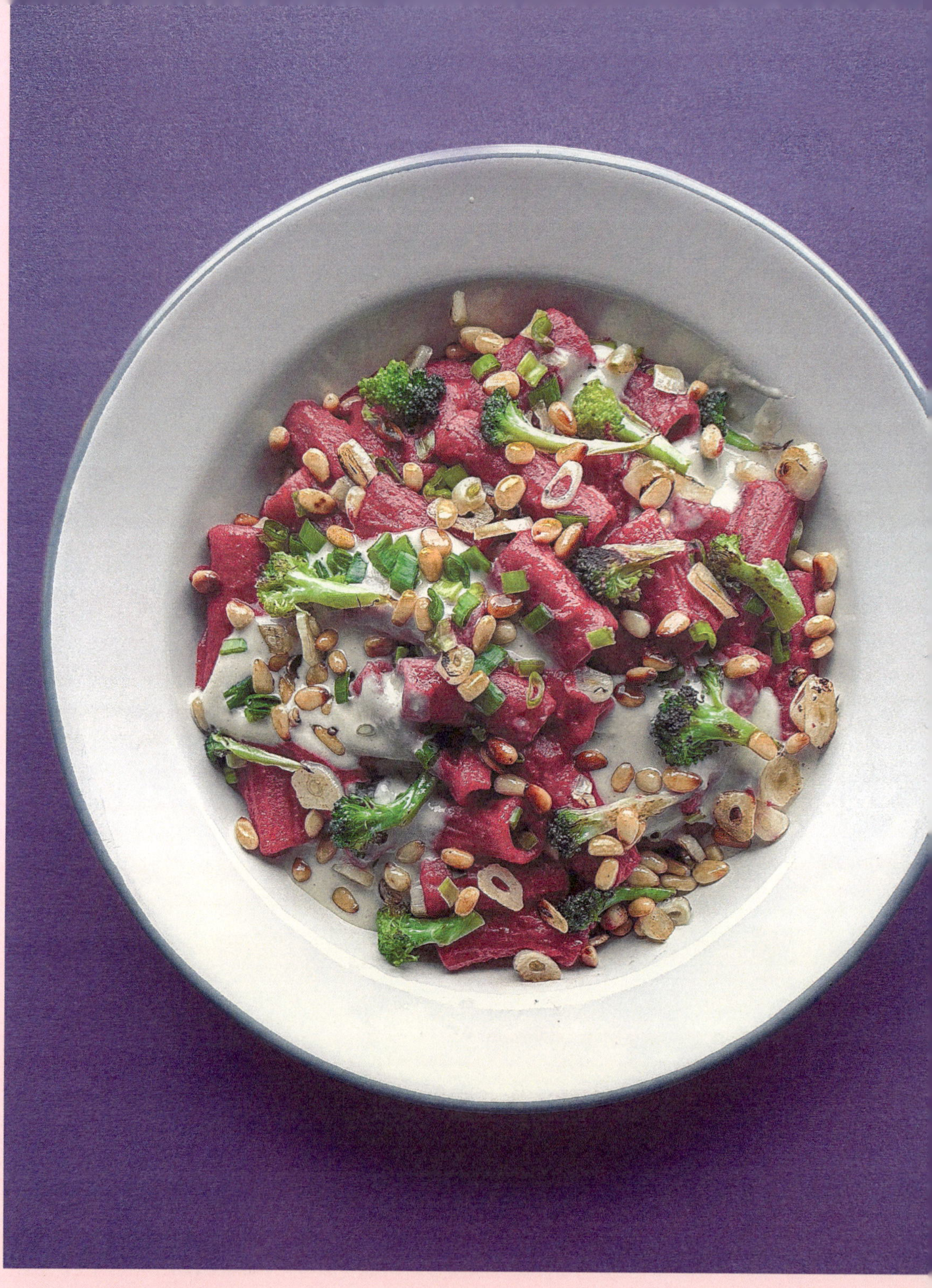

**Serves: 2-4**

*A comforting hearty pasta dish, perfect for cold winter days.*

**Ingredients**

200 g pasta of your choice
250 g beetroot
200 ml plant based milk
1 large onion
30 ml vodka
1/4 cup hemp hearts
2 tbsp nutritional yeast
2 tsp salt
1/2 tsp black pepper
1/4 cup olive oil
1/2 lemon juice
2 tbsp toasted pine nuts
1/4 cup chopped scallions
4 garlic cloves sliced and toasted
1/2 cup broccoli roasted
Plant based yoghurt to serve

1. Preheat oven to 200 degrees. Peel and wash your beets and onion. Roughly cut in chunks. Place the beets and onion into a pyrex, pour vodka and 1 tbsp olive oil over the beets and let roast in the oven for 20 minutes.
2. Place roasted beets, hemp hearts, plant based milk, green onion, lemon juice, nutritional yeast, pepper and salt in a food processor, mix on high until get completely smooth mixture.
3. Transfer mixture in a large pan, add another tbsp olive oil, stir on medium heat for 5-6 minutes.
4. Add your pasta into the sauce. Toss well until all pasta coated with the sauce.
5. Serve with roasted broccoli, pine nuts, garlic and plant based yoghurt.

# LASAGNA WITH HOLLANDAISE AND ASPARAGUS

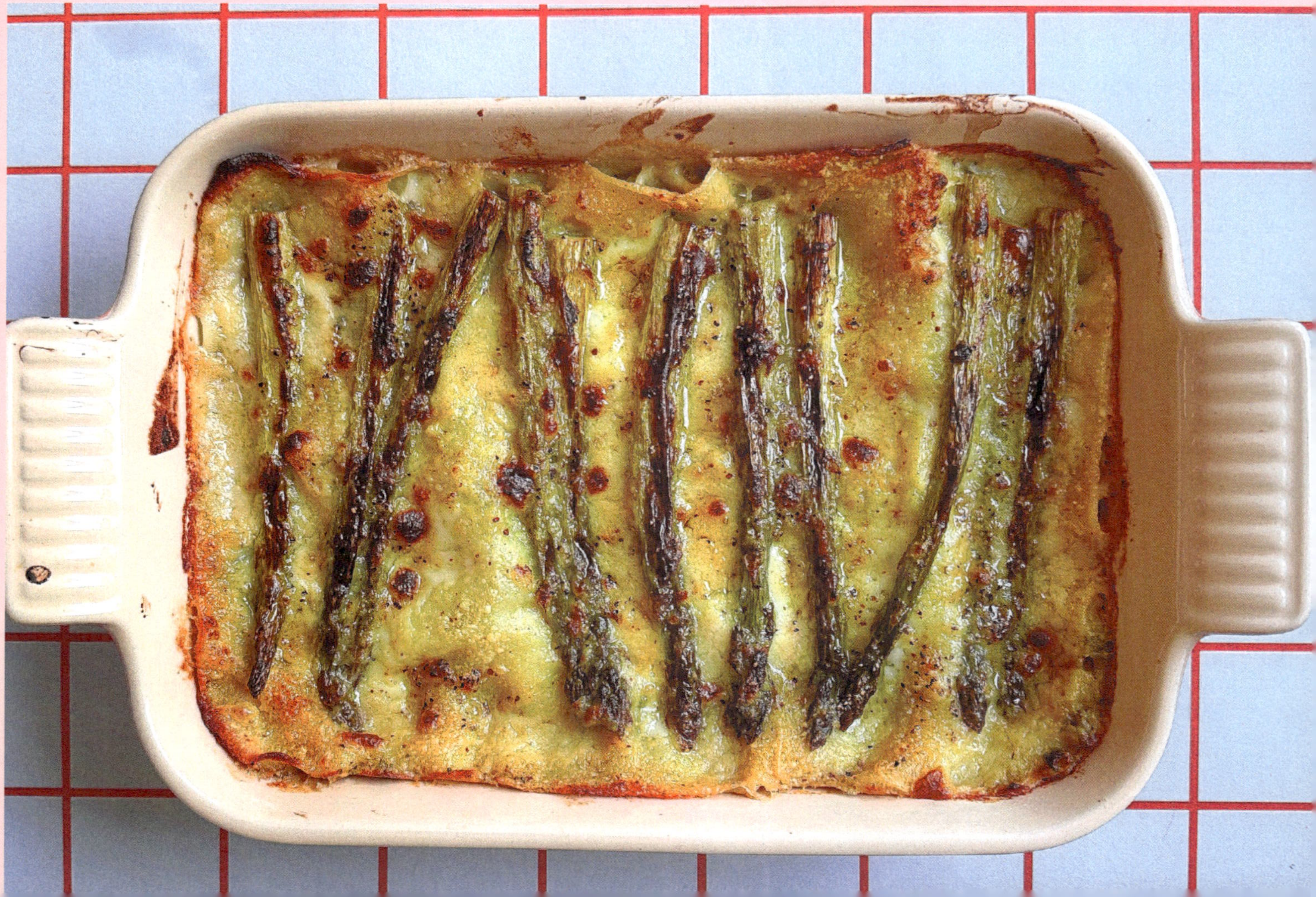

**Serves: 3**

**Hollandaise Sauce**

4 tbsp olive oil
2 tbsp oat flour
200 ml oat milk
1.5 tsp mustard
1 tbsp vegan white wine
1 tsp lemon juice
1/2 tsp turmeric powder
Salt as needed

**Top Layer**

8-10 chopped asparagus
6 slices vegan mozzarella
Lime wedges for serving
Tagetes for serving

**Lasagne**

250 g lasagna of your choice

**Asparagus Leek Filling**

1 cup chopped asparagus
1 large chopped leek
2 chopped shallots
2 finely chopped garlic cloves
1 tbsp olive oil
1/4 cup water as needed

**Béchamel Sauce**

4 tbsp olive oil
3 tbsp oat flour
1 tbsp tapioca flour
500 ml oat milk
150 ml water
Salt and black pepper

**Hollandaise**

1. Pour olive oil into a saucepan and stir in oat flour. Continue stirring to keep the mixture smooth.
2. Add oat milk and water. Bring to a simmer. Then add white wine, mustard and lemon juice. Season with salt and pepper.
3. Cook your hollandaise sauce for about 4-5 minutes until it thickens to the desired consistency. Season to taste and set aside.

**Top Layer**

1. Thinly slice the mozzarella and set aside.
2. Separate 8-10 asparagus spears from the filling and sauté in a pan with a little olive oil and water until slightly softened.

**Asparagus Filling**

1. Slice onion, garlic, asparagus, and leek thinly. Place in a saucepan with a little olive oil and sauté over medium heat for 4–5 minutes. Then add chopped fresh dill and mix. Set aside.

**Béchamel Sauce**

1. Pour olive oil into a saucepan over medium-low heat. Stir in the oatmeal and tapioca, stirring constantly to avoid lumps in the sauce.
2. Gradually stir in the plant-based milk, season with salt and pepper. Simmer until the sauce thickens.

**Assembly**

1. Preheat the oven to 180°C/355°F.
2. Spread a third of the béchamel sauce in the bottom of your baking dish (26 cm).
3. Top with a third of the asparagus filling and finish with a layer of lasagna sheets.
4. Repeat these steps three times until both the béchamel sauce and asparagus filling are gone.
5. When you have reached the last top layer, drizzle hollandaise sauce over it. Place vegan mozzarella slices on top of the sauce. Then top with whole sautéed asparagus. Pour the remaining hollandaise sauce over the asparagus.
6. Bake in the middle of the oven at 180°C for 40-45 minutes or until golden brown and cooked through.
7. Let the lasagna stand for 15-20 minutes before serving.
8. Sprinkle with a little black pepper and serve with tagetes and lime wedges.

# ROASTED CELERIAC SLICES

## WITH MUSTARD SAUCE & RICE

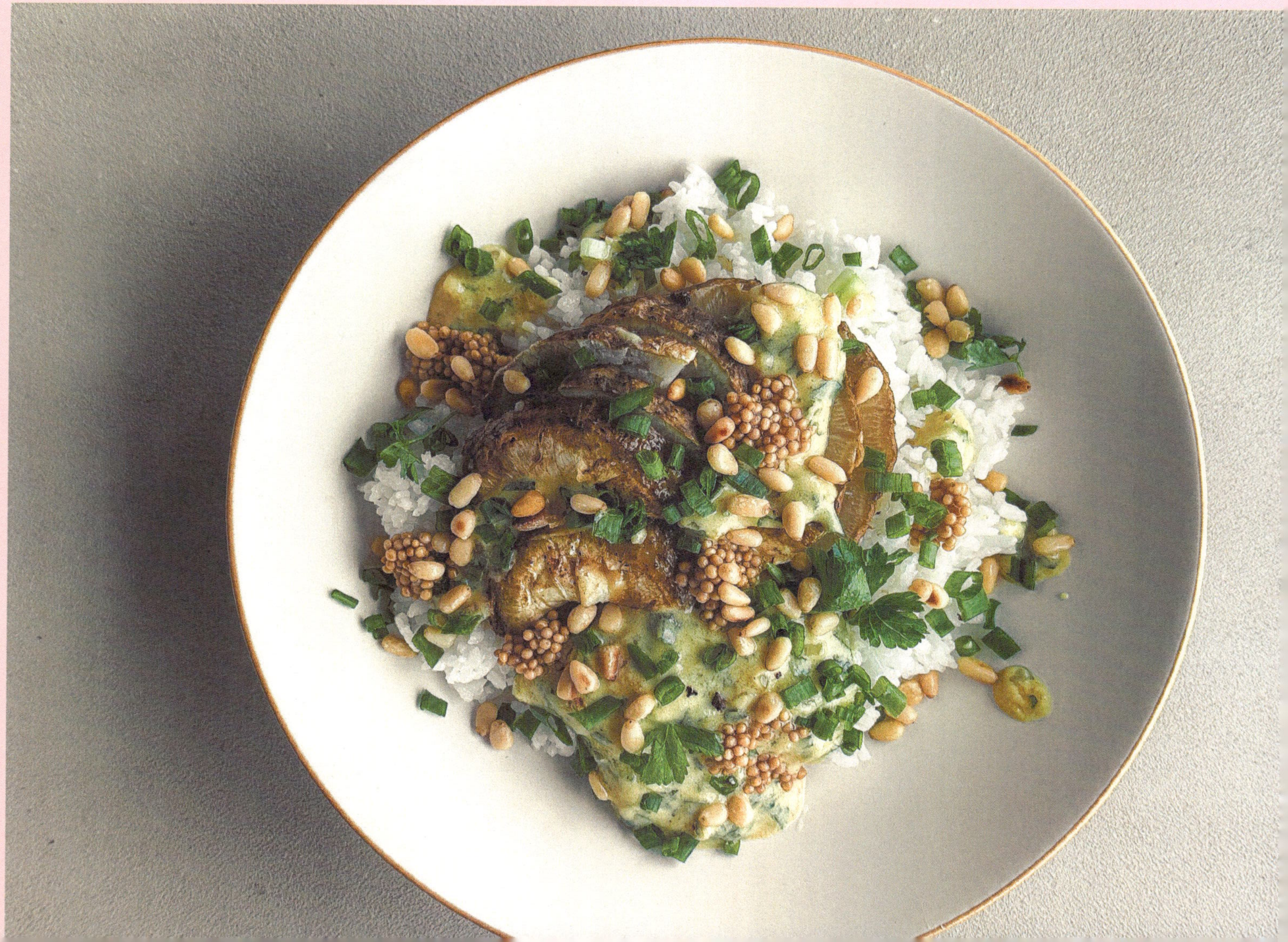

Serves: 3

**For the Celeriac**

2 whole celeriac, hairy roots discarded and scrubbed clean. No need to peel.
1 tbsp olive oil
1 tsp pink himalayan salt

**For the Mustard Sauce**

2 tbsp olive oil
1 small shallot, finely chopped
2 garlic cloves, crushed
3 tbsp dijon mustard
1 tbsp lemon juice
2 tbsp spring onions, finely chopped
1 tbsp parsley, finely chopped

**For the Serving**

1 cup rice + 2 cups water
3 tbsp toasted pine nuts
2 tbsp chopped parsley
Black pepper and salt to taste

**For the Celeriac**

1.Preheat the oven to 170°C fan.
2. Pierce the celeriac with a fork all over about 20-25 times and place in a baking bag on the tray.
3. Mix the olive oil and salt, then rub the celeriac generously with the oil mixture.
4. Roast for about 1.5 hours or so, until the celeriac is deeply browned, soft all the way through and oozes a celeriac caramel.
5. Leave to rest for 15 minutes, then cut widthways into 1 cm thick slices, brushing each cut side with the olive oil.

**For the Mustard Sauce**

1. Put the olive oil, garlic and onion with a pinch of salt into a small saucepan on a medium heat. Cook for about 6 minutes, swirling the pan until the shallots have softened and caramelised. Place them into a bowl.
2. Then add mustard, lemon juice, chopped spring onions and parsley. Mix together.

**For the Rice**

1. Wash and rinse the rice.
2. Add 2 cups water and 1 cup rice to a large pot.
3. Bring the water to a boil. Once it's boiling, add a big pinch of salt. Maintain a simmer.
4. Cook without peeking or stirring.
5. Let the rice rest covered.
6. Fluff the rice with a fork.

**Assembly**

1. Start plating with rice, roasted celeriac slices on the top and lastly pour the mustard sauce over the celeriacs.
2. Add some toasted pine nuts and fresh parsley, sprinkle some black pepper and salt. Serve warm.

# KITCHARI SPICED CAULIFLOWER

## WITH QUINOA, RED ONION, GARLIC MAYO

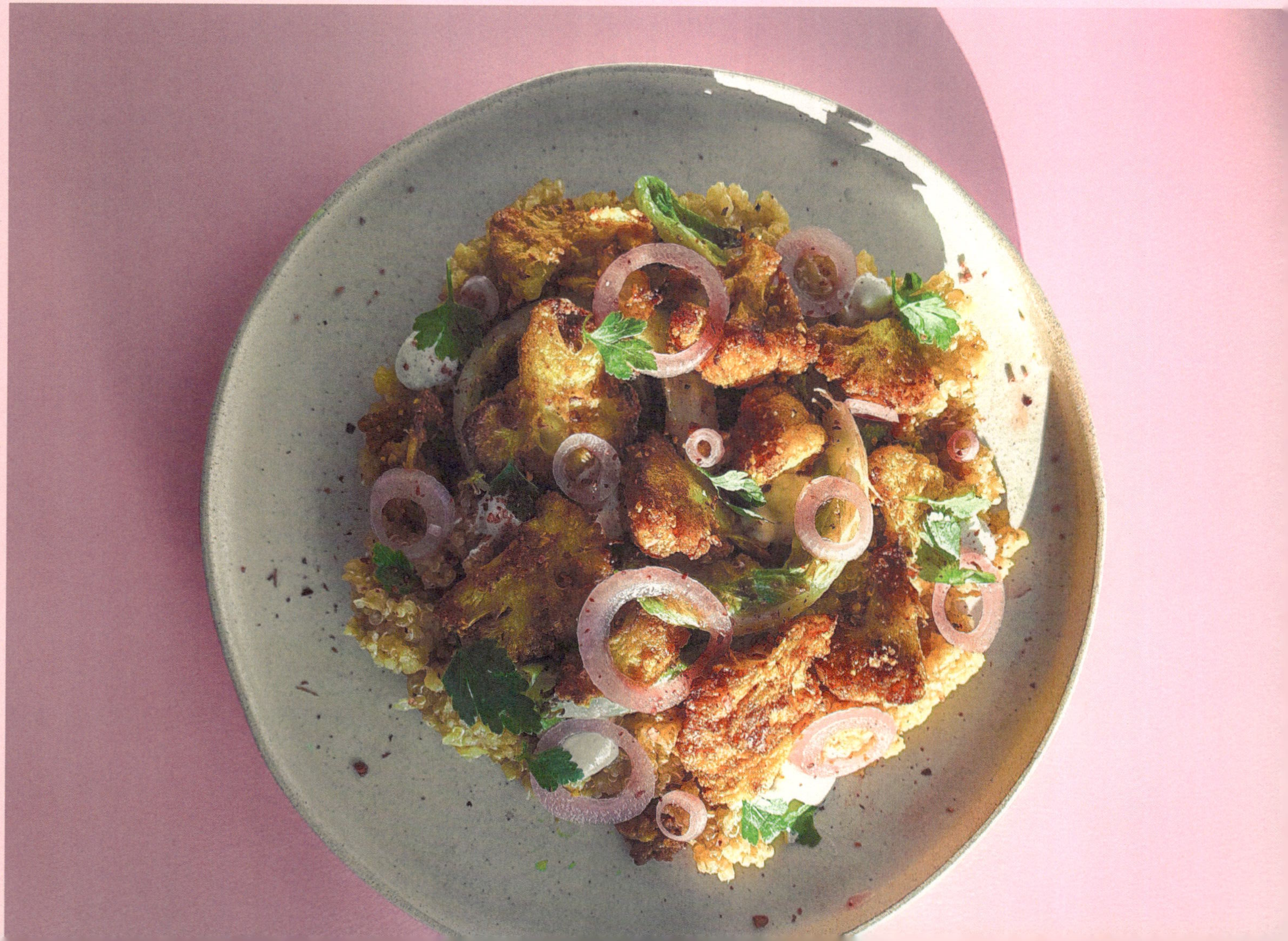

*Golden cauliflower florets roasted in warming kitchari spices take center stage in this vibrant dish. The cauliflower's earthy depth is lifted by a silky garlic mayo, bringing creamy richness to every bite. Served over fluffy quinoa, it gains a wholesome, nutty foundation, while the sharpness of pickled onion cuts through with a refreshing tang*

**Serves: 2-3**

**Ingredients**

400 g cauliflower
1 cup quinoa cooked
1/4 cup olive oil
1/2 cup garlic mayo
1/4 cup pickled red onion
Fresh parsley

**Kitchari Spice**

1 1/2 tsp ground turmeric
1 tsp ground ginger
1 tsp ground coriander
1 tsp cumin powder
1/2 tsp chili flakes
2 tbsp nutritional yeast
3 tbsp cashew flour
1 tsp ground coriander

1. Heat the oven to 200 C. Adjust the oven rack to the middle position. Line a baking sheet with parchment paper.
2. In a large bowl, add all kitchari spice ingredients. Mix everything very well. Then add olive oil, and mix again.
3. Place the cauliflower florets in the bowl toss with spices until everything is evenly coated.
4. Roast for about 25-30 minutes or until the cauliflower is tender and golden brown.
5. On a pan, on medium high heat, fry cauliflower leaves.
6. Serve your roasted cauliflower with pickled red onion, cauliflower leaves, cooked quinoa, garlic cashew cream and fresh parsley.

# AUBERGINE & BROWN LENTILS

## WITH BALSAMICO, MINT AND JUICY GRAPES

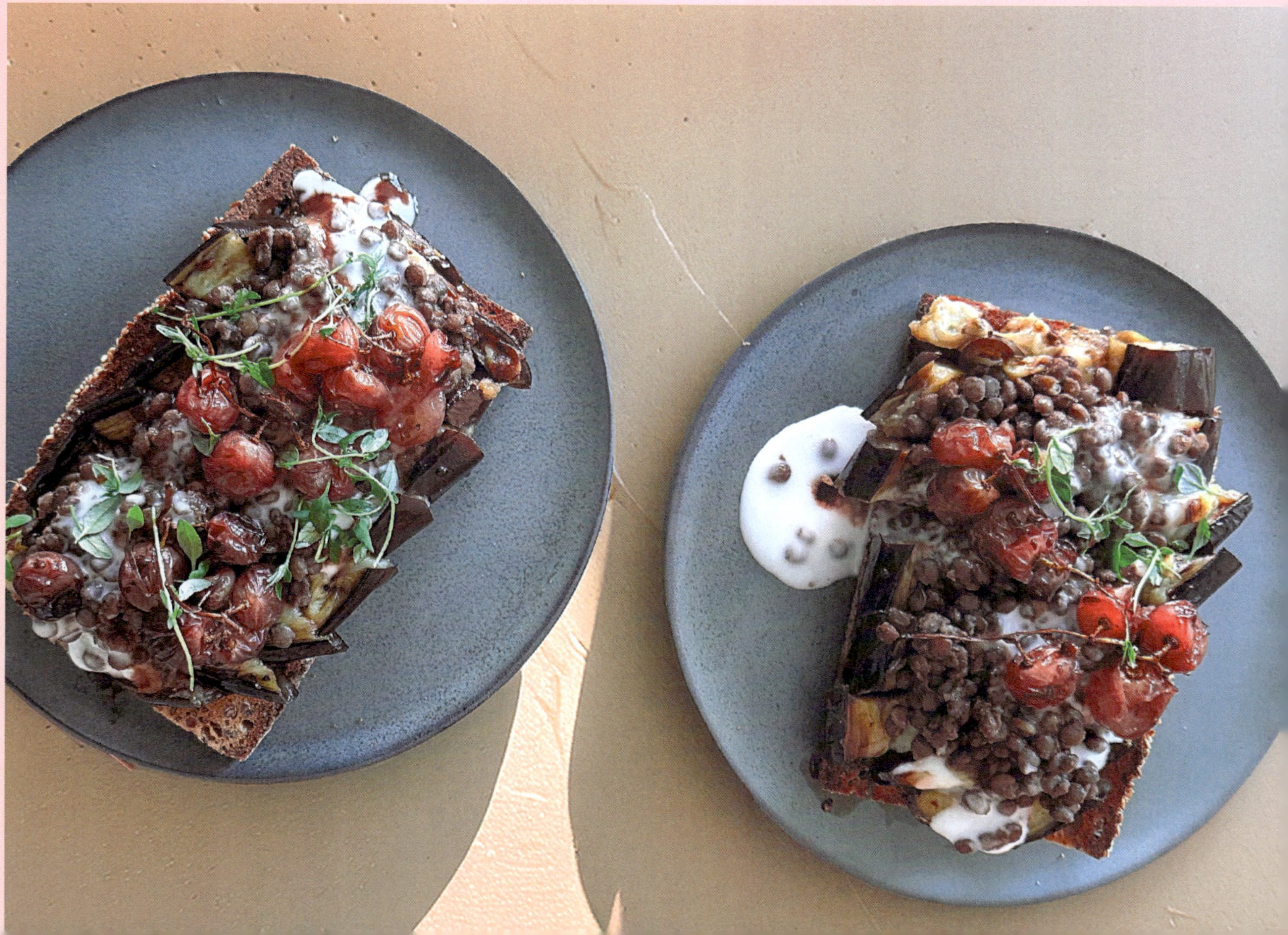

*This rustic open-faced sandwich layers silky roasted aubergine with hearty brown lentils, creating a satisfying balance of smoky depth and nutty earthiness. Juicy grapes and fresh thyme bring brightness and lift, while a drizzle of balsamic reduction ties it all together with sweet acidity. The result is a dish that's both comforting and refreshing, where Mediterranean warmth meets vibrant, plant-based simplicity.*

**Serves: 4**

**Brown Lentils**

150 g brown lentils
2 tbsp olive oil
1 tbsp coconut aminos

**Grilled Aubergine**

3 large eggplants
2 tbsp olive oil
Salt and black pepper
Juice of 2 lemons
1 cup fresh mint

**For serving**

Roasted grapes
Toasted Bread of your choice
Fresh thyme
Black Pepper
Balsamic vinegar
Yoghurt (page 17)

1. To make lentils, wash and strain, cover with water and cook for about 18-20 minutes or until all the water content is absorbed, you may need to add a little more water during the cooking process. When cooked, add coconut aminos and olive oil, mix well.
2. Cut your eggplants in half, drizzle with olive oil, salt and pepper. Place on a baking sheet with baking paper. Make small cuts on the eggplants with a fork. Bake in a preheated oven at 180 C for about 30-40 minutes or until both sides are brown, juicy and soft. It takes 15-20 minutes. Cut the eggplant flesh into cubes, transfer to a bowl, add lemon juice, olive oil, chopped fresh mint, salt and pepper. Mix well.
3. Bake the grapes in a 150 C preheated oven until soft.
4. Transfer lentils to eggplant bowl, add roasted grapes, toss everything together.
5. Toast your bread. Top with eggplant lentil mixture. Drizzle with cherry balsamic, yoghurt, a little more fresh thyme, black pepper and salt.

# GYOZA WITH SPICY TAHINI SAUCE

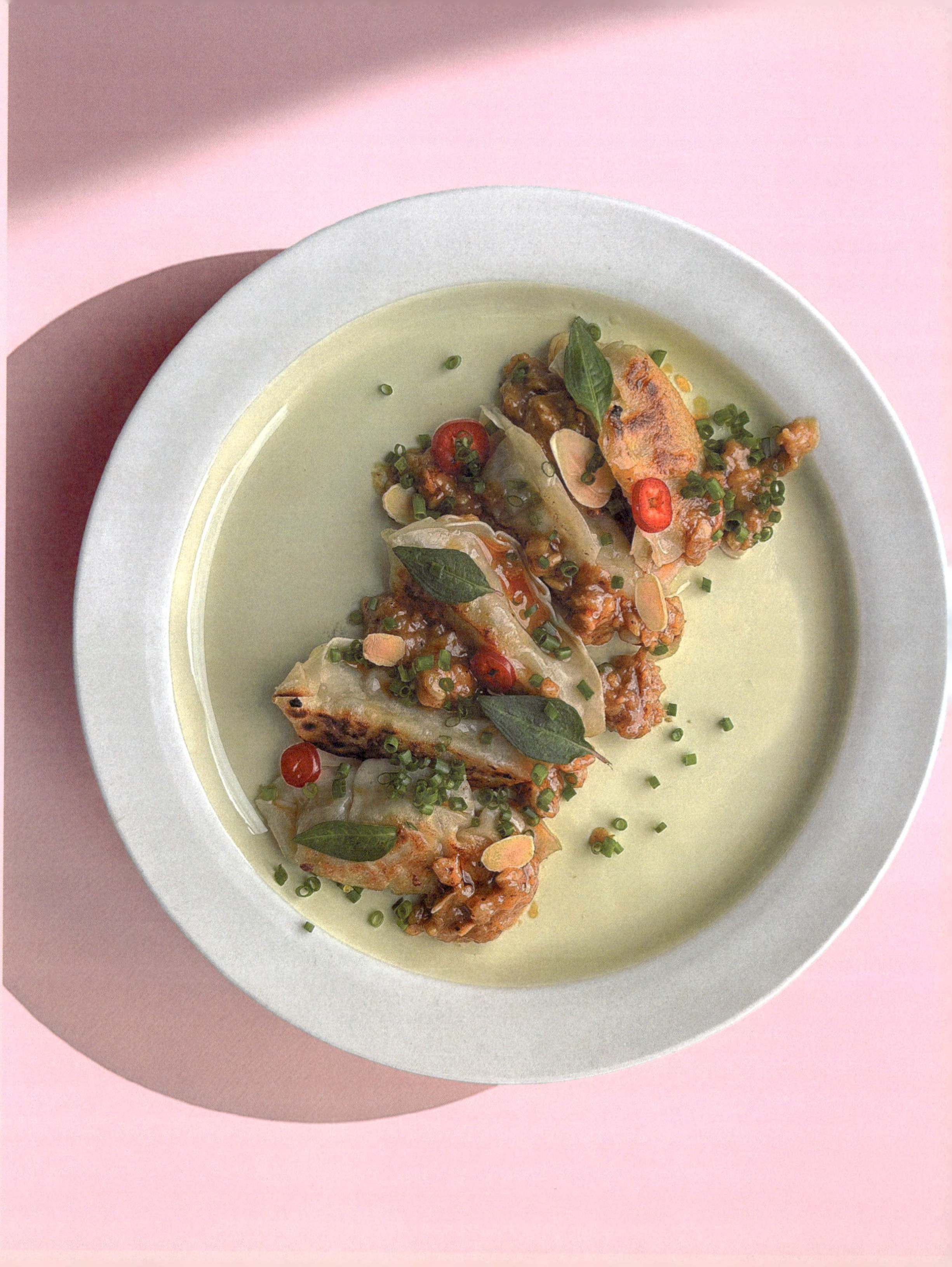

**Wonton**

150 g rice flour

70 g tapioca flour

10 g psyllium powder

140 ml warm water

15 ml olive oil

A pinch of salt

**Filling**

70 g finely chopped onion

3 cloves garlic, finely grated

1 tbsp olive oil

1 tbsp coconut aminos or mushroom sauce (page 22)

Equal amount finely grated ginger

1 tsp chili flakes

200 g finely chopped mushrooms

50 g finely chopped cabbage

Salt and pepper

**Tahini sauce**

3 tbsp light tahini

2 cloves garlic, finely grated

Equal amount finely grated ginger

2 tsp rice vinegar

2 tbsp coconut aminos

1 tbsp coconut nectar syrup or agave

2-3 tbsp water to thin

**For Serving**

2 tbsp chili oil

1/4 green onion, shredded

1/4 bunch Vietnamese basil

1/4 cup toasted almond flakes

1/2 thinly sliced fresh chili pepper

**Serves: 2**

1. To make the wonton, place all the wonton ingredients in a bowl except the oil and water, mix together. Then add the water and oil. Mix thoroughly with a spoon and then let sit for 2-3 minutes. When the time is up, knead the dough on a baking sheet with a little rice flour.
2. Wrap the dough in cling film and let it rest in the fridge for 30 minutes. Divide the dough into 4 equal pieces. Using a rolling pin, roll out the dough to about 2 mm. Cut the dough into rounds with an 8-10 cm round cutter. Repeat the process for the rest of the dough.
3. To make the filling, put the onion, garlic, ginger, olive oil and mushroom sauce or coconut aminos in a saucepan, cook until softened. Then add the chopped mushrooms, continue cooking, finally add the chilli, salt, pepper and cabbage, let it cook for just 1-2 minutes or until it absorbs all the water in the pan.
4. Add 1 tbsp of the filling to the centre of one dough. Use a finger dipped in water to run along the edges of the wrapper. Then fold the wrapper in half over the filling and pinch it together in the centre with your fingers, but do not seal it yet. Using the thumb and forefinger of your right hand, start making a crease about once every 6mm on the top of the wrapper from the centre towards the right side, making 4-5 creases.
5. Heat the oil and add 100ml of water to the pan. Immediately cover with a lid and steam the gyoza for about 3 minutes or until most of the water has evaporated.
6. When the pan is hot, place the dumplings in a single layer, flat side down, in a circular pattern.
7. Cook until the bottom of the dumplings turns golden brown and they have absorbed all the water, about 3-4 minutes.
8. Whisk together all the ingredients for the dipping sauce in a small saucepan, cook over medium heat until slightly thickened. Add a splash of water if you need to thin.
9. Place the dumplings on top and drizzle with the sauce followed by the crispa chili oil. Top with some spring onions, Vietnamese basil, chili and almond flakes.

# OAT RISOTTO

## WITH PLUM AND TOMATOES

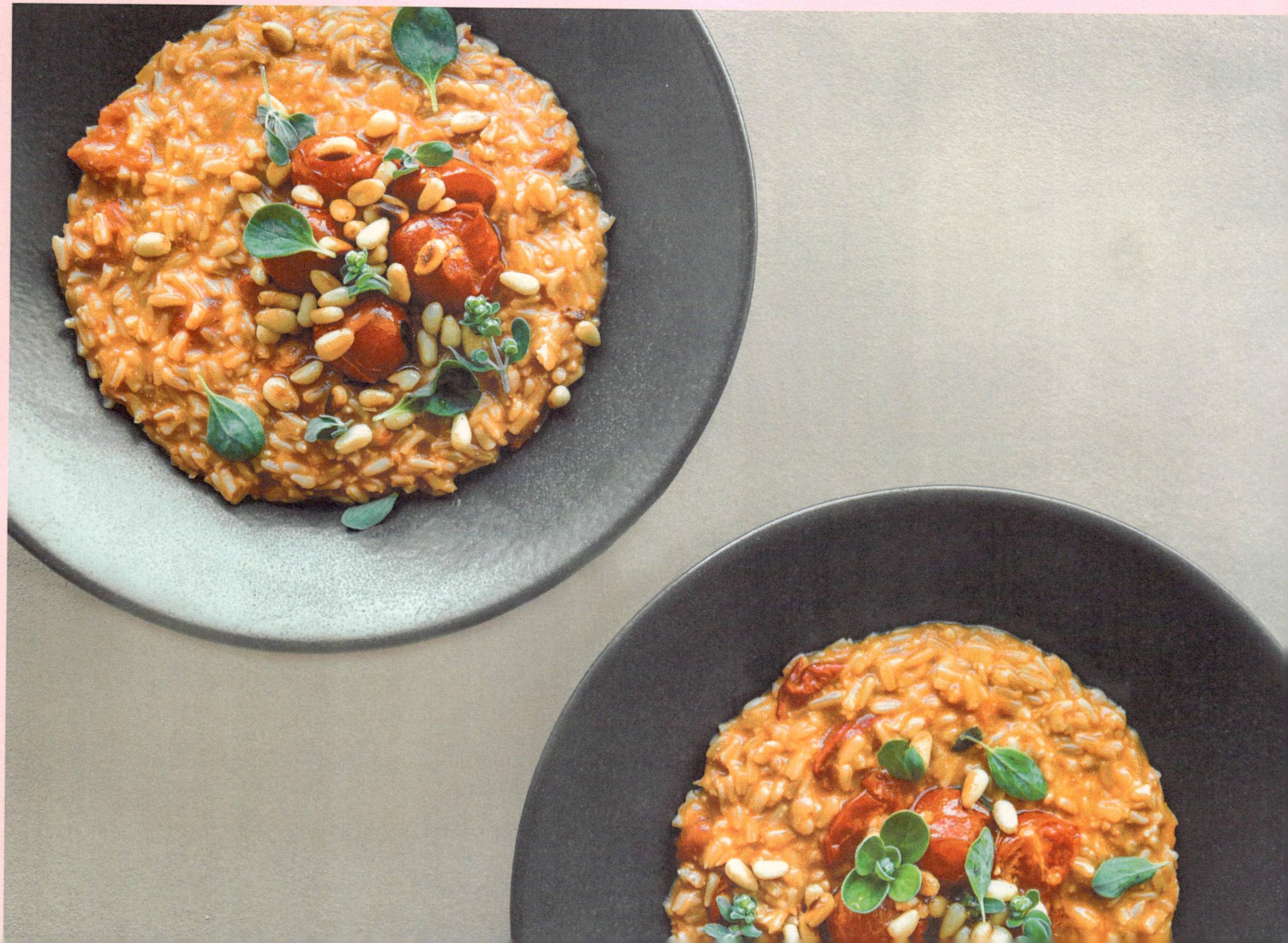

*Oats release a lot of starch as they cook, which is exactly what makes risotto so great, and if you follow the same procedure of making regular risotto and stirring constantly, you will end up with something of a similar texture as risotto.*

**Serves:** 2

500g ripe tomatoes
2 ripe plums
150g whole oats
1 cup filtered water
3 garlic cloves minced
1 tsp seaweed powder
1 tsp shiitake powder

**Add-Ons**

1 tsp salt
Freshly grounded blackpepper
Vegan parmesan topping to serve (page 23)
or toasted pine nuts to serve
Herbs of your choice (majoram, rosemary or basil. Use only one.)

1. Place whole oats in a bowl, wash and dry. Cover with water, let it sit overnight or for 10-12 hours.
Then strain the excess water. Set aside.
2. Wash and cut your tomatoes and plums, place in a deep pot, add the minced garlic, shiitake powder and seaweed powder.
3. Cook on medium-low heat for 15-20 minutes or until tomatoes leave their juice and they are soft enough.
Then add the whole oats, cook another 20 minutes until oats absorbs the water.
4. Add 1/2 cup to 1 cup filtered water as needed depending on water content in the tomatoes you might need to add more water. Taste it if it is too thick, add more water and continue to cook. It should be a bit juicy, not too thick.
Once cooked, let it sit for 8-10 minutes before serving.
5. Season with salt, seaweed and black pepper. Serve with parmesan topping or toasted pine nuts and herbs of your choice.

**TIPS** - If you can't find the whole oats, you can also use steel-cut oats, risotto rice or other types of rice you prefer.

# SKAGEN CAKE

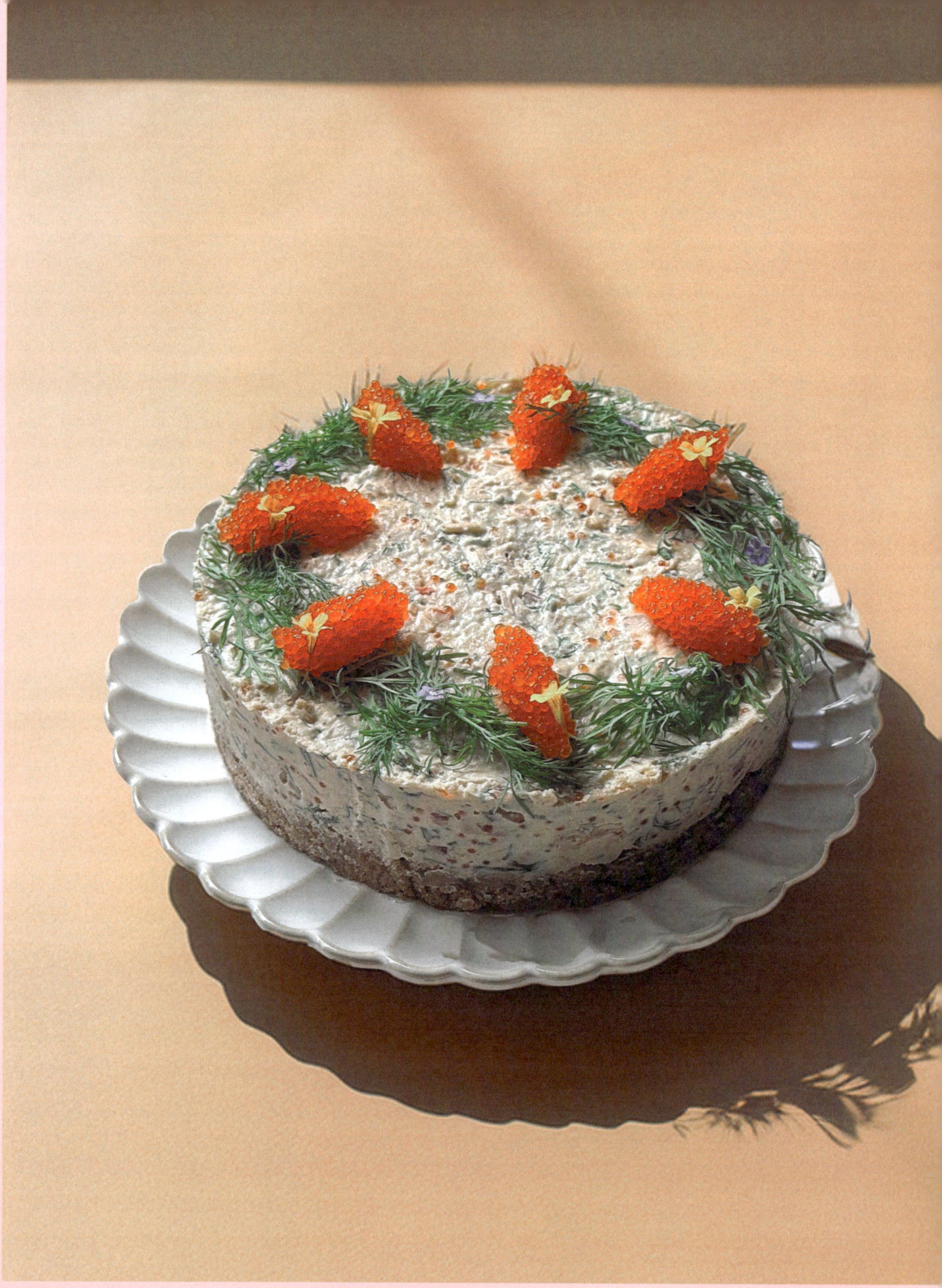

**Serves: 7-8**

**Ingredients**

200g gf breadcrumbs (on the next page)
75g melted vegan butter
or coconut oil

**Filling**

1 pack jackfruit (approx. 280 g)
1 batch cashew fraiche (see below)
250 g vegan cream cheese
2.5 tbsp agar agar flakes + 1 dl water
3 tbsp grated horseradish
1 bunch fresh dill
1 red onion (finely chopped)
1 lemon (zest + juice)
80 g seaweed caviar (on the next page)
1/2 tsp salt
1 pinch pepper

**Cashew fraiché**

100 grams of natural cashew nuts (soaked for at least 6 hours)
1 dl water
1 large pinch of salt
2 tbsp lemon juice
1 tbsp olive oil
2 tbsp coconut oil

*Skagentårta is a luxurious variation on the sandwich cake with delicious pieces of the sea. It is traditionally made with kavringe, but use whatever you like. Remember that it should be refrigerated for 3 hours before serving!*

1. Blend the crumbs in a food processor until crumbly. Melt the butter and add to the food processor.
2. Press the crumbs into the bottom of a springform pan. Leave it in the fridge while you make the skagen mixture.
3. Cut the tofu into small cubes and chop the dill and place in a bowl.
4. Take 1 dl cashew fraiche and pour it into a saucepan together with the agar agar. Pour in the water and continue stirring so that everything is mixed, and heat until it simmers for a couple of minutes.
5. Mix in the rest of the cashew fraiche, seaweed caviar, red onion, lemon zest and lemon juice in the bowl, stir carefully so that it is distributed properly. Season with salt.
6. Then pour the agar agar cashew fraiche into this bowl and mix everything.
7. Take the base out of the fridge and add the filling.
Refrigerate for 2–3 hours before serving. Decorate with flowers, dill and seaweed caviar.

**Cashew Fraiché**

1. Start by soaking the cashews in water for at least 6 hours or overnight.
2. Strain the water and rinse the nuts before adding them to a powerful blender with 1/2 cup water, salt, lemon juice, olive oil and coconut oil.
3. Blend on high speed until you have a smooth batter, which usually takes at least 5-6 minutes.
4. When the consistency is smooth, pour it into a jar and use as you would regular creme fraiche. For the Skagen cheesecake, use the entire batch.

# GLUTEN-FREE RYE BREAD

**Ingredients**

25 g fresh yeast
1 tbsp olive oil
1 1/2 dl almond milk,
1 1/2 dl brewed coffee, cooled
2 dl water
1 dl dark agave
3 tbsp finely ground psyllium husks
3 dl teff flour
1 dl buckwheat flour
3 tbsp whole flaxseeds
1 tbsp anise, ground
1 tbsp fennel, ground
2 tsp bicarbonate of soda
1 1/2 tsp salt

*A crusty bread for those who want to eat purely vegan gluten-free. So easy to make if you have guests who have special diets, for example. The best thing is that it still tastes great so everyone will be satisfied and want your recipe.*
*One of the ingredients is perhaps a bit unexpected, but the brewed coffee gives both a rich and spicy character to the bread.*

1. Crumble the yeast into a large bowl. Add the almond milk, brewed coffee, water, dark agave syrup and olive oil. Mix all the ingredients together to form a loose batter.
2. Add the rest of the ingredients and mix everything together.
3. Line a 1 1⁄2 liter loaf pan with baking paper.
4. Pour the dough into the pan, smooth the surface and dust with a little teff flour. Cover with a baking cloth and let rise for 1 hour.
5. Preheat the oven to 225 degrees. Place the bread on the lowest rack and bake for 60–70 minutes.
6. Remove the pan, tip the bread out and let the bread cool completely before cutting.

# SRIRACHA CAVIAR

**Ingredienser**

0.6 dl sriracha sauce (page 17)

0.6 dl water (boiled with 1 tbsp dulse and strained)

1 tbsp agar-agar

**Other components**

1 dl cold olive oil

1 dl cold water

*Sriracha Caviar is a fun and easy way to enhance any dish. We use simple molecular gastronomy techniques to create these little flavor gems, perfect for sprinkling on sandwiches, pasta, salad or rice.*

1. Pour oil into a tall glass and chill in the freezer until slightly lumpy (about 3-4 hours).
2. In a small saucepan, bring sriracha, 1/2 cup water, and agar-agar to a slow simmer over medium heat, stirring constantly. If mixture starts to smoke, remove saucepan from heat, reduce heat, and continue cooking.
3. Simmer for about 5 minutes, then remove from heat and pour mixture into a small bowl.
4. Draw up sriracha mixture into your small syringe. Drop sriracha dulce pearls, one drop at a time, into the cold oil from about 5 inches above the surface of the oil.
5. Once you have used all of the mixture, strain the caviar by pouring the oil through a strainer.
6. Place strained caviar in a bowl of ice cold water to remove any remaining oil, then strain the water and serve!

# JACKFRUIT BAO BUNS

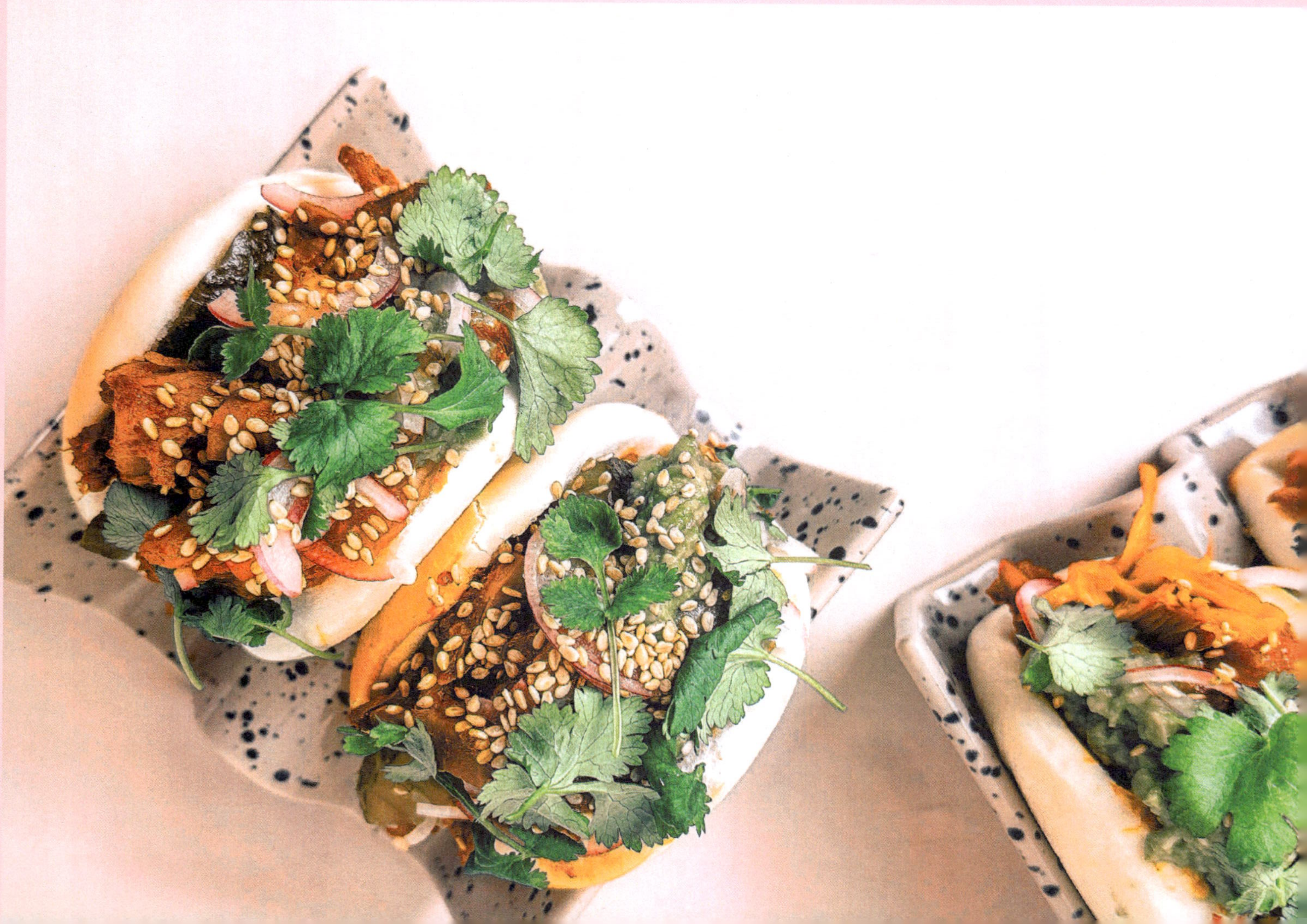

**Serves: 3**

**Ingredients**

350 g young jackfruit
1 cup mushroom sauce (page 22)
1/2 cup olive oil
2 tbsp tomato paste
1 tbsp sriracha
2 tbsp finely diced fresh ginger
1 tbsp finely chopped garlic

**For serving**

6 bao buns (see below)
1 cup fresh coriander
1 small red onion, finely sliced
1/2 cup pickled cucumber
2 cups guacamole
1 cup tomato salsa
White sesame seeds

**Bao Buns**

10 g instant yeast
15 g coconut sugar
2-4 tbsp warm water
250 g tapioca flour (set 30-40 g aside to dust your buns later)
100 g rice flour
90 g glutinous rice flour
2 tsp baking powder
1/2 tsp salt
Approx. 150 ml water (start with about 60 ml of it and gradually add as you need)
50 ml olive oil

1. Mix tomato paste, mushroom sauce, olive oil, sriracha, minced garlic and ginger in a large bowl.
2. Add the jackfruit, mix together. Let it marinate for at least 2-3 hours or overnight.
3. Put a large frying pan on the stove, add the marinated jackfruit and 2 dl water. Cook until the jackfruit absorbs all the water.
4. To make bao buns,start by activating the yeast. In a bowl, add the instant yeast, 15 g of coconut sugar, 2-4 tbsp water. Mix together. Let it sit for 8-10 minutes. The mixture should be foamy and bubbly.
5. Meanwhile, in a mixing bowl, mix the tapioca, rice flour, baking soda, salt, turmeric if using and glutinous rice flour together.
6. Knead the dough in the bowl. The dough should moist and a bit wet but not sticky. If the dough feels dry add a bit of liquid.
7. Place the dough in a lightly oiled bowl and cover with cling film. Leave the dough in a warm place for an hour.
8. Put a small cup of water next to you in case you need it to help you shape the dough. Divide the dough into equal sized small pieces and roll each ball between your hands before flattening it and pressing it into an oval shape and folding it over. Repeat with the remaining dough balls.
9. Set the shaped buns in a warm area for a second rise, allowing them to expand to roughly 50% beyond their starting size (they won't fully double). This rise tends to be quicker around 20 to 35 minutes but try not to judge by the clock. What matters is the feel; the dough should seem lighter when you pick up a bun and appear about half again as puffy.
10. Place each bun on a piece of baking parchment paper and place in a bamboo steamer.
11. Steam for about 10- 12 minutes, or until the buns have puffed up and are firm and cooked through.
12. Take them off the baking parchment, open its lid and fill with pulled jack.
13. Add guacamole and tomato salsa.
14. Top with pickled cucumber, red onion, coriander and sesame seeds.

# SWEDISH SANDWICH CAKE

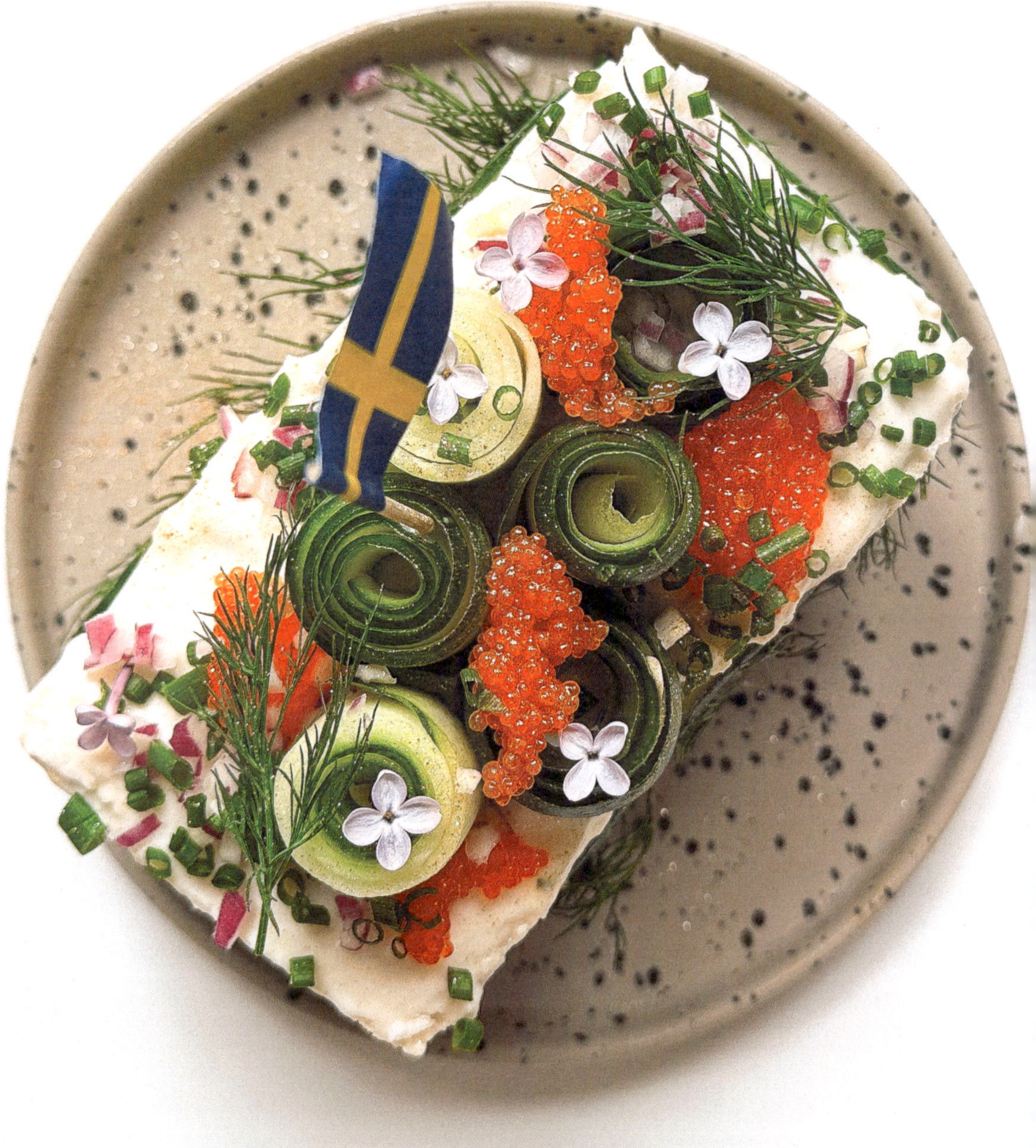

**4 Servings**

*A truly luxurious and creamy swedish sandwich cake that fits perfectly at all celebrations and summer gatherings.*

**Jackfruit Filling**

2 small mashed avocados
½ dl (about 3 ½ tbsp) vegan crème fraîche (or use multifunctional cashew cream in the pantry chapter)
150 g jackfruit, finely diced
1 tbsp agave syrup
2 tbsp mushroom sauce
1 tbsp paprika powder
½ tsp ground ginger
¼ tsp cayenne pepper
1 tbsp olive oil
1 scallion, finely chopped
½ lemon, zest and juice
Salt and black pepper, to taste

**Sandwich**

12 slices gf sandwich bread, crusts removed

**For the frosting**

1 dl vegan cashew fraîche (page 157)
½ dl vegan mayonnaise

**Toppings**

A large cucumber
A small bunch of fresh dill
One small red onion, finely chopped
Edible flowers, optional
Vegan sriracha caviar

1. Start by cooking the jackfruit. Place it in a saucepan and add paprika powder, ground ginger, cayenne pepper, mushroom sauce, agave syrup, olive oil, and a splash of water. Let it cook until softened and all liquid is absorbed. Allow to cool for 30 minutes.
2. Prepare the jackfruit filling by first mixing the mashed avocado with the crème fraîche until smooth. Add the remaining ingredients and mix well. Finally, fold in the jackfruit and stir. Chill in the fridge while preparing the other components.
3. For the frosting, combine vegan cashew fraîche, and mayonnaise in a bowl. Whisk until smooth and free of lumps. Place in the fridge until ready to use.
4. Prepare the garnishes. Slice the cucumber into long ribbons with a vegetable peeler. Cut the ribbons in half and roll them tightly to form cucumber rolls.
5. To assemble, place three slices of crustless sandwich bread side by side on a serving platter or board to create a loaf shape.
6. Spread a 1 cm thick layer of jackfruit filling over the bread, all the way to the edges. Add another three slices of bread on top and spread another layer of filling. Repeat once more, then finish with the last three slices of bread to form the "lid."
7. Spread the frosting evenly over the top and sides of the cake. This takes a little patience, but it doesn't need to be perfect as most of it will be covered with decoration.
8. Once the cake is frosted, decorate with seaweed caviar, cucumber rolls, dill, and edible flowers of your choice.

Store in the fridge until serving – or slice and enjoy right away.

# TEMPEH WITH PUMPKIN CURRY & BASIL PESTO

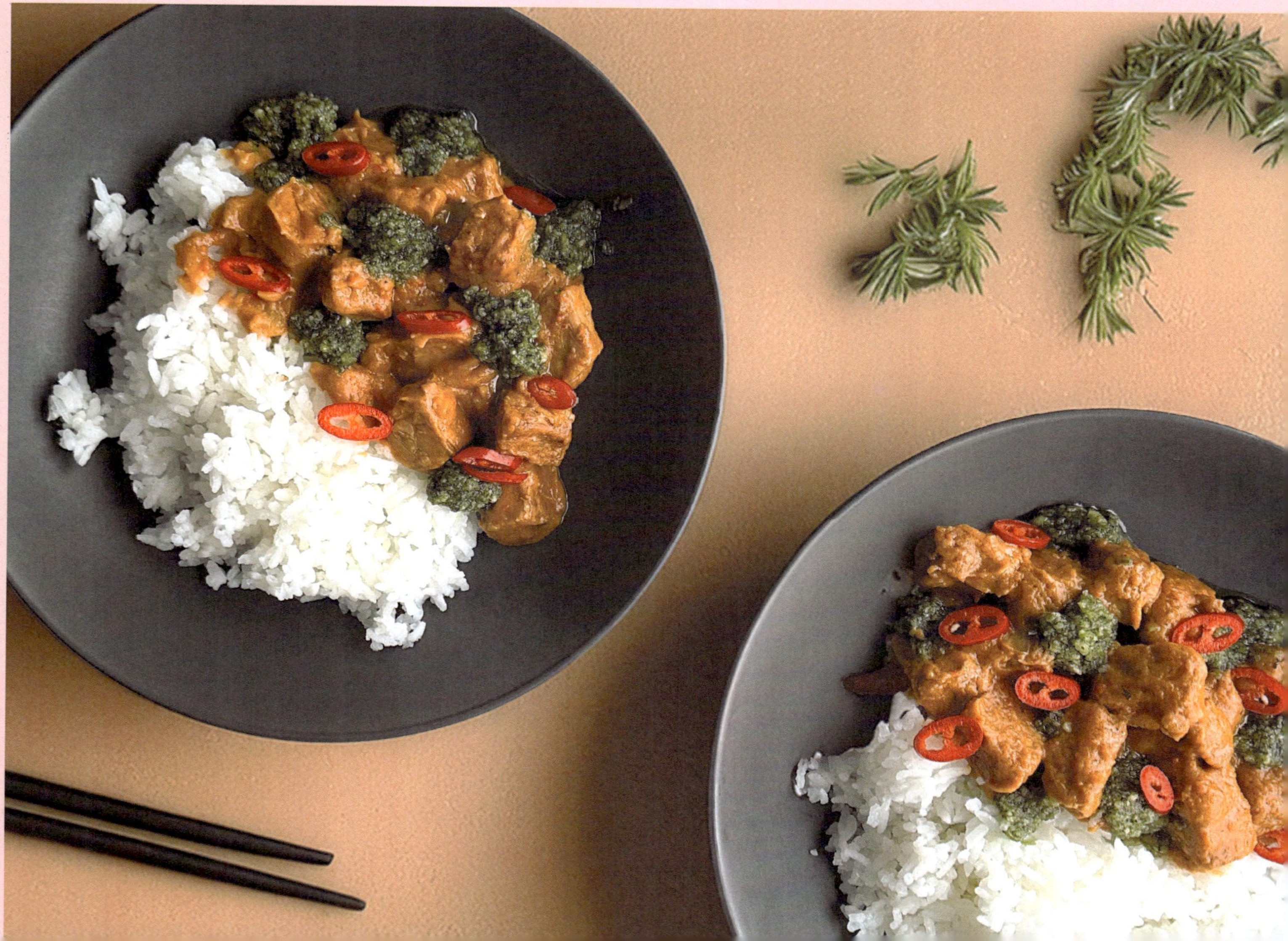

**Serves: 3**

**Ingredients**

250g tempeh

1 cup rice + 1 1/4 cup water

1 sliced chili pepper to serve

**Tempeh Marinated**

1 cup water

2 tbsp coconut aminos

1 tbsp agave

1 tbsp grated ginger

**Pumpkin Curry**

200 g diced pumpkin

2 tbsp olive oil

1 chopped onion

3 chili peppers

4 cloves garlic

1 cup water

1 tsp yellow pea miso

1 tsp ground coriander

1 tsp Himalayan salt

**Basil Pesto**

50 g basil

2 tbsp olive oil

1 tbsp lemon juicea

1/4 cup pine nuts or cashew nuts

3 minced garlic cloves

1/2 tsp Himalayan salt

*Seasoning pumpkin puree with spices is a surefire way to enhance the flavor. Pumpkin works wonders with basil and subtle pine nut flavors along with full of bold flavors that come from birds eye chili and coriander, can be served with plant-based meat alternatives, and common base ingredients can be oats, rice, or pasta.*

1. Mix the marinade ingredients in a deep container. Cut your tempeh into cubes. Add in the marination sauce. Refrigerate overnight.
2. Place all pumpkin curry ingredients except water in a saucepan, cook over medium heat for 2-3 minutes until it starts to color. Then add the water and cook until the pumpkins absorb the water content and are soft enough. Transfer the mixture to a blender, blend until smooth. Transfer back to the pot.
3. Place the tempeh along with the marinade in a pan, cook until all the water has evaporated, then lightly brown the tempeh on all sides in the pan.
4. Cook your rice according to the package directions.
5. To make the pesto, blend the pine nuts or cashews, salt, lemon juice and garlic in a small food processor until finely chopped. Add the basil and pulse again. Then drizzle in the olive oil with the food processor blade still running. Transfer mixture to a small pan, heat for 2-3 minutes.
6. Pour pumpkin sauce over tempeh and stir to coat.
7. Serve your rice with pumpkin coated tempeh, basil pesto and hot chili pepper on top.

# ROASTED CABBAGE

## WITH MUSTARD & BELUGA

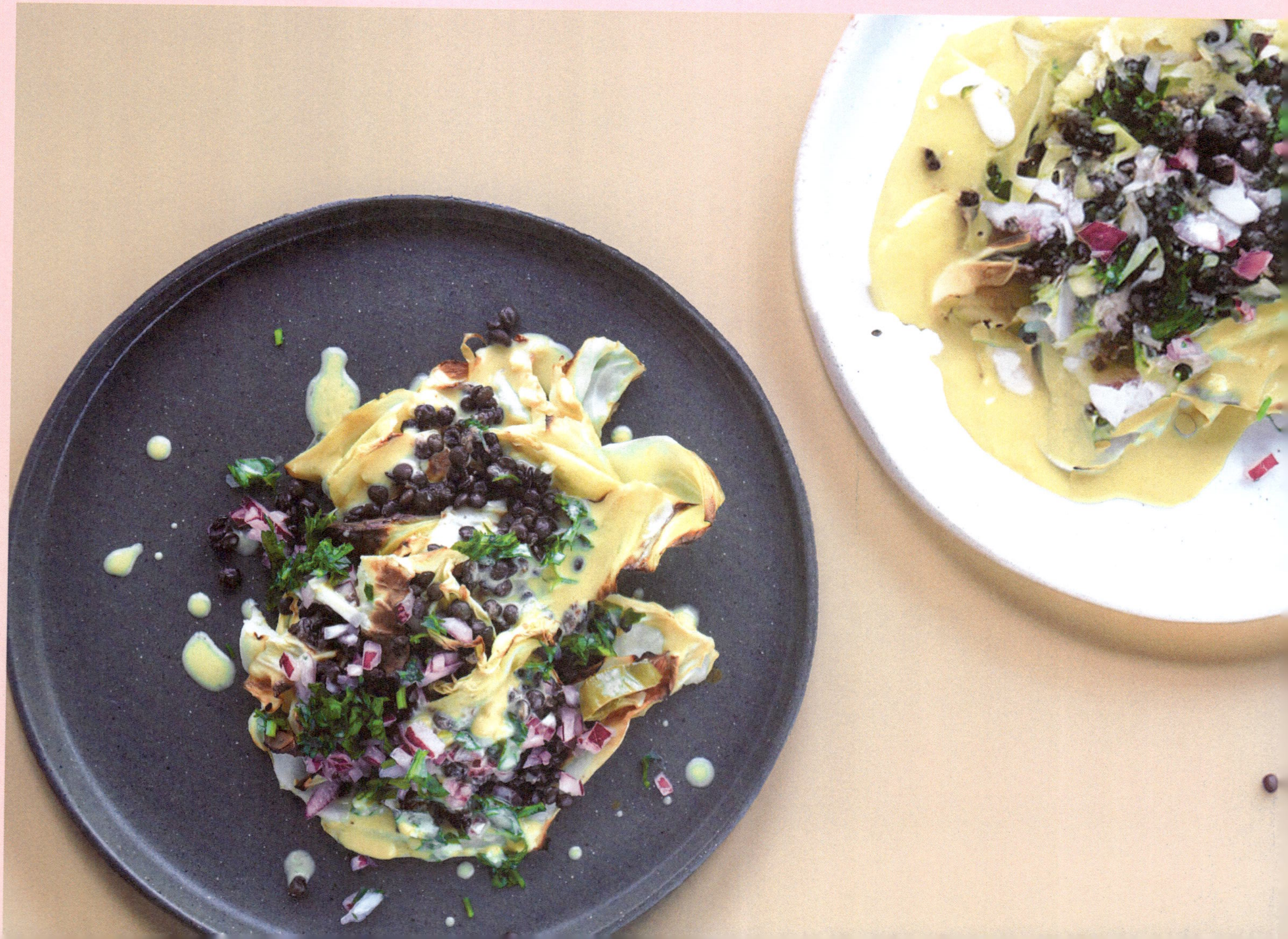

*Charred wedges of roasted cabbage bring a smoky sweetness that pairs beautifully with the sharp bite of a silky mustard sauce. Earthy beluga lentils add depth and heartiness, while fresh parsley and crisp red onion lift the dish with brightness and crunch.*

**Serves: 2-3**

**Ingredients**

1/2 medium green cabbage
1 vegetable broth
Salt and pepper to taste
Lemon wedges to serve
Chopped parsley to serve
Cooked beluga to serve (1 cup beluga cooked in 1 3/4 cup mushroom stock)

**Mustard Sauce**

Juice from 2 whole lemons
1 large red onion, finely chopped
2 cloves garlic, finely chopped
2 tbsp Dijon mustard
1/4 tsp salt

1. Preheat oven to 220° C. Line a baking sheet with parchment paper.
2. Cut cabbage half into four equal wedges and set on prepared baking sheet. Use a pastry brush to coat the cut side of each wedge with vegetable broth and sprinkle with salt and pepper.
3. Turn wedges and repeat.
4. Place the baking sheet in the oven and cook for 10-12 minutes. Flip the wedges and roast until nicely browned, 8-10 minutes more.
5. Meanwhile, make the sauce by adding all the sauce ingredients to a small pan and mix until combined well.
6. Cook the beluga until absorbs all the water.
7. To serve, place the wedges on a plate, whisk sauce again and drizzle over wedges. Add 2-3 tbsp beluga lentils over the cabbage. Sprinkle some chopped red onion and parsley. Serve with lemon wedges.

# GREEN CURRY

## WITH TEMPEH, BAMBOO SHOOTS & PEAS

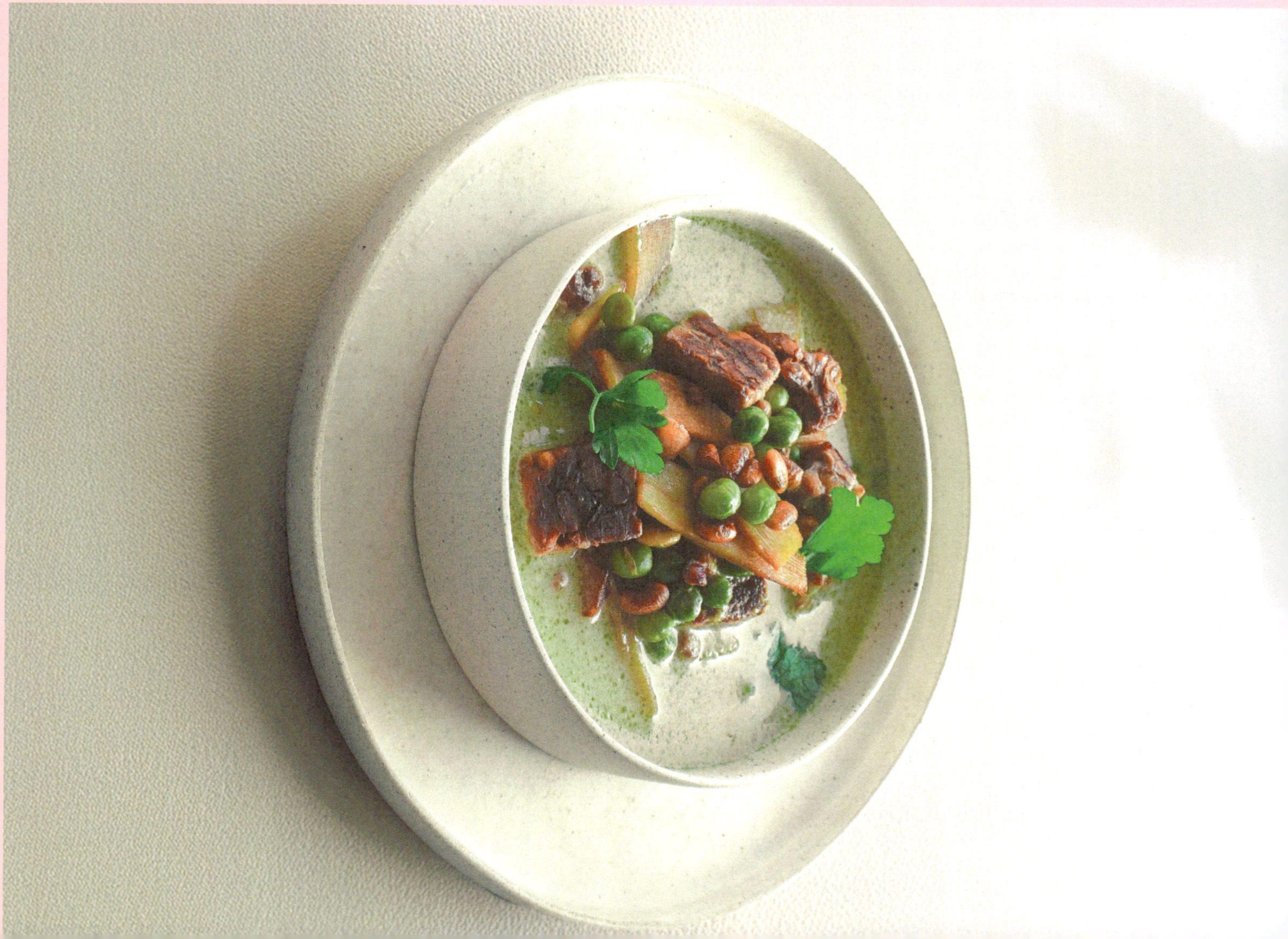

*A thoughtful blend of Thai aromatics and herbs, green curry paste and silky coconut milk deliver bold and fragrant flavours that will make your taste buds dance, while a mix of tempeh and vegetables makes this a complete dinner. Serve it with rice if you like.*

**Serves: 3**

**Curry Paste**

2 medium shallots
5 garlic cloves
4 cm ginger
2 stalks of lemongrass, soft inner part chopped
5 thai green chilies
1 tsp ground coriander
1/2 tsp ground cumin
1/4 tsp white pepper
1 tsp salt

**For the Soup**

3 tbsp vegetable oil
400 ml full fat coconut milk
6 fesh kaffir lime leaves
250 ml vegetable stock
1 tbsp coconut aminos + 1 tsp nori powder or 1 tbsp vegan fish sauce (page 20)
1/2 lime juice
2 tsp coconut sugar

**Vegetables**

200 g tempeh cubed
1 cup bamboo shoots chopped
1 cup green peas
Fresh thai basil leaves
1/4 cup winter melon cut in 1-inch chunks

1. In a food processor, combine all the paste ingredients until finely chopped.
2. Heat up oil in a heavy-bottomed casserole dish on a low heat.
3. Add curry paste to the hot oil and fry it off gently, for 10 minutes, stirring the entire time. Stir in coconut milk. Lastly add in the lime leaves and veg stock.
4. Allow the sauce to come to a gentle simmer. Simmer for 10-15 minutes on a low heat.
5. Season with coconut aminos and nori flakes or vegan fish sauce, lime juice and a touch of coconut sugar.
6. Allow the curry flavours to develop overnight as it always tastes better the day after it has been made.
7. In terms of the veggies, you could simply cook them in the simmering curry, or stir-fry in the pan first with little olive oil and a dash of coconut aminos.
8. Serve on top of plain rice if desired.

PLANT BASED UMAMI

# TOM YUM

## WITH MAYO, CAPERS AND CHILI

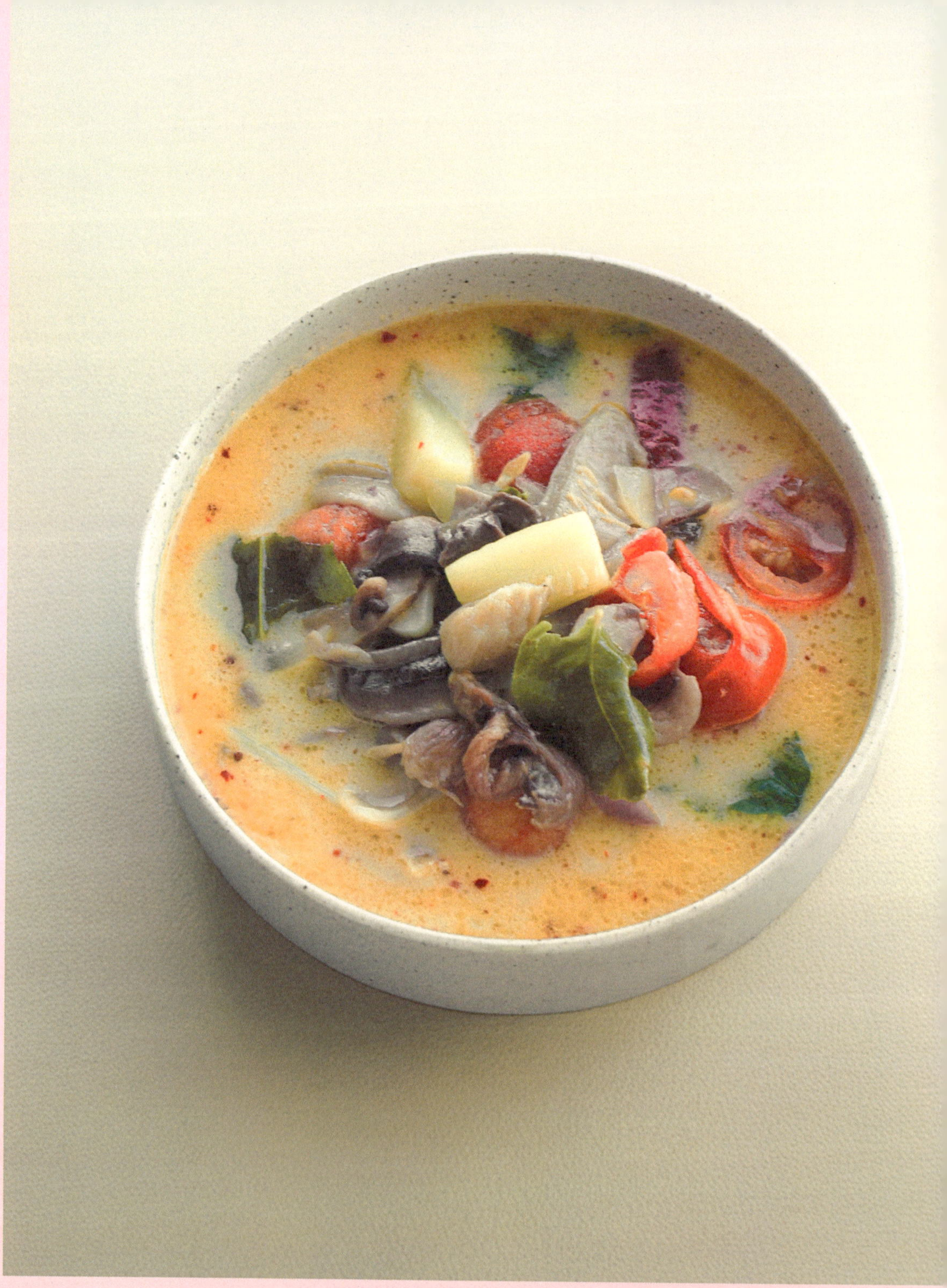

*A classic Thai soup celebrated for its bold, aromatic balance of hot and sour flavors. The broth is infused with lemongrass, kaffir lime leaves, galangal, and chili, creating a fragrant base that is both invigorating and comforting. Notes of lime juice and tamarind bring refreshing acidity, while a touch of chili heat lingers on the palate.*

**Serves: 2**

**Ingredients**

1 lemongrass stalk cut in 4 pieces
1 tsp galangal grated or 1 tsp galangal powder
3 garlic cloves minced
2 tbsp tamarind paste
1 tbsp chili oil
1 tbsp coconut sugar
4-5 kaffir lime leaves
6-7 cherry tomatoes
1 large silver onion
2 whole red chili peppers
1/2 tsp chili flakes
1 tsp freshly ground coriander seeds
1 tbsp mushroom sauce
1 cup coconut milk
1 cup vegetable stock
1 cup water
500 g assorted mushrooms chopped
100 g bamboo shoots (or inner parts of zucchini) -optional but goes so well in this dish.
3 tbsp lime juice

1. Crush the lemongrass to release the oil and aroma. Slice the stalks into 3-4 inch pieces, add to your pot.
2. Crush the garlic as well add to the pot.
3. Add the chili pepper, coconut sugar, halved tomatoes, chopped onions, kaffir lime leaves, galangal and tamarind paste as well.
4. Heat the pot on medium heat. Sauté the aromatics for 2 to 3 minutes over medium high heat until the onion is translucent.
5. Then add the mushrooms, bamboo shoots (or zucchini) continue to sauté for 4-5 minutes.
6. Add the mushroom sauce, vegetable stock, water and coconut milk.
7. Cover and simmer on low heat for 10 minutes.
8. Remove from the heat and add the lime juice as well as salt and chili to taste.
9. Serve in small bowls and garnish with fresh cilantro (if desired).

PLANT BASED UMAMI

# KHAO SOI

## NORTHERN THAI SOUP

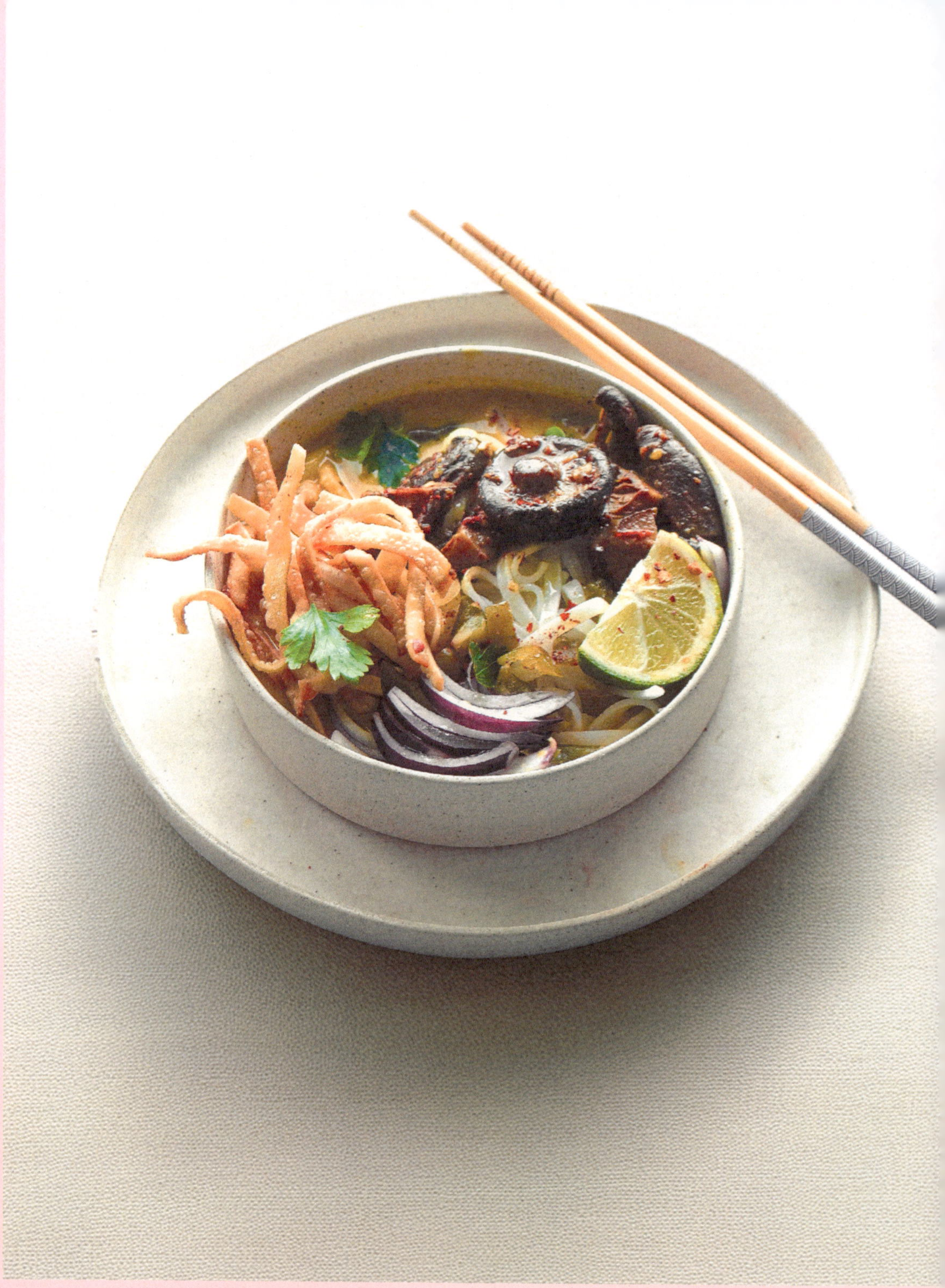

**Serves: 3**

**Khao Soi**

150 g rice noodles

1 lt water

4 tbsp vegan fish sauce (page 20)

1 tbsp coconut sugar

40 g dried shiitake mushrooms soaked or

200 g fresh mushrooms of your choice

400 ml coconut milk

1/2 tsp salt

**Chili Paste**

70 g chiles chopped

75 g shallots about chopped

3 garlic cloves roughly chopped

1 stalk lemongrass white parts only, chopped

4 kaffir lime leaves

5 slices galangal or 1 tsp galangal powder

1 small fresh turmeric (5 g) chopped or

1/2 tsp turmeric powder

1 tsp coriander powder

1 tsp salt

**Garnish**

A handful of wonton strips (page 153)

Chopped shallots

Pickled sour mustard leaves thinly sliced or pickled jalapeno

A few lime slices

A handful of chopped cilantro

**Wonton Strips**

Cut wontons into thin strips. Fill a small pot with enough oil and turn on the heat. Once the oil is heated, quickly fry the wonton strips until golden brown. Remove and drain on a paper towel to absorb excess oil. Set aside until ready to use.

**Curry Paste**

Place the chiles, shallot, garlic, lemongrass, lime leaves, galangal, salt, plus coriander, and turmeric in a food processor. Add a drizzle of oil, then blend into a fine paste. You can also use a mortar and pestle to pound the ingredients if you prefer.

**Cooking**

Heat up a large wok and add a little bit olive oil (use water if you are avoiding the oil). Add the chile paste and stir-fry over medium-low heat until fragrant. If it appears dry, add a little more water or oil. Do not over-fry the paste or it will turn bitter.

Then add the mushrooms, coconut sugar, vegan fish sauce or protein of your choice (tempeh, jack fruit etc would work. Just cook the tofu or tempeh in the oven or pan before adding to the curry paste at this stage ) and continue to stir-fry until they release their aroma. Now add the water and half of the coconut milk. Bring it to a boil and leave it simmering for 20-25 minutes.

**Noodles and Garnish**

Meanwhile cook your noodles of choice as directed by the package, then evenly divide the cooked noodles between three bowls.

Prepare the toppings and side ingredients.

**Serving**

Back to the soup, turn down the heat and add the rest of coconut milk. Let it simmer for another 5 minutes.

Ladle the hot curry over the noodles. Garnish with fried wonton strips, shallots, sour mustard, lime wedges, and cilantro.

# OKONOMIYAKI

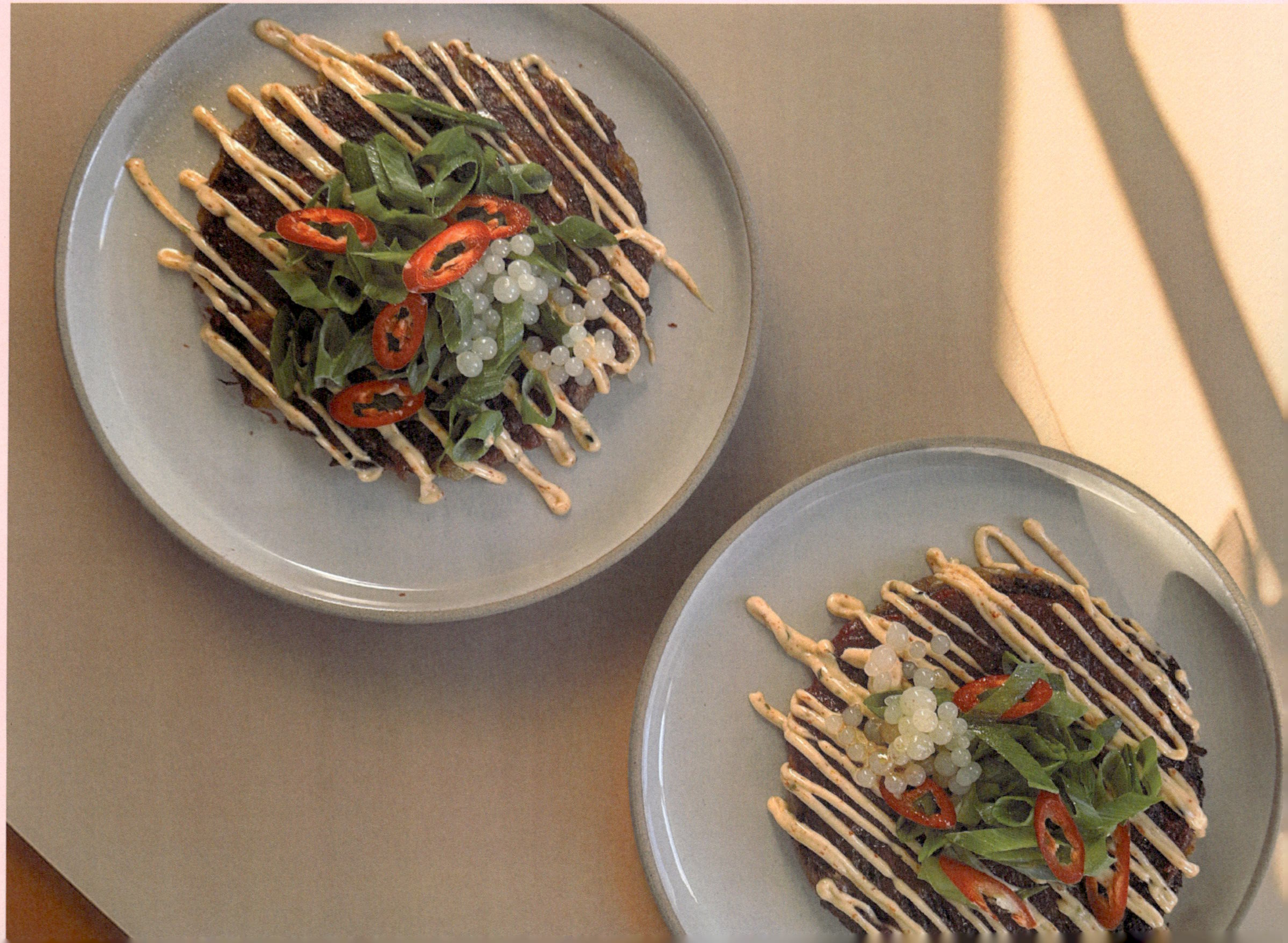

**Serves: 4**

*Jackfruit Okonomiyaki offers a rich balance of umami, sweetness, and gentle heat, led by the miso-caramelized jackfruit and aromatic ginger–cabbage mixture. The pear adds a subtle fruity lift, while the okonomiyaki sauce and togarashi mayo bring tangy, creamy, and lightly spicy depth.*

**For the Jackfruit**

400 g young jackfruit
1 tbsp coconut sugar
1 tbsp minced garlic
1 tbsp fava bean or chickpea miso

**Okonomiyaki stir-fry mixture:**

100 g thinly sliced white cabbage
4 green onions chopped
1/2 pear thinly sliced
1 yellow onion finely chopped
1 tbsp minced fresh ginger
1 tbsp olive oil
1-2 tbsp coconut aminos

**Okonomiyaki batter:**

50 g gluten-free oat flour
40 g tapioca flour
2-3 tbsp psyllium husk powder
100-120 ml water

**Okonomiyaki sauce:**

1/4 cup tomato paste
2 tbsp red wine vinegar
1 tbsp coconut aminos
1 tbso olive oil
1 tbsp agave syrup
1 tbsp coconut sugar

**Togarashi mayonnaise:**

1 cup plant based mayonnaise
1 tsp nanami togarashi

**Toppings:**

Green onions & chili finely sliced
Pickled ginger-agar pearls (page 49)

1.Rinse the jackfruit, cut into small pieces and transfer to a pan. Add olive oil, miso, garlic and coconut sugar and cook until caramelized and gets some color. Remove from the pan, transfer to a large bowl and set aside.
2. In the same pan, add shredded white cabbage, onion, green onions, pear and ginger. Add some olive oil and miso or other fermented liquids according to your choice; like fava bean sauce, coconut aminos etc. Saute until everything nicely caramelized. Once done, transfer mixture over the jackfruits in the bowl.
3. Then add all ingredients for the okonomiyaki batter, mix together until everything combined together. Set aside for 5 minutes so the mixtures comes together.
4. Heat a large non-stick skillet over medium heat. Add 1 tbsp olive oil. Place a round mold in the middle of pan or randomly pour about 3-4 tbsp okonomiyaki batter into the skillet in a pancake shape. Cook for about 5 minutes or until the bottom is golden brown.
5. Carefully flip, cover, and cook for another 5-6 minutes. Once both sides are golden brown, transfer to your plate.
6. To make okonomiyaki sauce, mix all ingredients in a small pan and cook until bubbled. Remove from the heat, brush your okonomiyaki with okonomiyaki sauce on top.
7. In a bowl, mix mayonnaise and togarasi spice together. Transfer to a piping bag, make a small cut in the end. Drizzle your okonomiyaki with togarashi mayonnaise.
8. Serve immediately topped with thinly sliced chili and chopped green onions, additionaly with ginger pearls if desired.

# STUFFED SAVOY CABBAGE

## WITH CHILI TOMATO SAUCE & YOGHURT

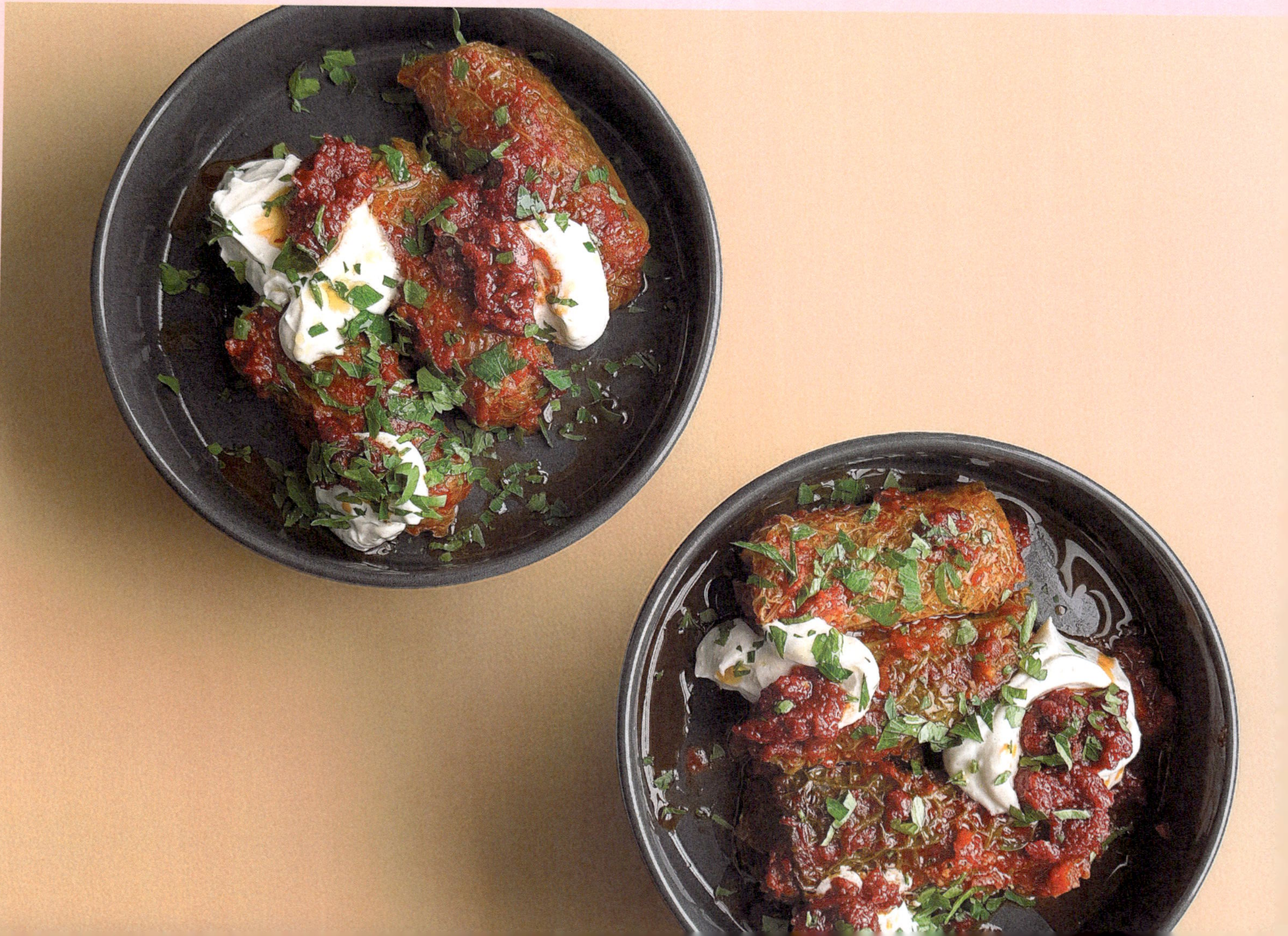

**Serves: 16 rolls**

**Ingredients**

1 medium head savoy cabbage , approx 16 -20 leaves

**For the filling**

300 g jackfruit mince (or use pea mince)
65 g oatmeal + 120 ml water
1 large yellow onion grated
4 garlic cloves minced
1 carrot diced
1/4 cup chopped fresh parsley
3 tbsp fermented fava bean liquid or (2 tsp miso)
3 tbsp tomato paste
1 tbsp coconut sugar
1 tsp shiitake powder
1/2 tsp chili powder
1 tsp salt

**For the sauce for cooking**

1 can crushed tomatoes + 1 cup water
3 bay leaves
1-2 tbsp tomato paste
1 tsp garlic powder
Salt and pepper

**For serving**

Freshly chopped parsley or dill
Plant based yoghurt
Chili oil

**Chili sauce to serve**

4 tbsp olive oil
3 tbsp tomato paste
1 tbsp coconut aminos
1/2 tsp garlic powder
1 tsp chili flakes and salt as needed

1. In a frying pan heat olive oil. Cook the grated onions and minced garlic over low heat for 3-4minutes until tender.
2. Dice the carrots. In a large bowl combine soaked and rinsed minced jackfruit or pea mince, parsley, onions, coconut sugar, carrots, rice, salt and pepper.
3. Add the rice and add 1/2 cup water, cook until the mixture absorbs all water content. Add the parsley, stir together. Set aside.
4. In a medium bowl whisk together miso, olive oil, crushed tomatoes and tomato sauce, salt and pepper.
5. Place your head of cabbage on a cutting board, cut off the bottom and pull the leaves away from the stalk. Repeat with the second head of cabbage. Place cabbage leaves in a pot with boiling water. Boil for about 3-5 minutes until cabbage leaves becomes softer to work with. Strain and let them cool for 2-3 minutes.
6. Preheat your oven to 350F/180C.
7. Take a cabbage leaf and cut the rib down, so it's not too thick. Put 2-3 tbsp of filling at the bottom of the wide part of a leaf and roll it like a burrito, tucking sides in. Your cabbage rolls will vary in size slightly depending on the size of cabbage leaves.
8. Pour a cup of the sauce on the bottom of your cast iron casserole or any other heavy bottom casserole dish and start stacking your cabbage rolls. Half way through add a couple of bay leaves and 1/3 of the sauce and continue stacking until all cabbage rolls are gone.
9. Pour the remaining sauce over cabbage rolls, put the bay leaves in the sauce and cover with a lid and bake in the oven for 1 hour. Then take the lid off and bake for 30 more minutes.
10. To make chili sauce, in a small sauce pan, cook all ingredients until bubbled.
11. Serve with plant based yoghurt, chili sauce and fresh herbs such as dill or parsley.

# I LOVE IT RAW

# STRAWBERRY CHEESECAKE

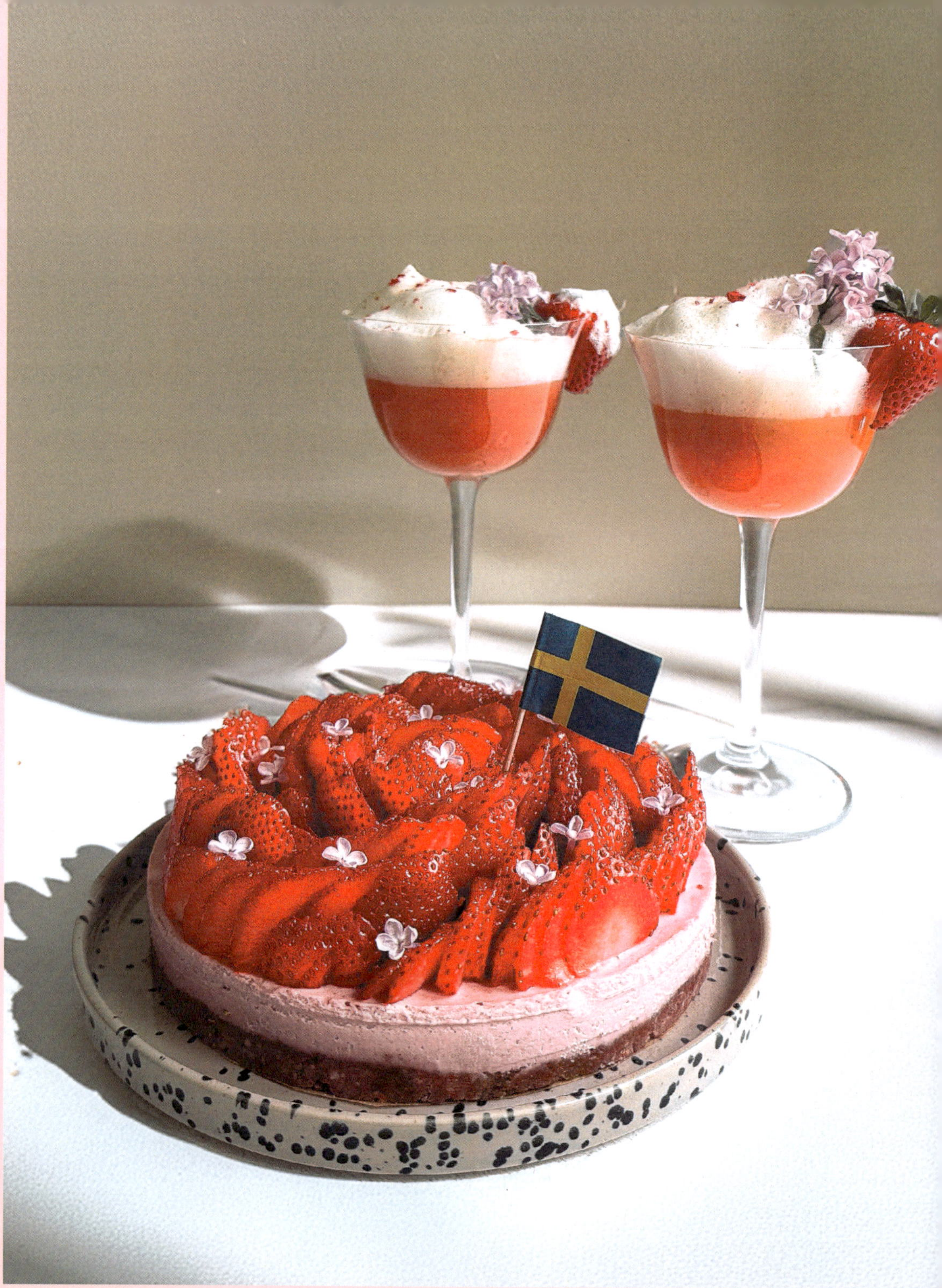

*The best cheesecake of the summer is made with a delicious nut and almond base, a delicious creamy filling of both fresh and freeze-dried strawberries. Then you top the whole thing off with even more heavenly fresh strawberries. It doesn't get any more summery than this delicious cake! And best of all - it's completely raw and vegan.*

**Serves: 6-8**

**Bottom**:

45 g coconut sugar
80 g almond flour
10 g coconut flour
25 g pistachios
20 g almond butter
15 g coconut oil
15 ml almond milk
1 tsp coconut aminos
A pinch of pink Himalayan salt

**Filling**

80g soaked cashews
90g coconut cream
40ml maple syrup
20ml lemon juice
15g freeze-dried strawberry powder
40g fresh strawberries
40ml melted extra virgin coconut oil

**For serving**

250g thinly sliced fresh strawberries
Lilac flowers or edible flowers

1. Place all base ingredients, except almond milk, coconut oil and coconut aminos, in a food processor. Blend well.
2. Add remaining ingredients and continue to blend until combined and a dough-like consistency is achieved.
3. Remove from food processor. Pour batter into a 18cm round cake tin lined with baking paper.
4. Press down with your hands until you have a flat, smooth base. Set aside.
5. Place all cheesecake filling ingredients, except coconut oil, in a high-speed blender. Blend until smooth.
6. Add coconut oil and blend again.
7. Pour batter over cake base. Freeze for 3-4 hours.
8. Remove from pan. Garnish with thinly sliced strawberries and edible flowers. Cut and serve.

# AVOCADO CHOCOLATE MOUSSE

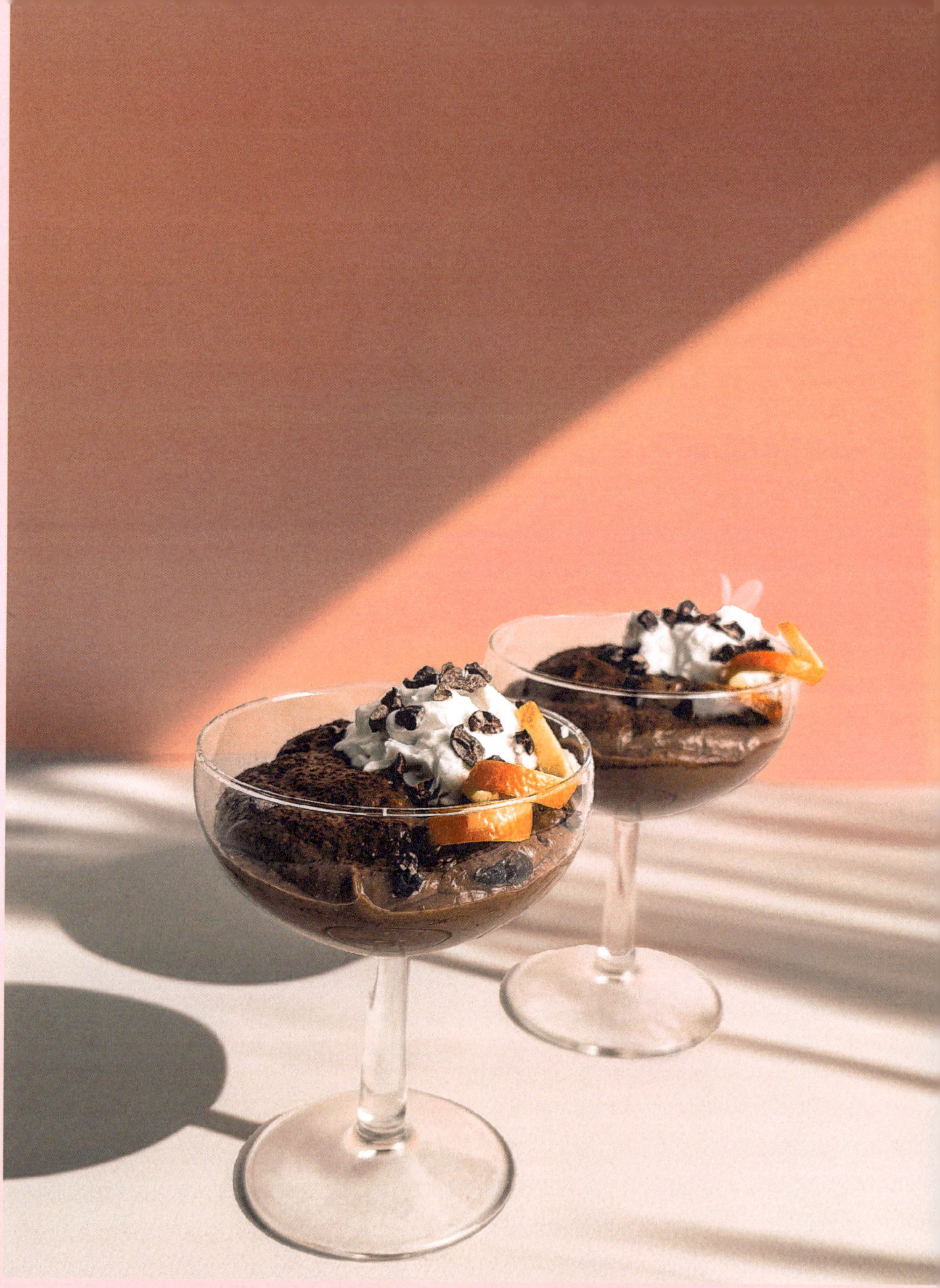

*In addition to being wonderfully healthy, this pudding requires no baking. Your preparation tool will be a food processor or blender, and once chilled, the mousse will be everything you'd expect from the regular version of the decadent dessert; fluffy, with a deep chocolate flavor and high enough fat content to give the same mouthfeel you'd expect from a chocolate pudding.*

**Serves: 2-3**

**Ingredients**

110g ripe avocados (1 ripe avocado, measured after pitting)
160g ripe bananas (1.5-2 small bananas, measured after peeling)
1/2 cup unsweetened almond milk (4 almond pieces + 1/2 cup water mixed)
1/4 cup raw cocoa powder
6 fresh dates pitted and chopped + 1 tbsp maple syrup if needed
1 tsp orange or lemon zest plus more for garnish
A pinch of salt
1/4 tsp ground cinnamon

**Toppings**

Coconut cream
Raw cacao nibs
Orange slice

1. Place all ingredients in a food processor and blend until smooth. Divide between jars.
2. Top with coconut cream, cacao nibs and orange swirls.

# LINGON SEMLA

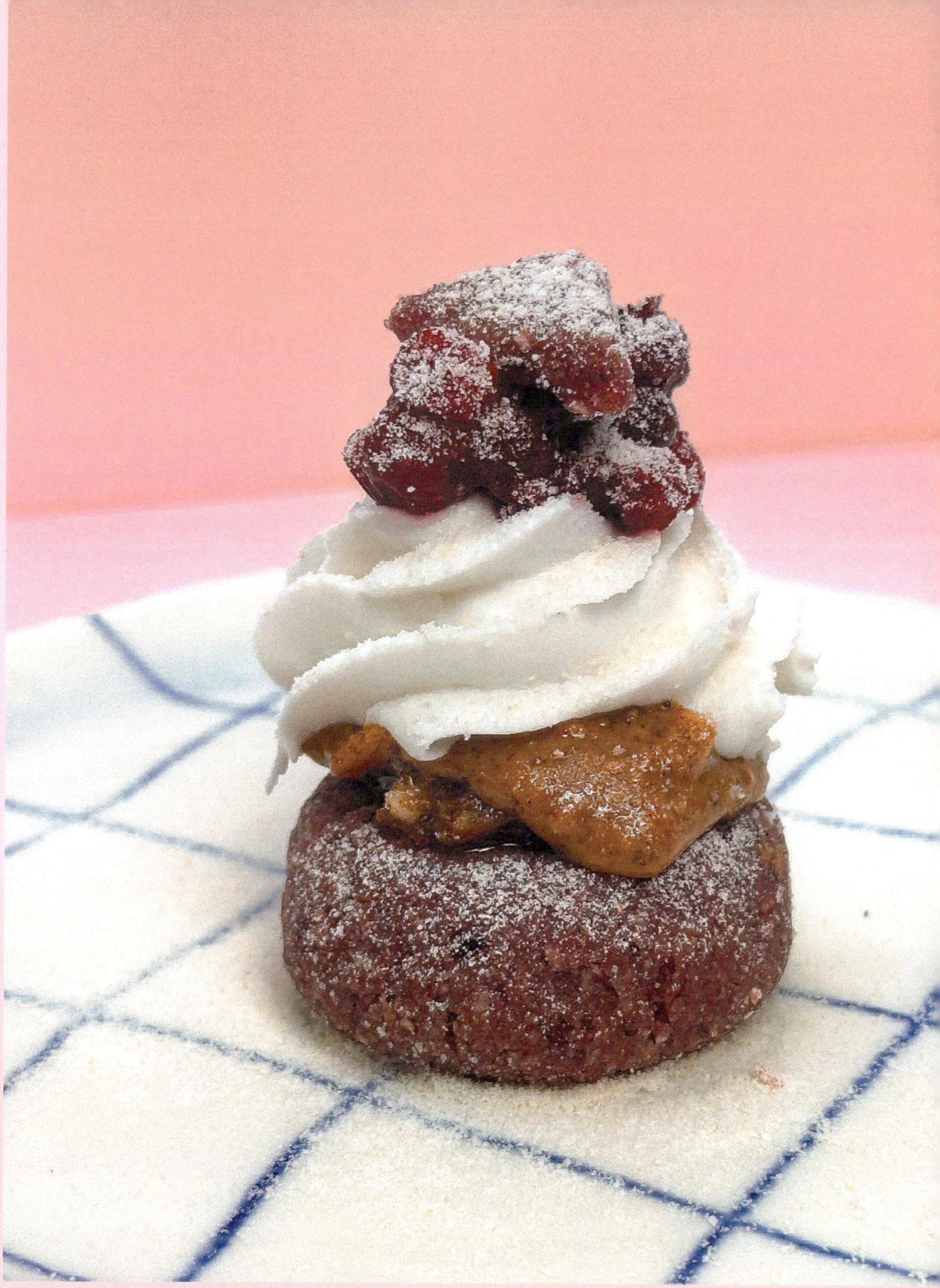

*A guilt-free twist on the classic Swedish treat, this raw semla features a soft, nutty base filled with luxuriously creamy almond and topped with coconut whipped cream and lightly sweetened with natural flavors. Aromatic hints of cardamom give it the signature semla warmth, while the raw preparation keeps it fresh, wholesome, and melt-in-your-mouth delicious*

**Serves: 6-7**

**Coconut frosting**

500 ml coconut cream (fatty part only)
1 tbsp coconut nectar syrup
2 tsp vanilla powder

**Lingon Jam**

70 g frozen lingonberries
2-3 tbsp coconut nectar syrup

**Bottom (Buns + Lid)**

45 g almond flour
70 g oat flour
30 g coconut oil
20 g frozen lingonberries
2 tbsp freeze-dried mixed berries
80 g pitted medjool dates
1/2 tsp cardamom
1 pinch himalayan salt

**Almond mass:**

1 dl almond butter
2 tbsp chopped almonds
15 g coconut sugar
15 g coconut nectar syrup or agave
A pinch of Himalayan salt
A little almond milk or water

**For dusting:**

2 tbsp coconut flour

1. Whip your coconut cream. Then add the coconut nectar syrup and vanilla, whisk together. Place the cream in the fridge until it is thick enough.
2. Place the frozen lingonberries and coconut nectar in a small saucepan and cook over medium heat until thickened. You can also do this in a food dehydrator at 46 C if you want to keep it completely raw.
3. To prepare the base, place all the base ingredients in a blender and blend until you get a sticky consistency. Scoop the mixture into a bowl and mix in the coconut flour, a tablespoon at a time.
4. Once you have mixed everything together, moisten your hands a little and roll into about 9 balls, cut the tops of the balls into a hat, set aside and then press down into the middle of the base.
5. To make the almond paste, place all the ingredients in a blender and blend until you get a creamy consistency.
6. Fill the bottoms with almond paste.
7. Use a piping bag and spread the coconut cream on the almond paste.
8. Add 1 tsp of lingonberry jam on the coconut cream (make sure the jam is cooled enough otherwise your coconut cream will start to melt)
9. Place the lid on top of the lingonberry jam.
10. Finish by dusting with some coconut flour if desired.

# CITRON VERBENA CHEESECAKE

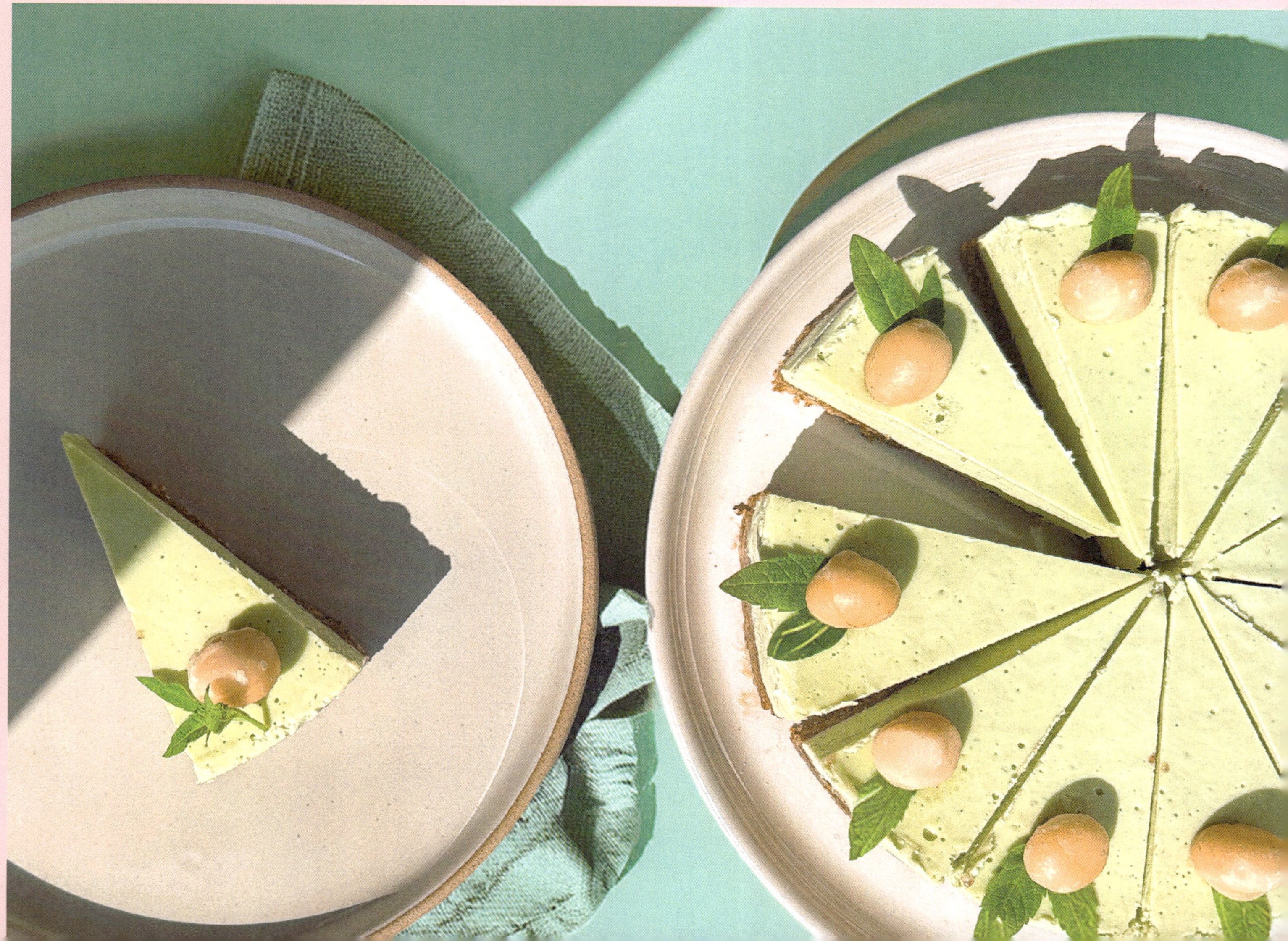

*A refreshingly light and zesty dessert, this raw citron verbena cheesecake combines a creamy, velvety cashew-based filling with the bright, lemony aroma of citron verbena. The natural sweetness of coconut and nuts in the crust perfectly balances the delicate tang of the citrus herb, while the smooth, luscious texture melts in your mouth.*

**Serves: 10-11**

**Bottom**

50 g almonds
20 g gf oatmeal
35 g almond butter
40 g coconut sugar
15 g maple, agave or coconut nectar
20 g extra virgin coconut oil melted
7 ml coconut aminos

**Filling**

150 g macadamia
140 g coconut cream
45 ml lime juice
7 g lemon verbena leaves
30 g extra virgin coconut oil
40 g seamoss gel

**For Decoration**

Lemon Verbena
Macadamia

1. Blend the almonds, oats and coconut sugar in a food processor until you get a fine powder. Then add the rest of the ingredients and mix well until combined. Add a splash of water if you need to.
2. Pour the mixture into a 18 cm round cake pan, pressing down with the back of a spoon to flatten as much as possible. Dip the spoon in the coconut oil and continue to flatten until the crust is smooth and shiny. Set aside.
3. Soak the macadamias for 3-4 hours. Then strain and transfer to the blender. Add the rest of the ingredients except the coconut oil. Blend until smooth.
4. Finally add the melted coconut oil and sea moss, blend until the mixture is silky smooth.
5. Pour the cream over the crust.
6. Freeze for at least 4-5 hours or overnight.
7. When ready, cut into slices, decorate with macadamia and small lemon verbena leaves.

# PRALINE CAKE WITH HAZELNUTS

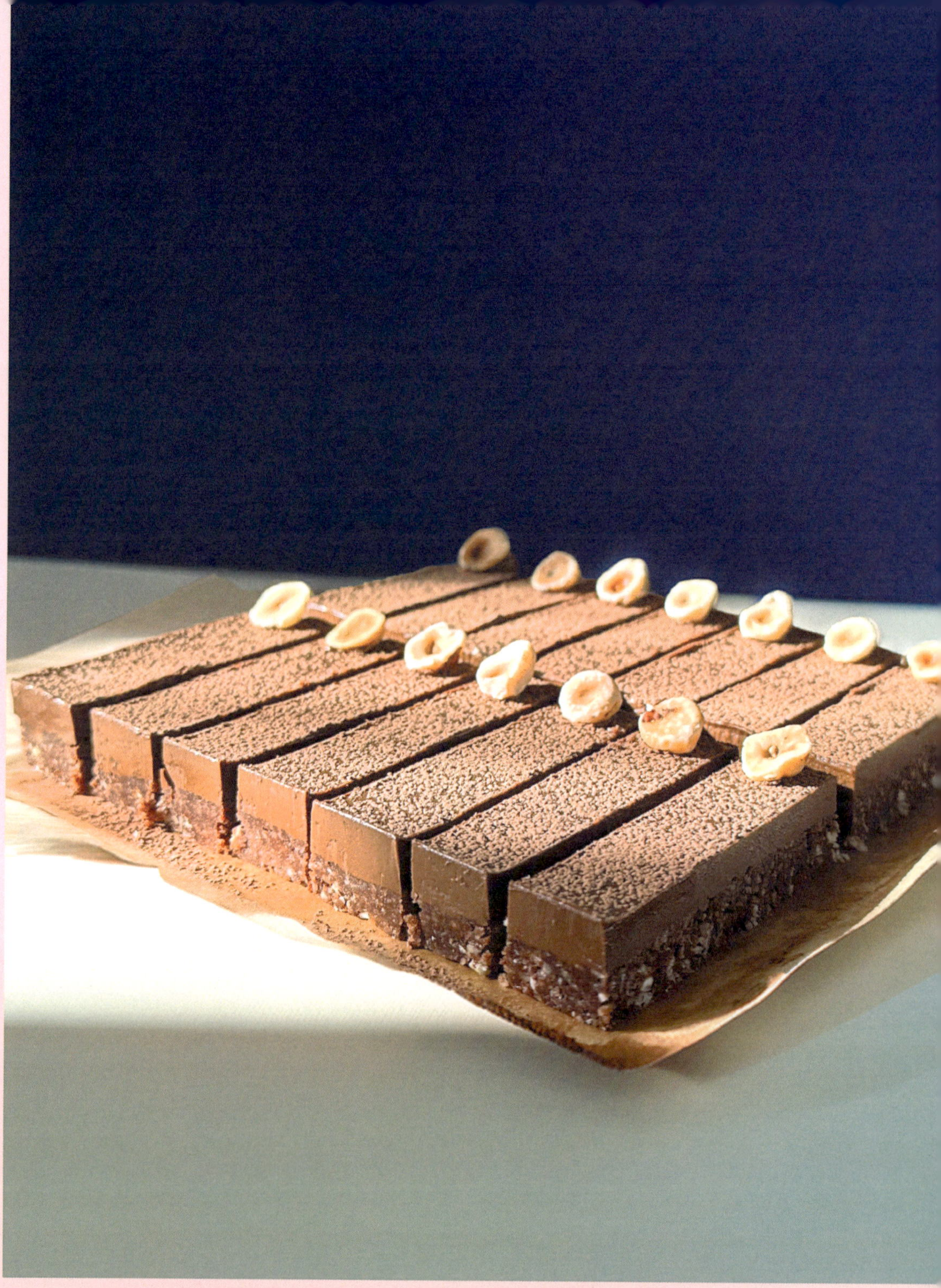

*Nothing tickles the memory buds like a childhood experience.*
*And who can forget childhood sweets like Toblerone, KitKat and Ferrero Rocher, among others, which were the answer to all our sugar cravings as a young person without us knowing. As an adult, you can now relive those childhood memories with our tempting raw sweets sprinkled with a little fairy dust and a healthy dose of nostalgia. These indulgent praline cake slices are the perfect answer to KitKats.*

**Serves: 14**

**Wafer Crust**

60 g hazelnut flour
50 g buckini
20 ml virgin coconut oil melted
15 g coconut flour
40 g powdered coconut sugar
15 ml maple syrup
35 ml coconut milk
10 g raw cacao powder
7.5 ml coconut aminos

**Praline**

70 g hazelnut butter
60 g raw chocolate
15 ml coconut oil melted
A pinch of pink Himalayan salt

**Crust**

1.Put hazelnut flour, buckini, coconut flour, coconut sugar and raw cacao in a mixing bowl, mix together.
2. Then add the water, melted coconut oil and coconut aminos.
3. Mix everything well with a spoon.
4. Knead the dough with your hands.
5. Line a 15×15 cm square baking sheet with baking paper.
6. Press the dough into the pan, flatten.

**Praline**

1. Melt the chocolate in a bain-marie: Heat water in a saucepan, a few centimeters from the bottom is enough. Chop or break the chocolate into smaller pieces and place in a heat-resistant bowl or, preferably, a bain-marie insert. Place the bowl or insert over the saucepan. The water should simmer but not boil. Let the chocolate melt slowly.
2. Once the chocolate has melted, stir in the coconut oil, salt and hazelnut butter until well combined and remove from the heat.
3. Pour the mixture over the base.
4. Freeze for 30-40 minutes. Then remove from the jar.
5. Using a sharp chef's knife, carefully cut the cake into 10 equal length slices. Serve plain or sprinkle some raw cacao nibs on top if desired.

# CHOCOLATE COVERED PUMPKIN FUDGE

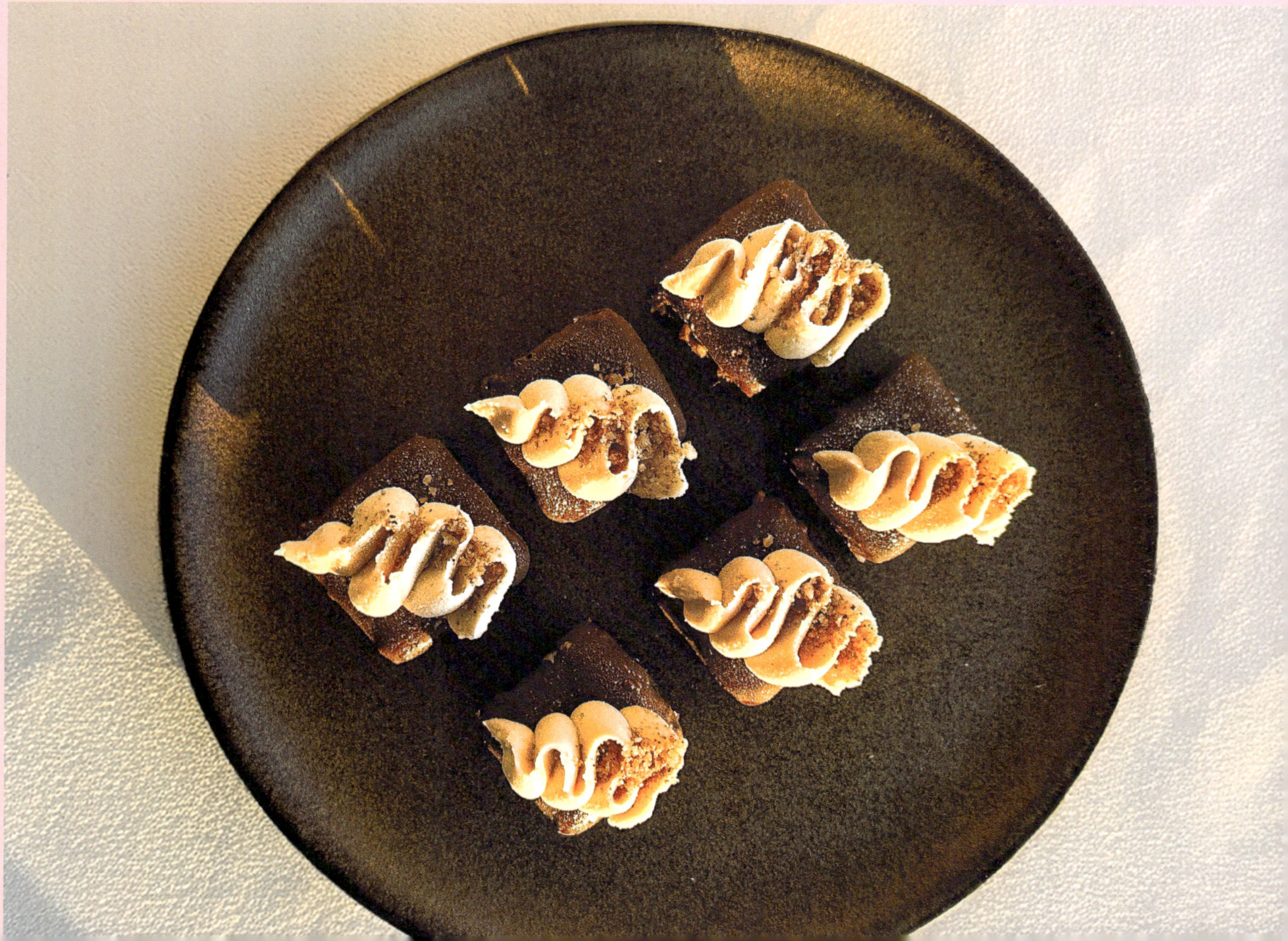

**Serves: 30**

### Ingredients

200 g shredded raw pumpkin
200 g medjool dates soaked
110 g almond flour
60 g desiccated coconut
50 g coconut sugar
45 g coconut oil melted
1 tsp chickpea miso
1 tbsp gingerbread spice
1/2 tsp pink himalayan salt

### Coating

150 g raw chocolate melted
1 tbsp coconut oil melted

### Topping

30 g walnuts roughly grinded
15 g coconut sugar
1 tsp gingerbread spice
A pinch pink himalayan salt

*This chocolate covered fudge features a creamy base of pumpkin , spicy gingerbread and rich sweetness of medjool dates along with caramel notes of coconut sugar. Make it for holiday season and enjoy with your family.*

1. Peel and thinly shred your pumpkin into a bowl. Soak medjool dates in warm water for 15 minutes, then strain and peel the skin. Pur your medjool dates into a food processor, process until puree. Then transfer to the bowl, mix together with shredded pumpkin.
2. Then add the almond flour, desiccated coconut, gingerbread spice, chickpea miso, melted coconut oil and pink himalayan salt. Combine together. Using your hands with gloves on, knead the dough until everything mixed well.
3. You will need 2 pieces 15x15 cm square cake mold or 30x30 cm 1 piece square mold for the dough. If you are going to use 15x15 cm, divide dough in two and transfer to the mold. Otherwise without dividing, just transfer to a 30x30 cm mold lined parchment paper, press down with the back of a spoon, flatten out as much as possible. Freeze for 2 hours.
4. Once the dough is firm enough, remove from the mold. Cut into small squares about 3x3 or 4x4 cm depending of your choice.
5. To make topping, place all topping ingredients in a food processor, grind at once, we want the topping a bit chunky, so not mix too much.
6. Using bain marie method, melt raw chocolate and mix with melted coconut oil. Using a dipping fork, dip each fudge into the chocolate. Make sure all parts of dough is covered. Tap to the edge of bowl to remove excess amount of chocolate.
7. Carefully transfer to a plate lined parchment paper, with a help of another fork. Sprinkle some topping on the squares.
8. Refrigerate for 20 minutes before serving. Keep in the refrigerator.

# RAW RASPBERRY TONKA CREAM SQUARES

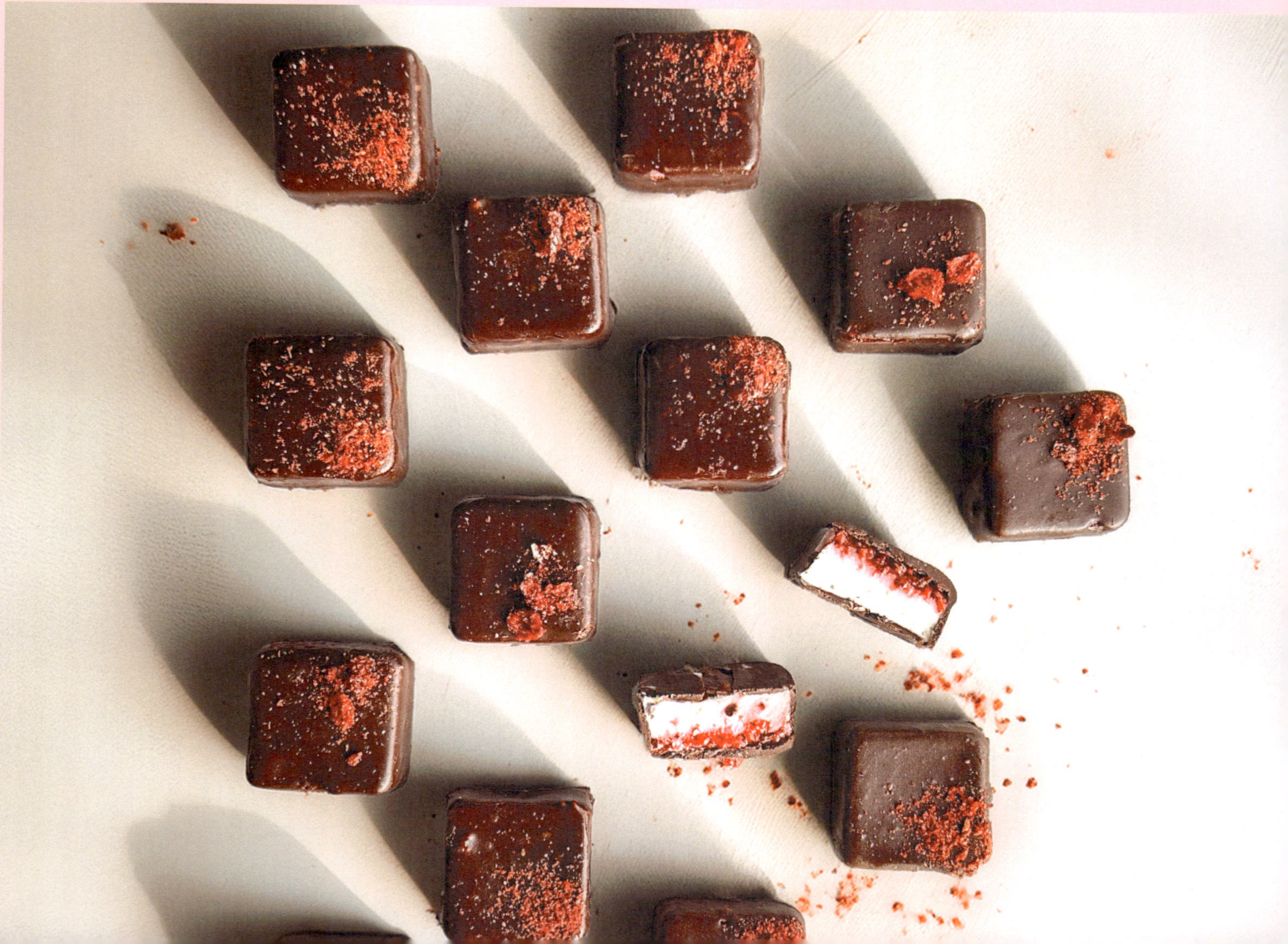

Serves: 24

**Tonka Cream**

120 g  cashews soaked
150 g coconut cream
60 g coconut oil
60 ml  maple syrup
30 ml lemon juice
1 g (5 capsules) lion's mane extract (optional)
1/2 tsp ground tonka beans
1/4 tsp pink himalayan salt

**Raspberry Jam**

200 g fresh or defrosted raspberries
7 g  chia seeds
15 ml lemon juice

**Coating**

100 g raw chocolate melted
15 g coconut oil melted
15 g smooth sesame butter (tahini)
1/4 tsp pink himalayan salt

**Raspberry Jam**

Add the raspberries and lemon juice to a saucepan and cook on medium heat for 5 minutes on until raspberries soften and begin to release their juice. Add chia and cook further 5 minutes, stirring occasionally. Turn off heat and set aside to cool. Once cooled enough, transfer jam between 24 x 3cm square silicon molds, flatten out with a back of a teaspoon. Make sure that the jam is distributed all the corners equally.

**Tonka Cream**

Soak your cashews for 4 hours, then rinse and dry, transfer to a high speed blender. Add remaining tonka cream ingredients except coconut oil  and blend until smooth. With the blender running, stream in melted (and cooled- it should be warm, not hot) coconut oil and continue to blend until completely incorporated. Use the blender tamper if necessary. Pour cream batter over the raspberry layer between 24 mini square molds. Then place in the freezer for 4-5 hours or overnight.

**Chocolate Coating**

Melt chocolate in a heat proof bowl, bain marie* method. Add the coconut oil and sesame paste and stir well until everything combined together. Once everything is melted, remove from heat.

**Assembly**

Remove the cream squares from the freezer and their moulds. Lay a small tray with parchment paper. Dip each square into the melted chocolate. Use 2 forks to do this, and allow excess chocolate to run off the dipped cup into the bowl. Place on lined tray then repeat with with all cups. Set in fridge for 1 hour, then store in an airtight container in the fridge (up to a week) or freezer (up to 1-2 months).

*Bain Marie method. This is the correct way to melt chocolate or cacao butter, and ensures you don't ruin the chocolate! Add 2-3 cm water to a saucepan and bring to the boil. Set a heat prod bowl on the top of the saucepan. The bowl should be resting on the saucepan rim and not touch the water. Keep heat on the lowest setting, melting slowly. Once melted, turn off heat and remove bowl from saucepan, setting aside.

# BALSAMIC BEET BALLS

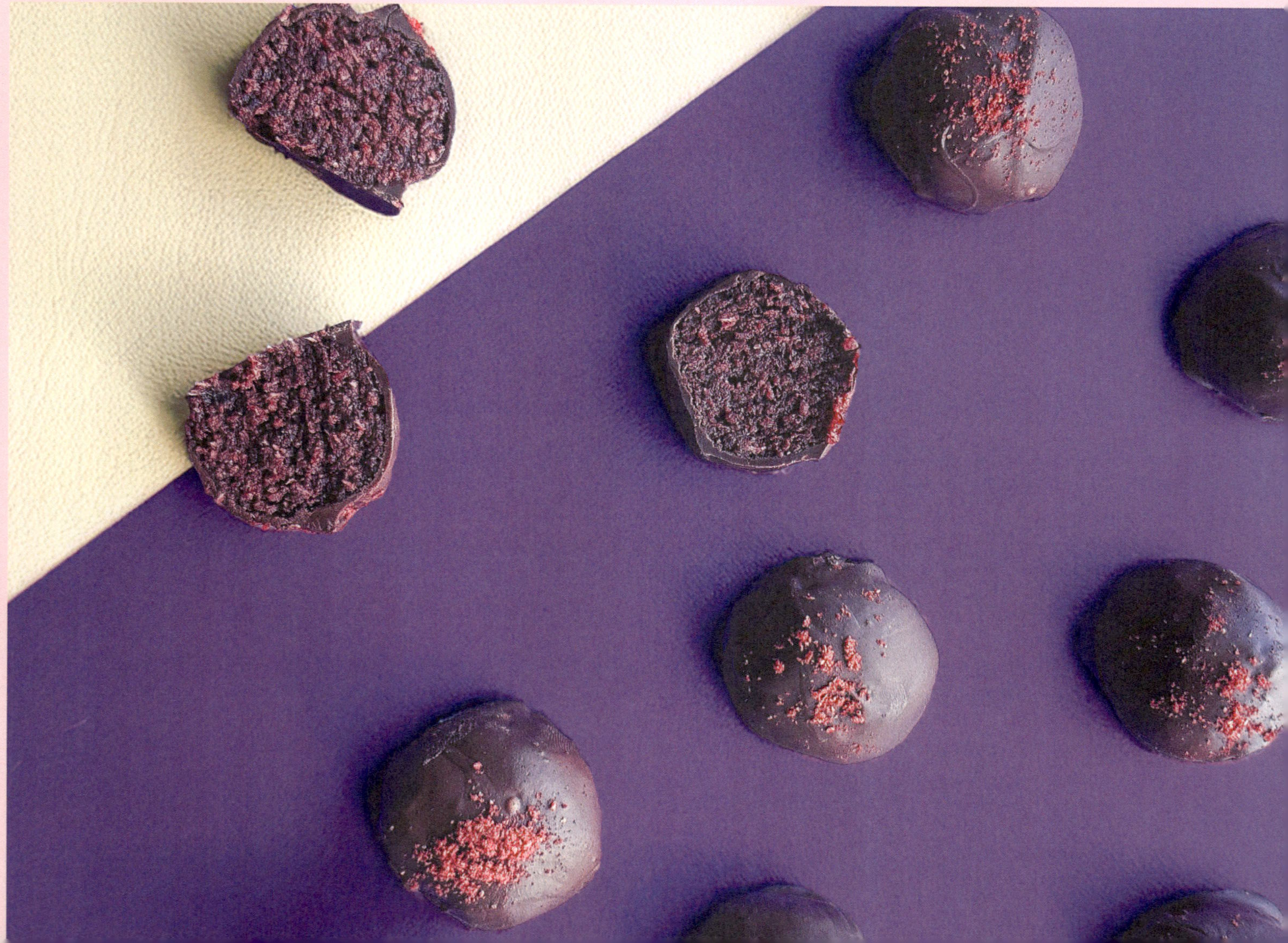

**Serves: 15 balls**

**Ingredients**

120 g dried raisins or dates soaked
100 g raw chopped beetroot
40 ml balsamic vinegar
20 g raw cacao powder
55 g desiccated coconut
90 g almond flour
20 g coconut oil melted
1/2 tsp pink himalayan salt

**For Dipping**

150 g melted raw chocolate
Freeze dried lingonberry or raspberry powder

*One of our most loved creations from our new raw vegan collection. The balsamic vinegar adds a nice tangy dimension to sweet beets, and creates a complementary flavor with chocolate.*

1. Place balsamic and beets in a food processor. Blend together until beet is chopped into very small pieces (rice-like).
2. Then add soaked raisins and continue to blend until you get a smooth paste.
3. Add the cacao powder, desiccated coconut, almond flour, salt and melted coconut oil. Blend together.
4. Transfer dough to a bowl, sit in the freezer for 30 minutes.
5. Once time is up, and the dough is thickened enough, roll the dough into small balls in desired size with your hands. Freeze for 10-15 minutes while you are melting the chocolate.
6. Melt the raw chocolate using bain marie, let it cool at room temperature for 10 minutes.
7. Remove the balls from the freezer. Dip each one in melted chocolate. Let it cool on a parchment paper.
8. Roll in edible gold powder and fd raspberry powder, or desiccated coconut according to your choice.
9. Place in the refrigerator for 15-20 minutes before serving.

# DAMMSUGARE INTENSO

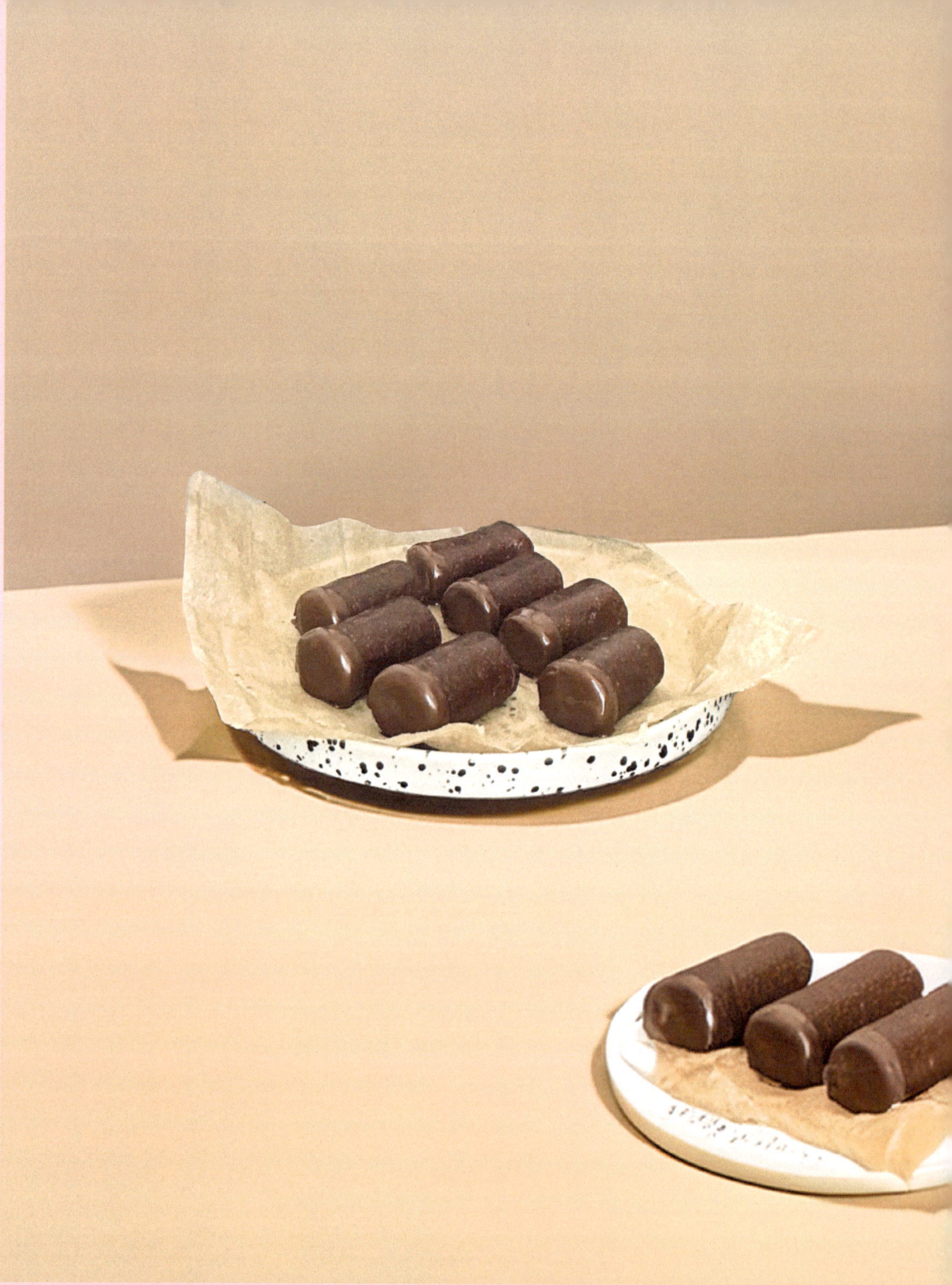

*Dammsugare Intenso is a bold reinvention of the Swedish classic. Instead of the traditional green marzipan, this version is wrapped in dark chocolate marzipan, giving it a deep, luxurious richness. Inside, the filling surprises with a touch of seaweed, adding layers of natural umami that balance the sweet, nutty, and chocolatey notes. The result is an elegant, modern pastry—familiar in shape yet unexpected in flavor—where Nordic tradition meets daring innovation.*

**Serves: 14**

**Chocolate Marzipan**

15g raw cacao powder
100g almond flour
100ml maple syrup or coconut nectar
35g coconut flour
A pinch of pink Himalayan salt

**Chocolate Punsch Dough**

100g almond flour
130g soft medjool dates (weight after pitting)
35 g desiccated coconut
30 g raw cacao powder
20ml virgin coconut oil melted
1/2 tsp sugar kelp flakes

**Chocolate Dipping**

160 g chocolate
20 g coconut oil melted

**Chocolate Marzipan**

1. Put the raw cacao powder and maple in a bowl, stir together. Then add the coconut flour, salt and almond flour, mix together and knead well until you get a very firm dough with a marzipan texture.
2. When the marzipan is ready, move it to a baking sheet and fold another baking sheet on top, roll the dough flat with a rolling pin and let it rest on the baking sheet in the fridge while you make the punch dough.

**Chocolate Punsch Dough**

1. Mix all the ingredients for the punch dough in a food processor and mix until you have a dough with the same consistency as raw balls.
2. Make three long rolls of the punch dough and place one on top of the marzipan and fold it in.
3. Then cut and roll until smooth. Repeat the process for the rest. Store in the freezer for 15-20 minutes before cutting to get a smooth nice shape.

**Assembly**

1. Using a rolling pin, cut 3-inch long punch rolls and set aside while you melt the chocolate.
2. Melt the chocolate with the coconut oil over a Bain Marie. Dip one side of the punch roll at a time, onto the baking paper and set aside in the refrigerator for about 10-15 minutes to set.
3. Then dip another side of the punch roll. Refrigerate again for at least 15-20 minutes before serving.

# DAMMSUGARE GOLD

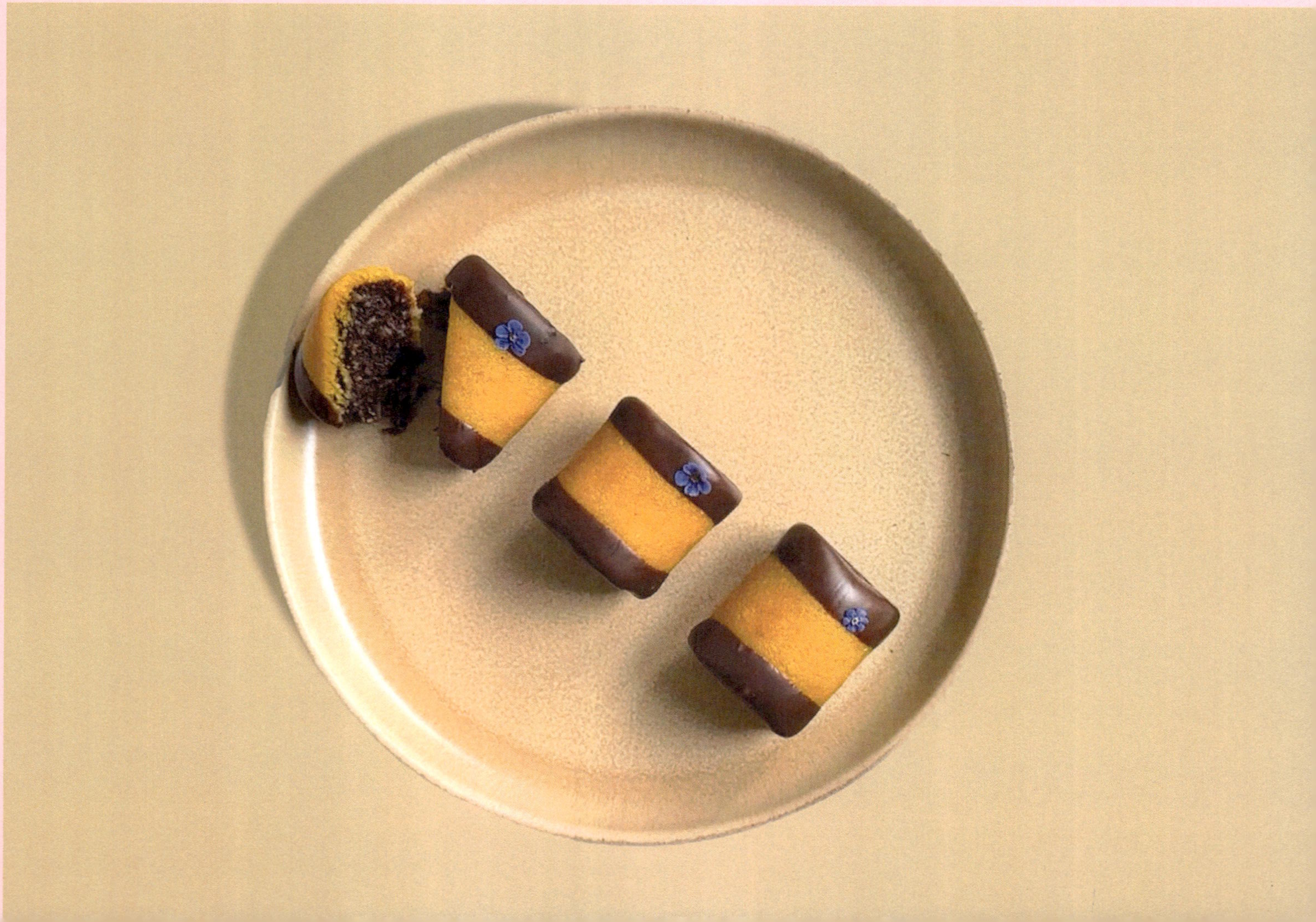

*A vibrant twist on the beloved Swedish dammsugare, this raw version shines with a zesty lemon filling wrapped in golden-yellow marzipan, naturally colored with turmeric. The brightness of citrus cuts through the sweetness, while the soft marzipan adds a delicate almond richness.*

**Serves: 14**

**Marzipan Dough**

1 tbsp turmeric powder
100 g almond flour
100 ml maple syrup or coconut nectar
35 g coconut flour
5-6 drops lemon essential oil
A pinch of pink Himalayan salt

**Chocolate Punsch Dough**

100g almond flour
130g soft medjool dates (weight after pitting)
35g desiccated coconut
30g raw cacao powder
20ml coconut oil melted
6ml arrack extract
1/4 tsp pink Himalayan salt

**Chocolate Dipping**

160 g chocolate
20 g coconut oil melted
Forget-me-not flower

**Marzipan Dough**

1. Put the turmeric powder and maple in a bowl, stir together. Then add the coconut flour, salt and almond flour and lemon oil, mix together and knead well until you get a very firm dough with a marzipan texture.
2. When the marzipan is ready, move it to a baking sheet and fold another baking sheet on top, roll the dough flat with a rolling pin and let it rest on the baking sheet in the fridge while you make the punch dough.

**Chocolate Punsch Dough**

1. Mix all the ingredients for the punch dough in a food processor and mix until you have a dough with the same consistency as raw balls.
2. Make three long rolls of the punch dough and place one on top of the marzipan and fold it in. Then cut and roll until smooth.
3. Repeat the process for the rest. Store in the freezer for 15-20 minutes before cutting to get a smooth nice shape.

**Assembly**

1. Using a rolling pin, cut 3 inch long punch rolls and set aside while you melt the chocolate.
2. Melt the chocolate together with the coconut oil over a Bain Marie.
3. Dip one side of the punch roll at a time, onto the baking paper and set aside in the fridge for about 10-15 minutes to set.
4. Then dip another side of the punch roll.
5. Decorate with Forget-me-not flowers. Refrigerate again for at least 15-20 minutes before serving.

# CINNAMON BUNS

## WITH CHOCOLATE, HAZELNUT & JERUSALEM ARTICKHOKE

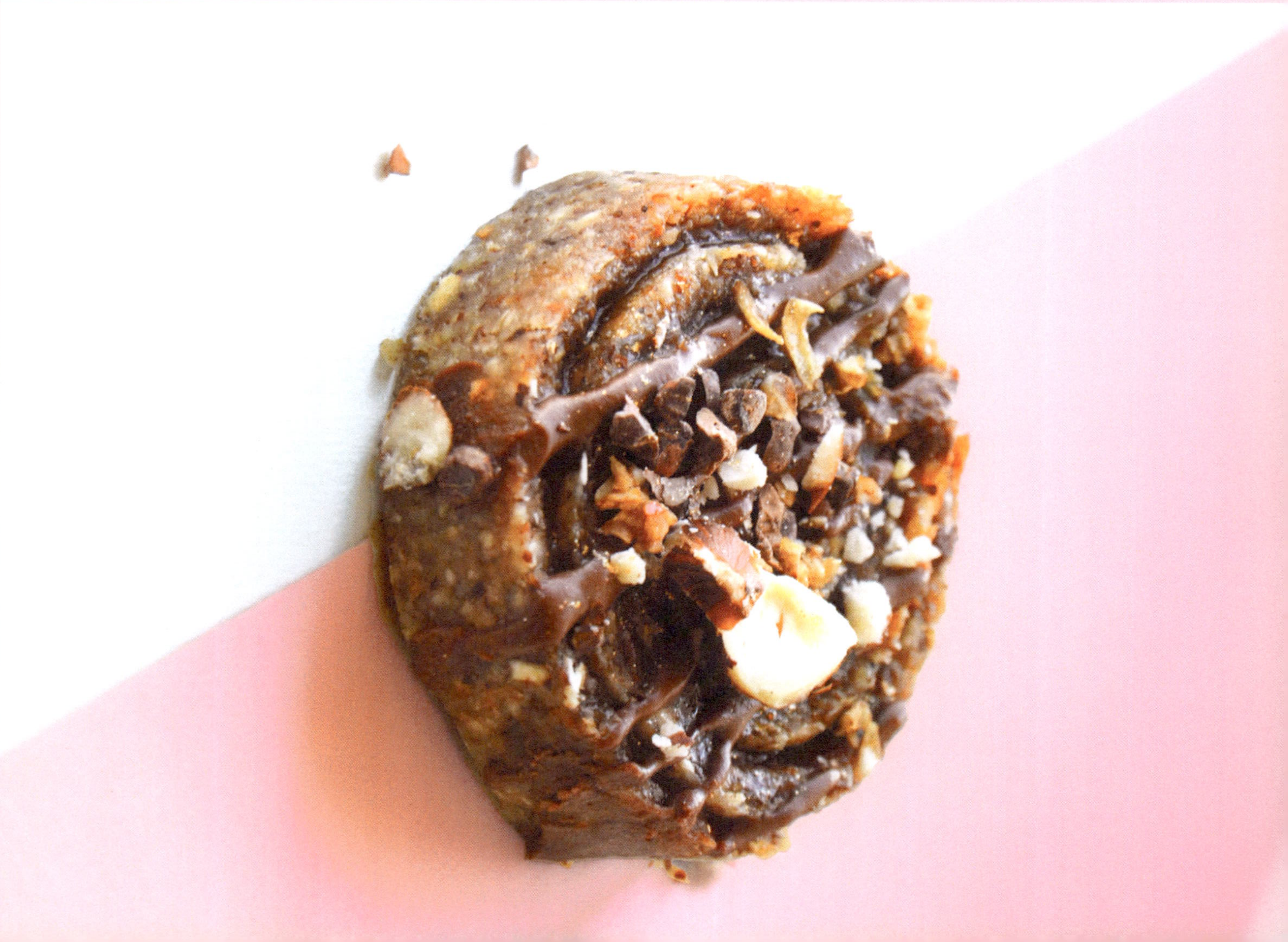

**Serves: 6-7**

**Cinnamon Bun Dough**

90 g hazelnut flour
55 g oat flour
100 g raisins
30 ml hazelnut milk
15 ml maple syrup
15 ml coconut oil
4 g ground cardamom
3 g vanilla bean powder
A pinch of pink Himalayan salt

**Filling**

1 tsp cinnamon
25 ml virgin coconut oil
15 ml maple syrup
30 g coconut sugar +10 ml water
A pinch of licorice or pink Himalayan salt

**Chocolate Sauce**

30 g coconut oil melted
25 g cup raw cacap powder
25 g powdered coconut sugar
1/2 tsp truffle mushroom powder
45ml filtered water
A pinch of salt

**Jerusalem Artichoke Topping**

1 large Jerusalem artichoke
1/2 tsp chickpea or yellow pea miso
1 tsp coconut sugar
1 tbsp olive oil

**For decorating**

Chopped hazelnuts
Jerusalem artichoke
Raw cacao nibs

**Cinnamon Bun Dough**

1. Put the flour and the rest of the other ingredients in a food processor and mix to a dough that holds together.
2. Roll the dough between two sheets of baking paper into a rectangle and place in the refrigerator to cool for about 15 minutes.

**Filling**

Place all ingredients in a small bowl and whisk well until smooth.

**Chocolate Sauce**

1. Melt the coconut oil using the bain-marie method. Transfer to a Blendtec Twister Jar or high-speed blendear. Add the remaining ingredients over the coconut oil. Mix well. Make sure the coconut sugar is incorporated enough to remove any graininess. Process until emulsified and thickened.
2. Pour into a squeeze bottle to use immediately. Otherwise, store in the refrigerator. Let it come to room temperature before using.

**Jerusalem Artichoke Topping**

1. Brush your Jerusalem artichokes, place them in a food processor and blend until they are rice-like. Mix 1/2 tsp miso, 1 tsp coconut sugar, 1 tbsp olive oil and 2 tbsp water in a small bowl. Mix.
2. Pour over the grated Jerusalem artichokes. Mix well until they are coated.
3. Place on baking paper and let dry for several hours until completely dry. Can also be baked in the oven at 60 degrees.

**Assembly**

1. Spread the cinnamon paste thinly on the bun dough.
2. Chill for at least 30 minutes or place in the freezer for 10-15 minutes.
3. Then cut strips about 1 cm wide with a sharp chef's knife. Roll each strip up like a bun.
4. Sprinkle cocoa nibs, Jerusalem artichoke and hazelnuts on top of the bun. Drizzle a little chocolate sauce over the buns. (If dehydrating, use after the dehydration process, if refrigerating, use before putting them in the fridge)

Alternative 1: Place the buns in the dehydrator at 42°C for 4 hours.
Alternative 2: Skip baking and place them in the fridge for an hour or so before serving.

# RASPBERRY LICORICE CAKE

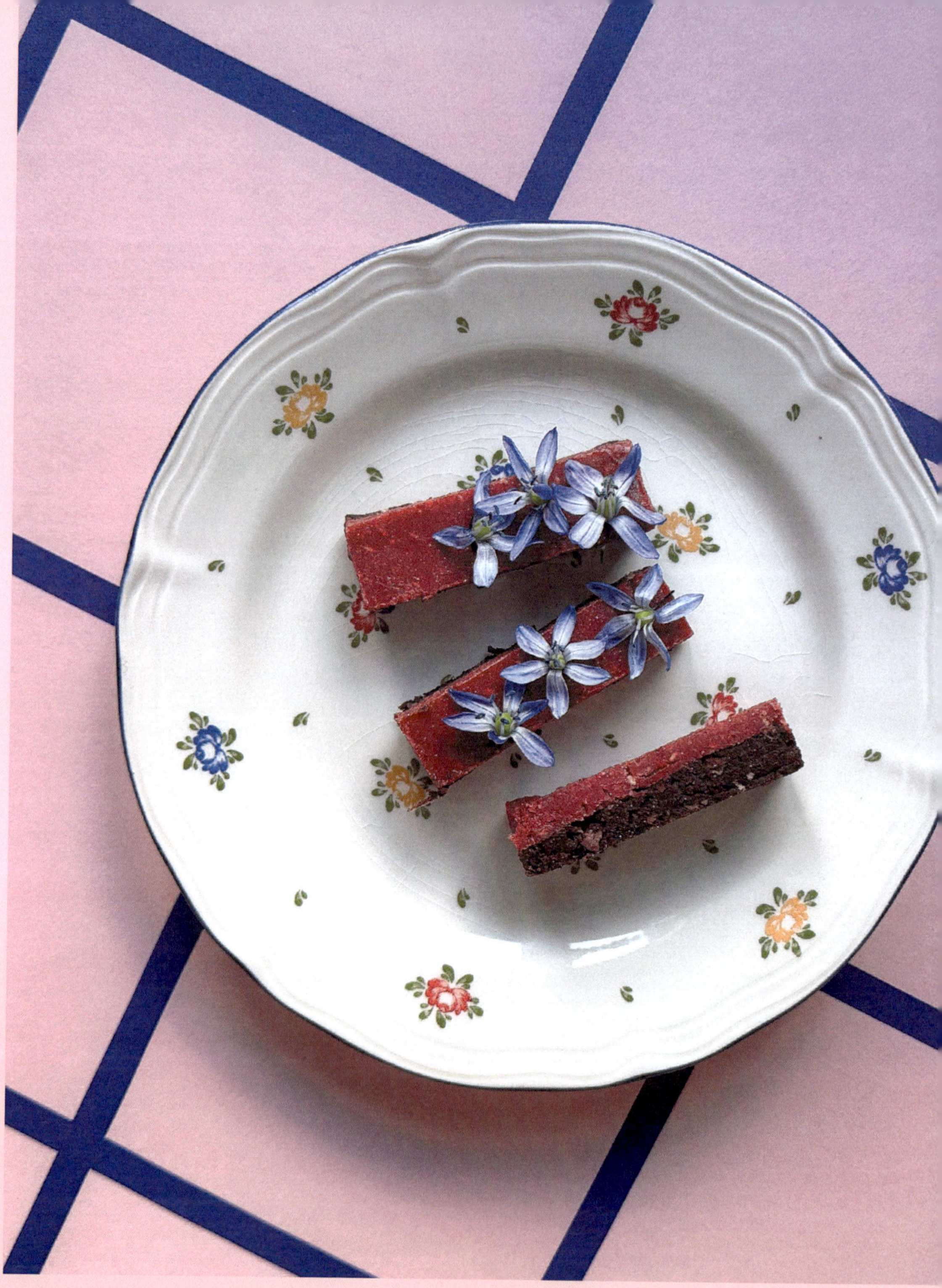

**Serves: 9**

**Licorice Crust**

140g soft dates soaked
1dl almond flour (45g)
20ml agave
15g cacao powder
15g cacao nibs (optional)
30ml cacao butter
1.5-2 tsp licorice powder
1/2 tsp vanilla extract
1/4 tsp salt

**Raspberry Filling**

20g freeze-dried raspberries, ground into powder
65g cashew butter or white almond butter
55g cacao butter, melted
15g coconut oil, melted
50ml agave
1/2 tsp vanilla extract
A pinch of salt

*Instead of sweets that consist of only empty calories, this cake is made from ingredients with a lot of nutrition in the form of vitamins and minerals, as well as good fats that strengthen the body. You can make it for Licorice Day or whenever you want when you want something sweet. It is best made a few days before it is to be eaten, the flavors will only be even better if it is left in the freezer for a few days.*

**Licorice Crust**

1. In a food processor, blend dates and agave together, then add the rest of the ingredients except for the cacao nibs. Mix until a dough forms. Finally, add the cacao nibs and mix together.
2. Place the dough in a square pan lined with parchment paper. Flatten it out with a spatula.
Dip the spatula in melted coconut oil to make the process easier.
3. Store in the freezer while you make the raspberry layer.

**Raspberry Filling**

1. Grind the freeze-dried raspberries into a powder in a high-speed blender.
2. Add the rest of the ingredients and blend until well combined.

**Assembly**

1. Pour the raspberry mixture over the base.
2. Freeze for 30 minutes or until it is the right thickness.
3. Then cut into long strips of squares according to your choice.
4. Decorate with flowers or freeze-dried raspberries.

# CHOCOLATE TRUFFLES

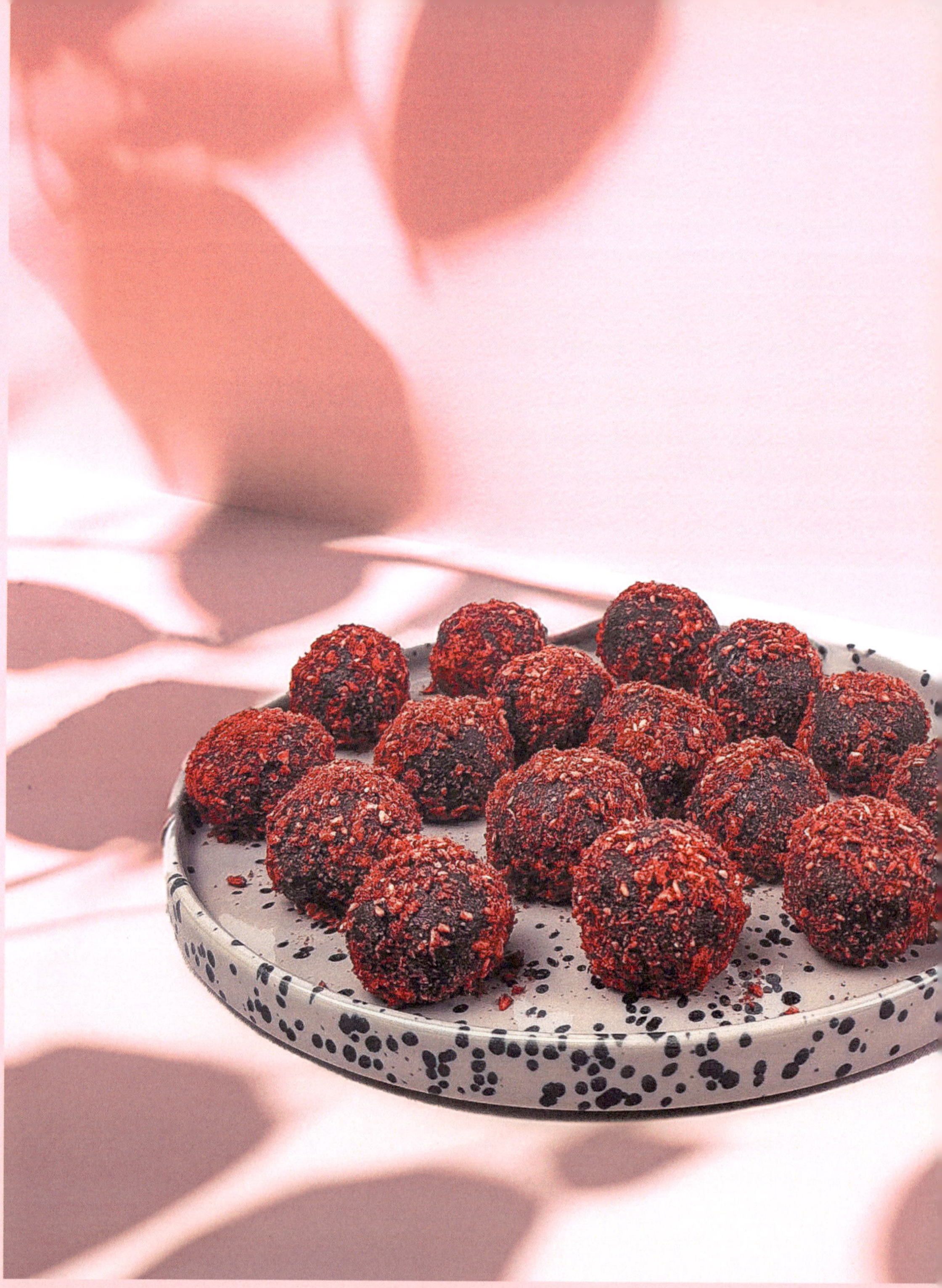

**Serves: 16**

*A classic confection but with natural ingredients and even more delicious. Smooth, creamy and rich, but just the right size.*

**Ingredients**

16 soft medjool dates
2 tbsp raw cacao powder
2 tbsp maple syrup
3 tbsp cacao butter melted
1/2 tsp sugar kelp powder
1 tsp vanilla bean powder
A pinch of pink himalayan salt

**Toppings**

1 cup freeze dried berry powder
1/4 tsp vanilla bean powder

1. Soak your dates for 15 minutes then strain and place in a food processor. Blend until soft and pureed.
2. Add the rest of the ingredients to the mixture, blend again until combined.
3. Mix the vanilla and cacao in a bowl.
4. Make small bowls and roll in the vanilla freeze dried berry mixture.

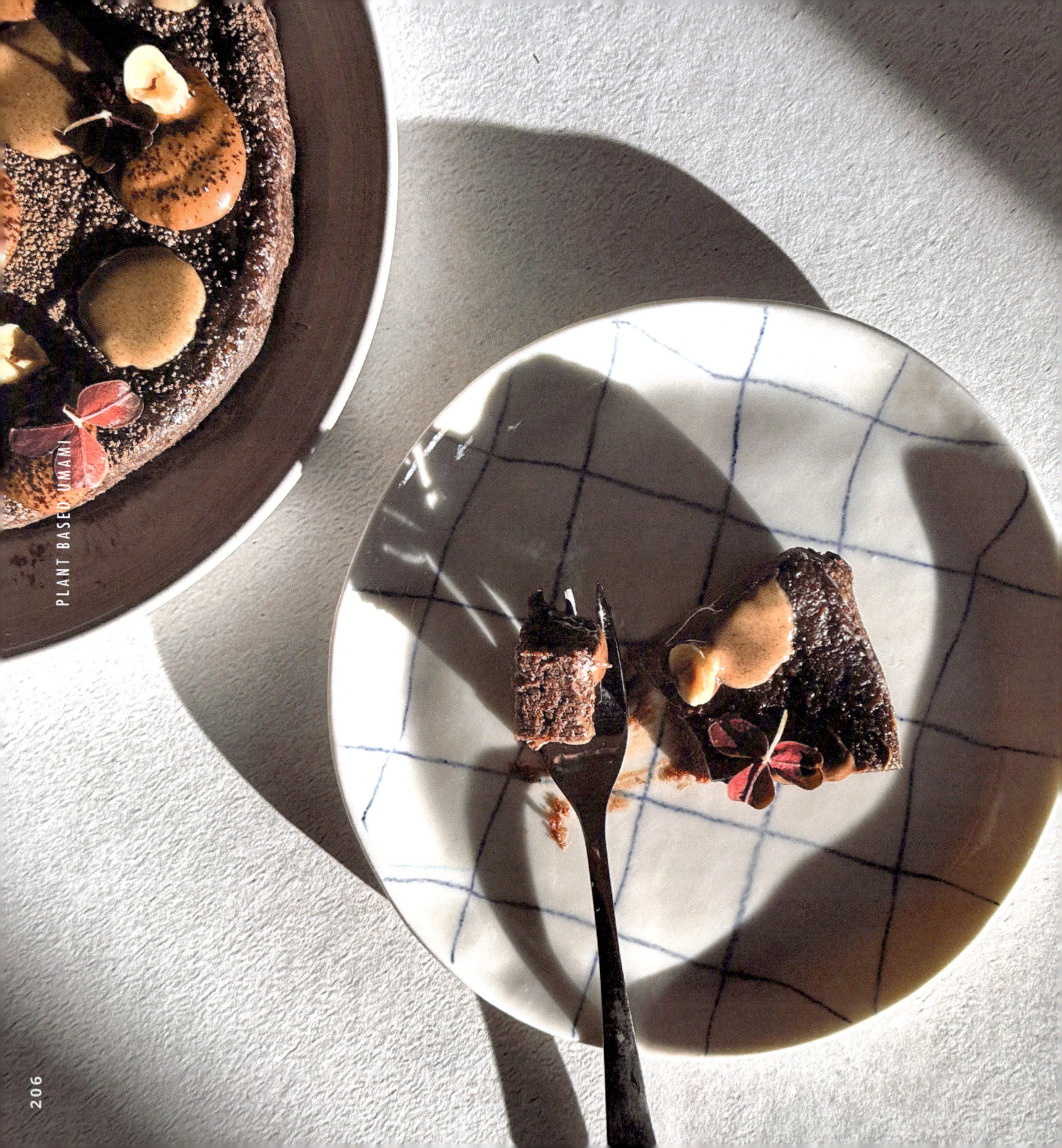

# GLUTEN-FREE BAKES

# CHOCOLATE CAKE WITH RASPBERRY

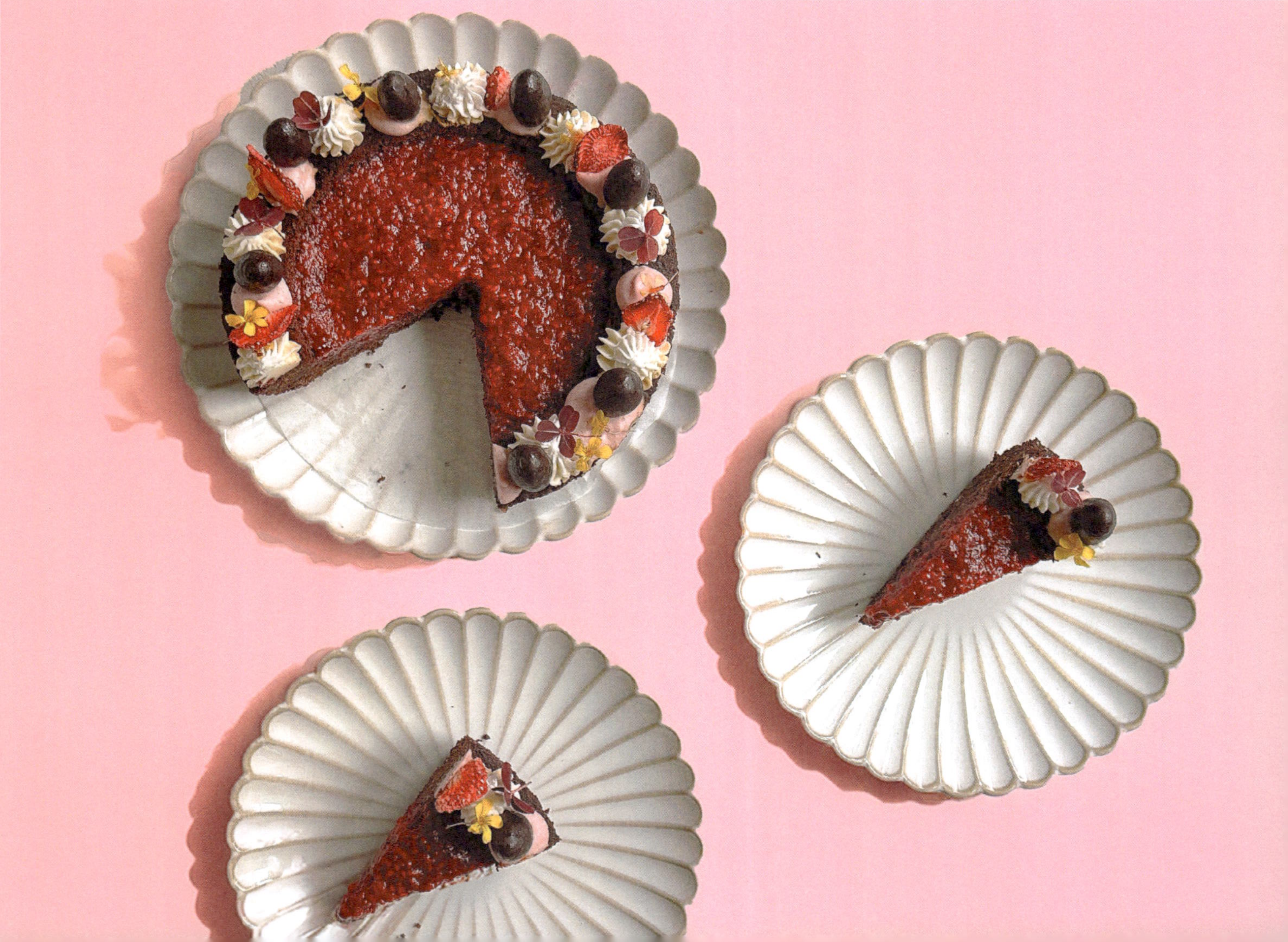

*Hop into Easter with this vegan, gluten-free chocolate cake Rich, fudgy, and chocolatey, topped with silky coconut cream and fresh raspberries for a burst of fruity brightness.*

**Serves: 2 x 16 cm**

**Wet Ingredients:**

100 g mashed banana
100 g applesauce
350 ml coconut milk
2 tsp vanilla extract
40 g cashew butter
165 ml maple syrup

**Dry Ingredients:**

140 g almond flour
140 g gf oat flour
90 g coconut sugar
76 g cocoa powder
4 g dark roasted ground coffee
75 g tapioca starch
50 g cassava flour
1 tbsp baking powder
1/2 tsp salt

**Filling**

400g raspberry or strawberry jam

**Strawberry Vanilla Frosting**

130 ml coconut cream
15 g erythritol or monkfruit powder
1/2 tsp vanilla extract
15 g freeze-dried strawberries

**Coconut Vanilla Filling**

200 ml coconut cream
30 g erythritol
1/2 tsp vanilla powder

**For Serving**

Red oxalis both flowers and leaves
Freeze-dried sliced strawberries
Chocolate-coated almonds

1. Preheat oven to 180C.
2. Mix wet ingredients in a large bowl until well combined.
3. Then add dry ingredients to wet ingredients and stir until well combined.
4. Pour into two cake tins. Bake in the oven for 30-35 minutes, or until a toothpick inserted into the centre of the cake comes out clean.
Allow the cake to cool completely before removing from the tin.
5. Cool for 5 minutes, then remove from pan. Allow to cool completely before moving on to the next step.
6. Using a 10cm round cookie cutter, slightly cut the centre of the cake. Do not cut through the entire base. There should still be some of the base left. Just remove the top. Use a tablespoon to cut out the centre of the cake.
7. Fill the cut centre with the jam.
8. Place the ingredients for the strawberry frosting in a blender, blend until fluffy. Freeze for at least 2-3 hours until firm enough.
Then transfer to a piping bag with a round nozzle. Decorate the edges of the cake by leaving a little space between them.
9. Place the ingredients for the coconut frosting in a blender bowl, mix together until the mixture is light and fluffy. Freeze for 2-3 hours. Then transfer
to a piping bag with a star nozzle. Drizzle a little cream between the strawberry cream.
10. Add freeze-dried strawberry slices and chocolate-covered almonds.
11. Garnish with oxalis.
Repeat the process for the second cake. You can also make it a two-layer cake if you wish.

# KLADDKAKA

## SWEDISH STICKY CAKE

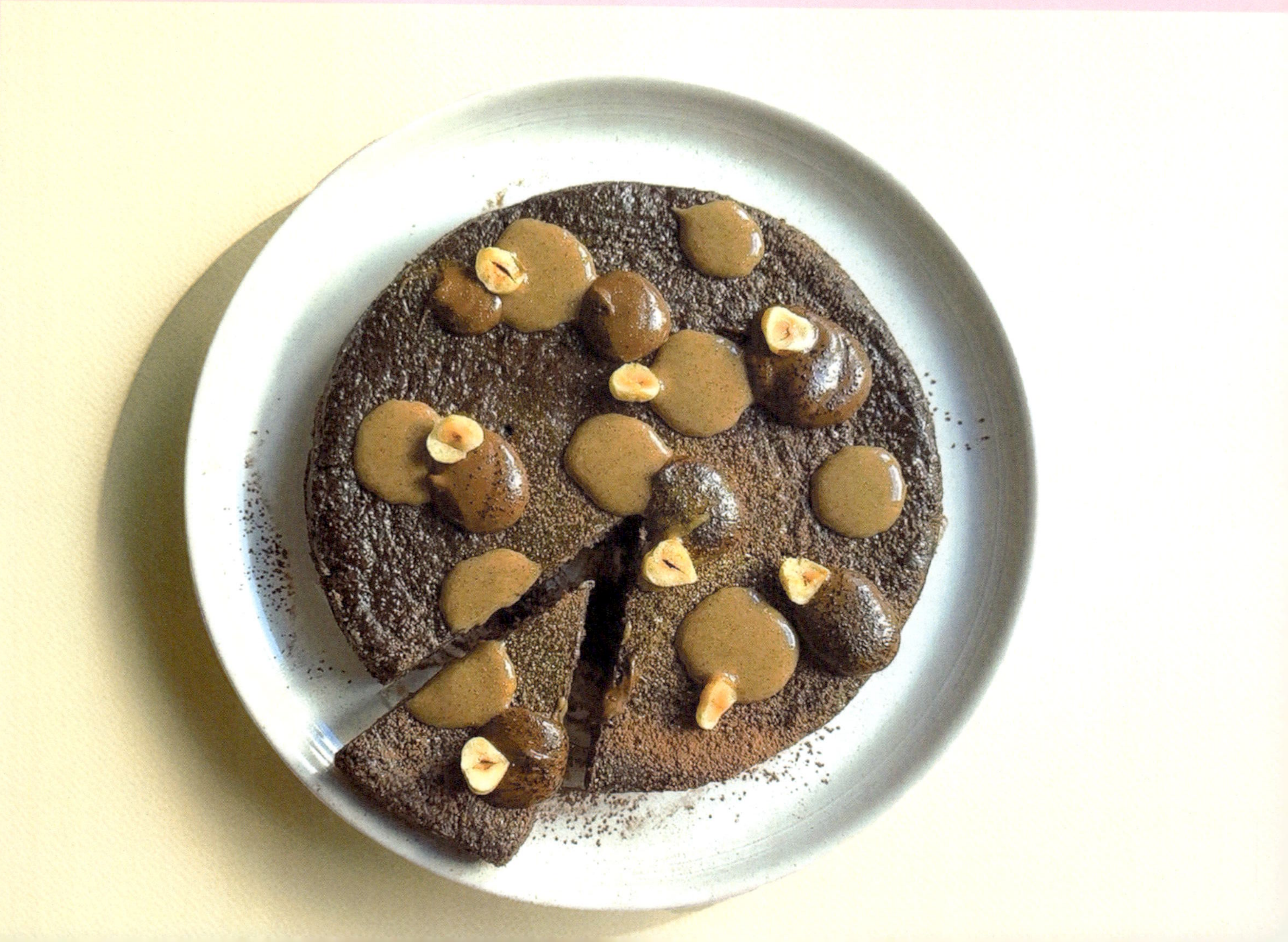

*This vegan kladdkaka is the ultimate rich, fudgy chocolate cake—dense, gooey, and irresistibly indulgent. Made without dairy or eggs, it relies on plant-based ingredients to create a deep chocolate flavor and perfectly sticky texture that melts in your mouth. Slightly crisp on the edges and decadently soft in the center, it's a simple yet show-stopping dessert for any occasion*

**Serves: 6**

**Ingredients**

90 g vegan butter (coconut, shea)
92 g 70% dark chocolate
2 tbsp ground flaxseed + 6 tbsp water
75 g coconut sugar
55 g almond flour

**Toppings**

Vegan hazelnut chocolate spread
Roasted hazelnut butter
Half-halved hazelnuts

1. Heat the butter in a bain-marie, pour into a bowl.
2. Melt the chocolate over a bain-marie and when it is very hot, pour it over the butter. Mix together.
3. Grind the flaxseeds, mix with water. Let it sit for 5 minutes. Then transfer to the bowl. Mix with the butter and chocolate mixture.
4. Add the coconut sugar to the mixture, whisk well until the sugar is well dissolved.
5. Add the almond flour, without mixing air into the mixture.
6. Pour into a round silicone mold or a 16 cm diameter cake mold. Cook for 25 minutes at 130 °C.
7. Let it cool for 30 minutes at room temperature. Then move to the refrigerator for 2 hours before cutting the cake. It can also be served warm.
8. Pour hazelnut chocolate spread into a piping bag, squeeze some drops onto the cake. Repeat the process for hazelnut butter.
9. Decorate with halved hazelnuts. Enjoy!

# CHESTNUT MUFFINS

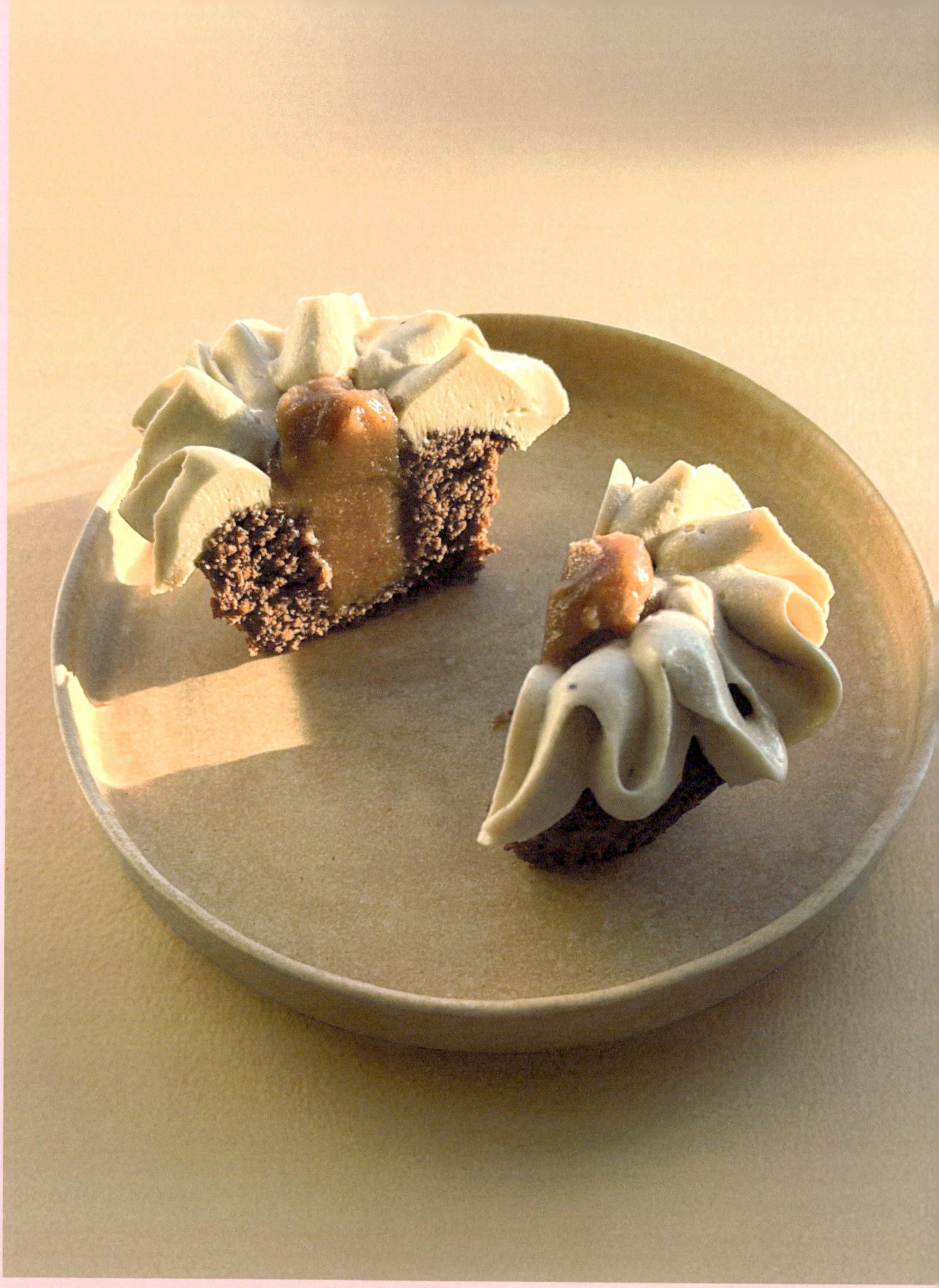

**Serves: 2**

**Ingedients**

100 ml almond milk
30 ml olive oil
15 ml lemon juice
100 g oat flour
50 g almond flour
70 g coconut sugar
20 g cacao powder
1 tsp baking powder
A pinch of salt

**Chesnut Marmalade**

500 g chesnuts
250 g coconut sugar
200 ml water
1 tbsp coconut aminos
1 tsp vanilla powder

**Frosting**

100 g cashews soaked
120 ml coconut milk
60 ml coconut nectar syrup
60 ml coconut oil melted
15 ml lemon juice
0.25 g (1/4 of a bean) tonka beans
1/4 tsp pink himalayan salt

**Chestnut Marmalade**

1.To make chestnut jam, Peel the chestnuts and roughly chop them. Boil in water for 15 minutes until soft.
2. Cut it into small pieces. Mix coconut sugar, vanilla, coconut aminos for increase the umami flavour of chestnuts and chestnuts in 200 ml of water in which the chestnuts were cooked. Mix and boil.
3. Cook at a high temperature until the jam becomes spreadable. Pour the hot jam into sterilized jars. We do this by heating the oven to 100 C and placing the washed ones in it for 15 minutes.
4. After marinating, close the jars immediately and let them cool down at room temperature. The shelf life of the jam is approx. half a year.

**Muffins**

1.To make muffins, reheat the oven to 180 °C and brush with oil 8 small muffin molds.
2. Process all dry ingredients in a food processor or bowl.
3. Add the wet ingredients and blend again until combined.
4. Pour the mixture into the ramekin and place the chocolate into the center.
5. Bake in the oven for about 20-22 minutes. If you use small molds, the baking time will be approximately 15-18 minutes.
6. Let cool for about 10 minutes before removing it from the mold.
Using an apple corer, open small holes in the middle of muffins.
7. Transfer chestnut marmalade in a piping bag, fill the holes with the marmelade.

**To make frosting**, place all ingredients expect coconut oil in a blender, mix together and silky smooth. Then add melted coconut and process again. Place mixture in a container and freeze at least 2-3 hours. Once cooled enough, transfer to a piping bag with Wilton 125 noozle, decorate the cupcakes by drawing a circle with the cream. Keep in the refrigerator before serving.

# PASSIONFRUIT POSSET

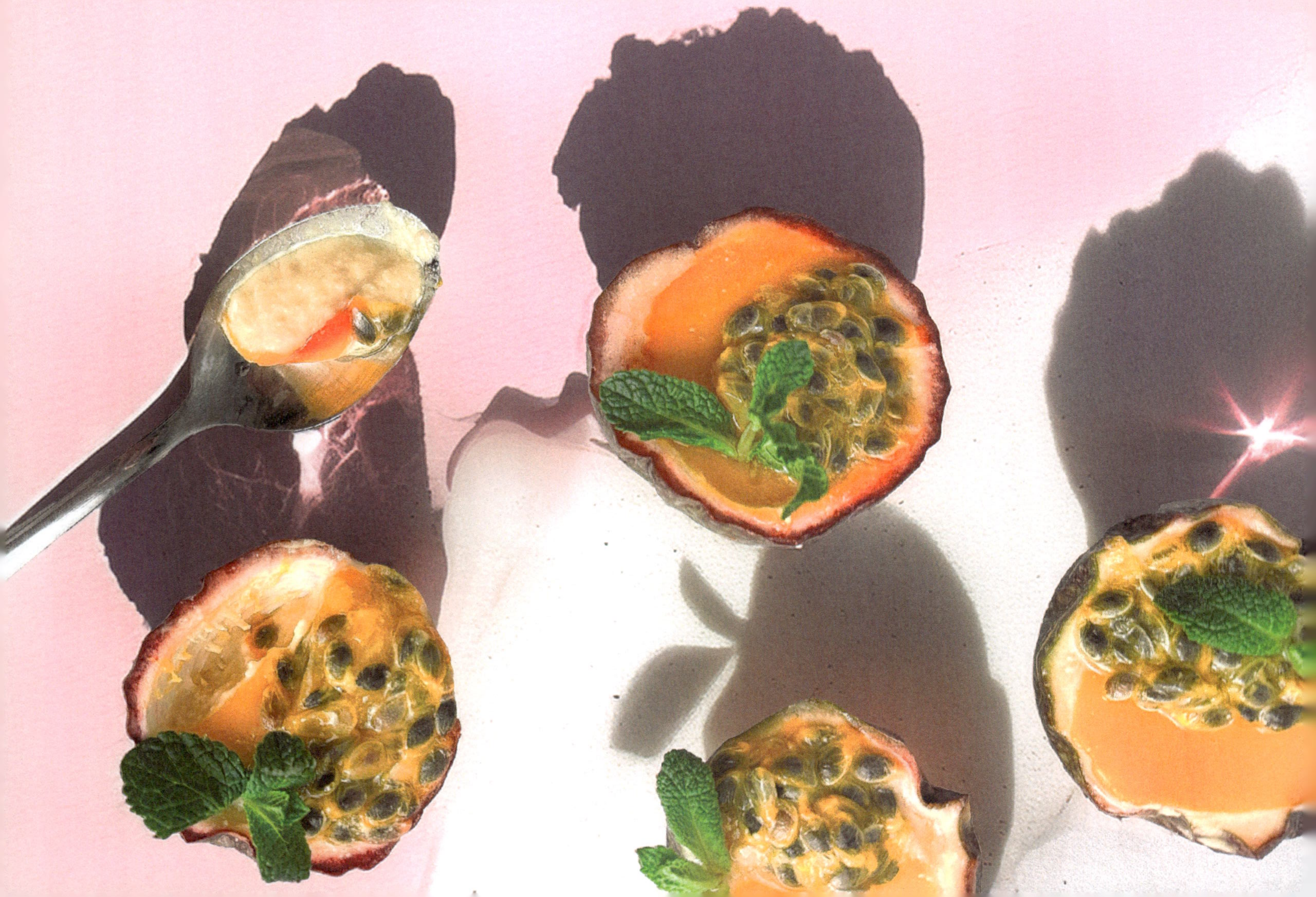

**Serves: 10-12**

**Ingredients**

300 ml coconut cream
60 ml coconut milk
2 g agar agar powder
1 tsp vanilla extract
3 tbsp maple syrup
1/2 lime juice (20 ml)
5-6 passion fruits (40 ml)
1/8 tsp salt
Fresh mint and pansies

*If you haven't discovered the greatness of passion fruit posset yet, now is the time to do so. This passion fruit posset is simple, sweet and tart, every creamy bite like a vacation on the sunny beach!*

1. Cut each passion fruit in half and spoon out the seeds and juice into a fine-mesh sieve over a bowl.
2. Run the back of a spoon over the seeds to press out the juice, you should end up with about 4 tablespoons of juice.
3. Place the remaining seeds in a small bowl, cover and refrigerate.
4. Place the empty passion fruit shells on a plate.
5. Place the coconut cream, coconut milk and agar agar in a small saucepan. Add the maple syrup and bring to a boil.
6. Bring to a boil for about a minute. Continue to simmer, whisking occasionally, for about 2-3 minutes.
7. Remove from heat, whisk in the passion fruit juice, vanilla extract, lime juice and salt.
8. Transfer the mixture to a dressing bottle or use a spoon to divide the mixture between the passion fruit shells.
9. Refrigerate for at least 4 hours or freeze for 30 minutes for a quick fix.
10. Place a spoonful of reserved passion fruit seeds on top of each posset.
11. Top with fresh mint leaves and pansies.

# TAU HU LA DUA

## VIETNAMESE PANDAN PUDDING

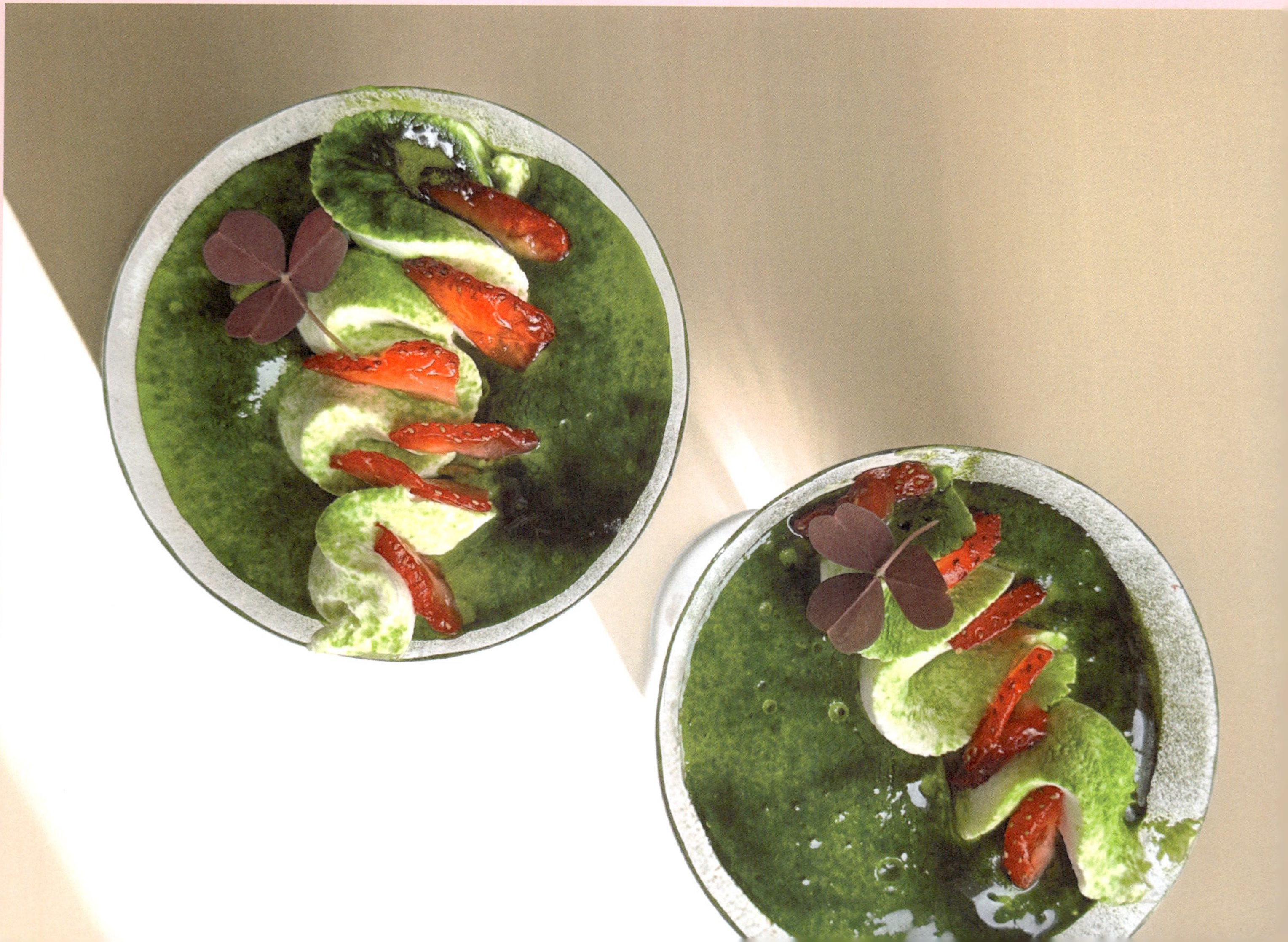

**Serves: 2-3**

**Ingredients**

300g silken oat tofu or vegan cream cheese
30g pandan extract powder
75g maple syrup
85g coconut cream

**For Serving**

Sliced strawberries
2-3 tbsp maple syrup
200 ml coconut cream

*A light, elegant Vietnamese dessert with strawberries, maple syrup and coconut – perfect for hot summer days. Not only does the pandan give the pudding a delicate green hue, but it also has that signature pandan aroma that feels like banana and vanilla that I absolutely love. Whether you have friends over or just want something refreshing after dinner, this is something you should try.*

1. Place all ingredients in a blender. Blend until smooth.
2. Divide the mixture into 3 glasses or bowls.
3. Let cool for 2 hours.
4. Then pour the coconut cream into a piping bag and decorate the pudding glasses.
5. Dust a little extra pandan powder over the cream.
6. Decorate with thinly sliced strawberries and oxalis.

Note: It should be in the refrigerator for at least 4 hours, preferably overnight.

# TOFU CHEESECAKE

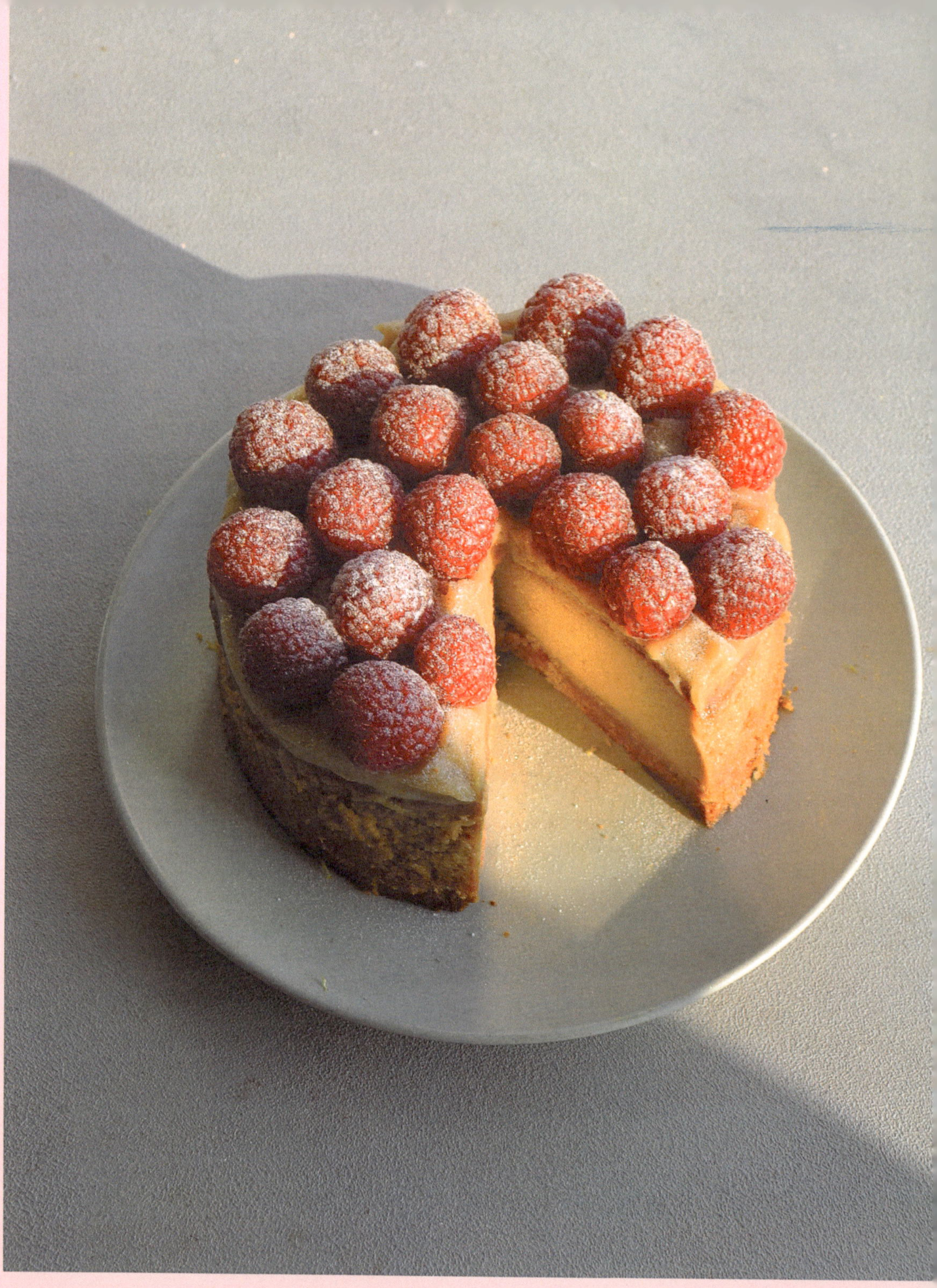

*A light, velvety, and tangy dessert, this silken tofu cheesecake balances the creamy smoothness of tofu-based filling with the vibrant sweet-tart flavors of raspberry and the subtle floral warmth of quince puree.*

**Serves: 2**

**For the Crust**

15 g coconut oil

45 ml grape molasses

75 g almond meal

40 g brown rice flour

A pinch of pink himalayan salt

**For the Filling**

300 g silken oat tofu or vegan cream cheese

100 g cashews soaked ( or use tahini, smooth almond butter, pine nuts, cashew butter etc. )

185 ml grape molasses

150 ml lemon juice

22 g tapioca flour

7 ml vanilla extract

A pinch pink himalayan salt

**For the Garnish and Serving**

1 cup quince purée (or apple)

125 g fresh raspberries

1 tbsp coconut flour

1 lemon zest

1. Preheat oven to 180 C.
2. Place all crust ingredients in a food processor. Blend until dough comes together.
3. Transfer to a 18 cm round cake mold lined parchment paper.
4. Press down with your fingers and then with a back of spoon. Flatten out as much as possible.
5. Bake the crust for 10 minutes in the preheated oven at 180 C.
6. Once done remove from the oven, set aside.
7. Set your oven to 160 C. Meanwhile prepare the filling ingredients.
8. Place all filling ingredients in a high speed blender. Blend until smooth.
9. Pour the filling over the half baked crust.
10. Place the cake in the oven and bake until the outside is set but the center is still a bit loose, about 1 hour.
11. Turn off the oven and leave the cake in for 15-20 minutes more.
12. Remove the cake from the oven and let it cool completely on a rack; cover and refrigerate overnight. About 30 minutes prior to serving, remove the cake from the refrigerator.
13. Top the cheesecake with fresh raspberries and quince puree.
14. Dust some powdered erythritol or coconut flour on the raspberries. Shred some lemon zest. Serve.

PLANT BASED UMAMI

# RUNEBERGIN TORTU

## FINNISH RUNEBERG CAKE

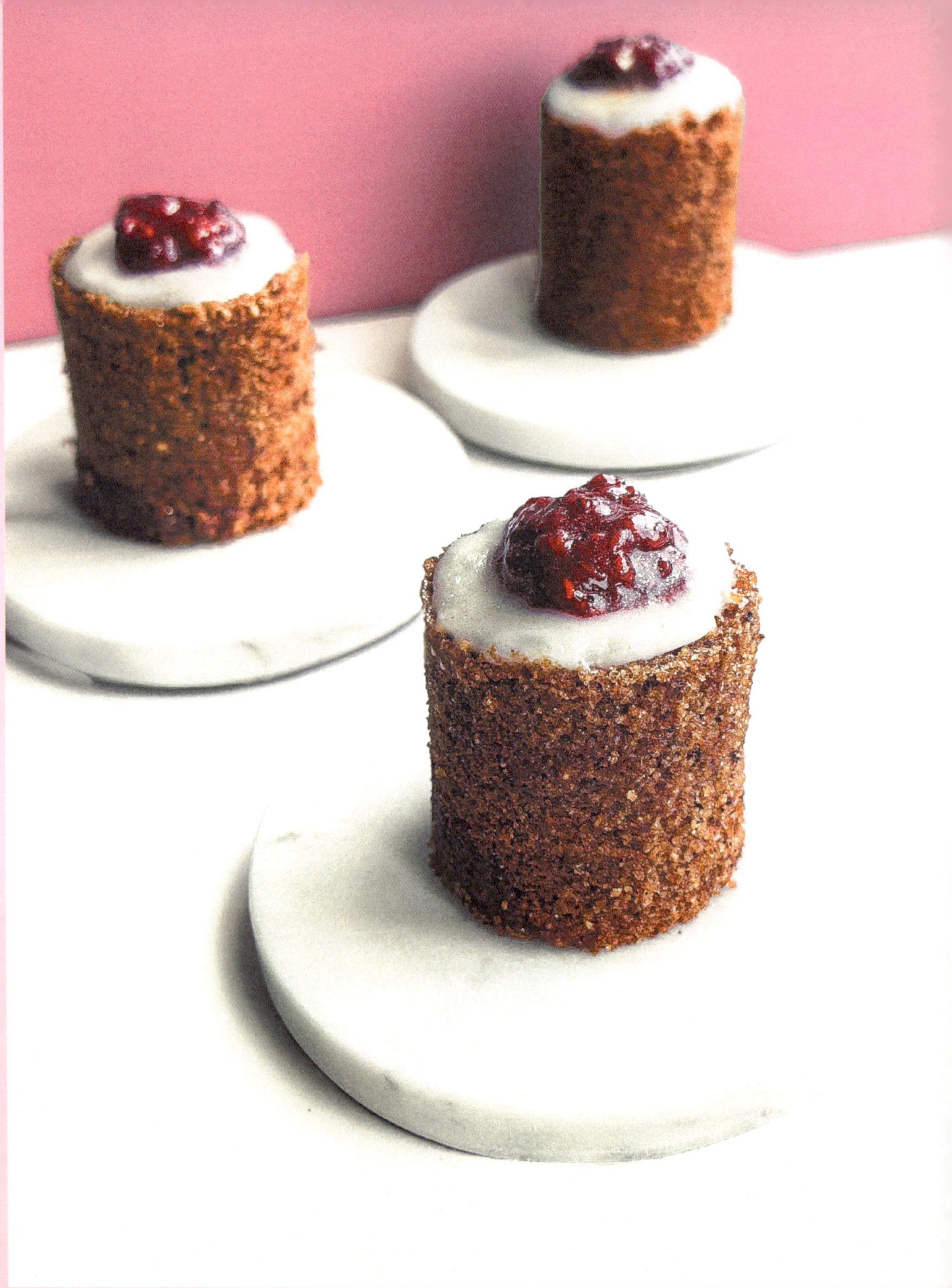

**Serves: 10-11**

**Dry Ingredients**

100 g oat flour
100 g coconut sugar
85 g rice flour
75 g almond flour
65 g tapioca flour
1 tsp cardamom
2 tsp baking powder
20 g almonds chopped
35 g walnut crumbs
1/4 tsp salt

**Wet Ingredients**

3 dl almond milk
55 g grapeseed oil
100 g coconut yoghurt or coconut cream + 1 tbsp lemon juice
55 g apple purée
6 g orange zest
2 tsp apple cider vinegar

**Raspberry Jam**

200 g raspberries
50 g maple
1 tsp chia seeds
1 tsp lemon juice

**Icing**

4 tbsp coconut milk powder
4 tbsp tapioca flour
2 tbsp maple syrup

*Runeberg Cake - A traditional Finnish sweet moist pastry (Runebergin Tortu in Finnish) are baked to celebrate the birthday of Finland's national poet Johan Ludvig Runeberg on 5 February. Every year around the date of his birthday, these exquisite little cakes are sold all over Finland and are hugely popular.*

1. Preheat the oven to 180 C and grease and line 10-11 pcs 5x5 cm loose bottomed tin. You will get 6 cakes from this batch.
2. Add all the dry ingredients to a large bowl and lightly mix.
3. In a separate bowl whisk together the wet ingredients and the coconut sugar until the sugar begins to dissolve.
4. Pour the wet ingredients into the dry ingredients and stir until fully combined. Pour into your prepared tins and bake in the oven for 20-25minutes, or until an inserted skewer comes out clean. The little cakes will rise quite a bit during baking.
5. Remove from the oven. Brush the most level ends of the cakes with a bit of Amaretto, for extra flavour. (optional)
6. Set to one side to cool completely before removing from the tin.
7. Meanwhile, prepare icing. In a bowl, mix tapioca and coconut milk powder together, Then add the maple anc stir well until everything combined well.
8. Cut a hole in the middle to fit approx. 1 tsp jam into each.
9. Use a spoon or icing bag to pipe out a thick circle of icing around the top edge of the cake.
10. Allow to set before filling the inner circle with jam.
11. Then fill with the jam.

# SEMLA

## SWEDISH FAT TUESDAY BUNS

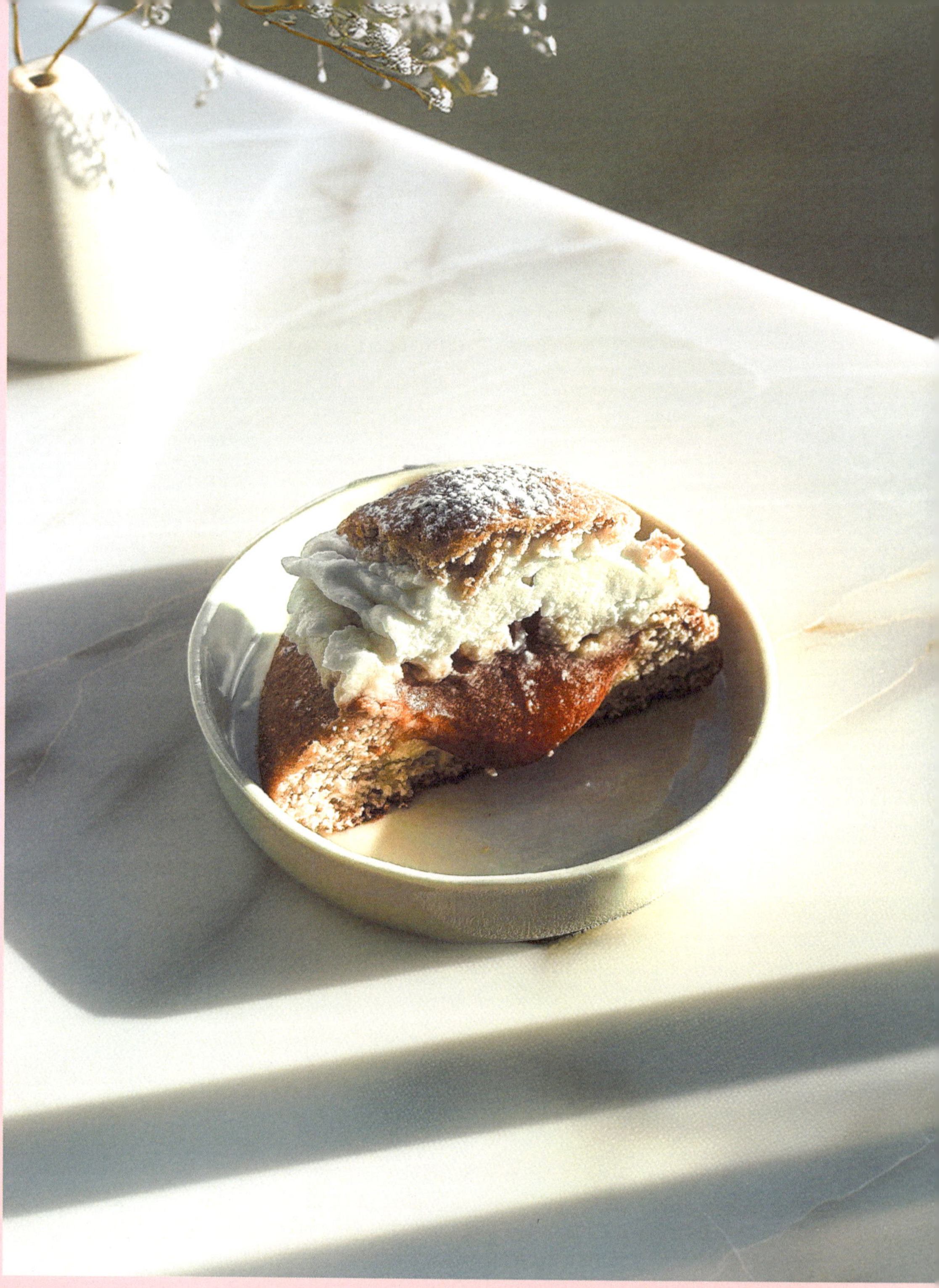

**Serves: 6**

**Dry Ingredients**

10 g instant yeast
120 g almond flour
80 g buckwheat flour
1 tbsp (8g) psyllium powder
18 g tapioca flour
1 tsp cardamom
A pinch pink himalayan salt
A pinch vanilla

**Wet Ingredients**

190 ml almond milk
35 g coconut oil
55 g agave

**Almond Filling**

55g (4 pcs) medjool dates
100 g almond butter
1 tbsp (15 ml) agave
1 tbsp (15 ml) almond oil
1/4 tsp salt

**Cream**

1 can coconut cream whipped

*On Shrove Tuesday, known as Fat Tuesday ('Fettisdagen') in Sweden and semlor (plural for semla) is hugely common all around the country. To eat it like local, start with the lid. Use it to scoop up some of the gooey contents. Proceed with the rest of the bun. The refined like to fork-it. Bohemians do it with a spoon. Tourists do it with confusion. And traditionalists order it in a bowl of warm milk. All are equally good.*

1. In a bowl, mix all dry ingredients expect yeast, and set aside.
2. Put the yeast in a bowl. Heat almond milk to 37 degrees in a saucepan. 3. Pour the almond milk over the yeast and stir until it dissolves. Then add the wet ingredients and stir.
4. Add the dry ingredients to the bun and mix together to form a dough.
5. Let the dough rest for approx. 30 minutes. The most important thing is to allow ample time for the buns to rise. Since you will probably be making these in a cooler February kitchen (on the semla week), leave plenty of time for the buns to rise. They will double and you will see the airiness
6. Set the oven to 175 C.
7. Divide the dough into 6 pieces and shape into 6 buns and place on a baking sheet lined with baking paper. As the dough is quite sticky, it is easiest to roll the buns by first dipping each piece of dough in a little buckwheat flour. Using your palm, press each ball of dough against the table and roll in circles until the bun is smooth and shiny, as if you are massaging it. Cup your hand around the bun without too much pressure and swirl it around in a circling motion to shape it into a round ball.
8. Cover with a tea towel and leave to rise for 40 minutes.
9. Bake in the middle of the oven for approx. 10 minutes.
10. Allow the buns to cool before cutting off the tops and spreading on almond paste and tops with whipped coconut cream using pastry bag with star tip. Dust with finely ground coconut milk powder or coconut flour.

# LAVA CAKE

PLANT BASED UMAMI

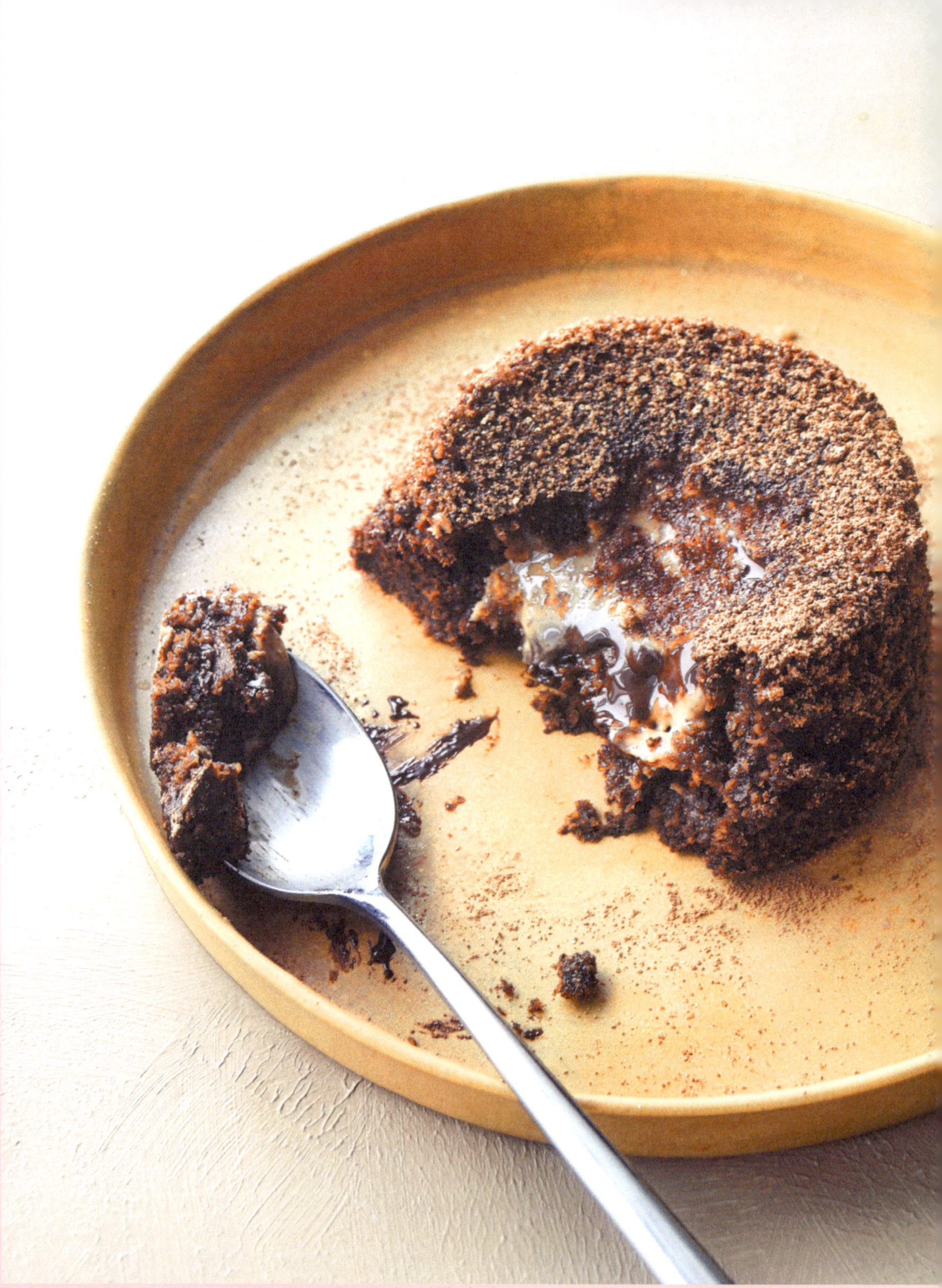

*This delicious lava cake with a gooey center is super simple and makes 2 individual chocolate lava cakes. Carob also can be used in the place of cacao.*

**Serves: 2**

**Ingredients**

50g cup oat flour
40g date paste
15g cacao powder or carob
1/2 tsp baking powder
60g banana
80g oat milk
25g almond butter
1/4 tsp apple cider vinegar

**Filling**

1/2 tbsp almond butter
1 square vegan chocolate or cherry jam

1. Preheat the oven to 180° C.
2. Mix the oat flour, cacao powder and baking powder together.
3. In another bowl, mash the banana with a fork. Then add the almond butter and date paste.
4. Add the oat milk and apple cider vinegar then mix well.
5. Pour some half of the batter into each soufflé mold ( about 3 inches in diameter, use the silicon one, otherwise you may need to grease the molds.)
6. Add the almond butter and a piece of chocolate on top. Cover with the rest of the batter.
7. Bake for 18 minutes. Once baked, remove the mold by inverting it onto the plate.
8. Dust some cacao on top. Serve immediately!

# INDEX

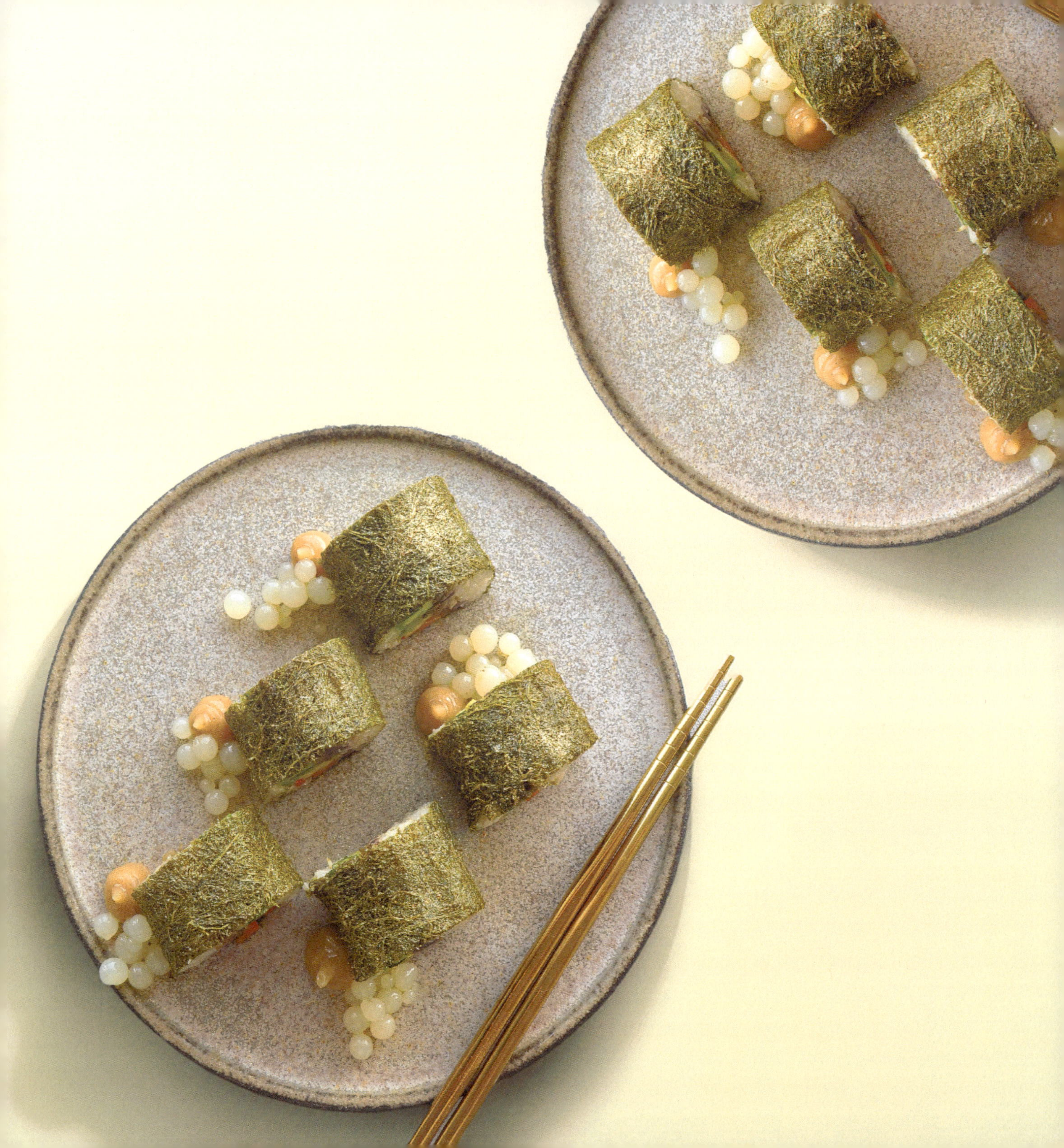

PLANT BASED UMAMI

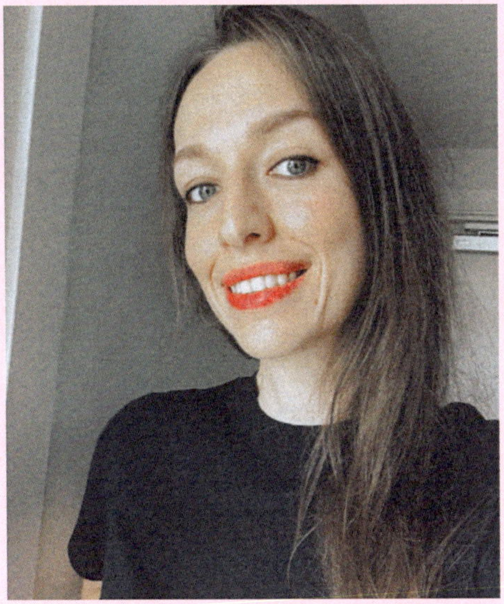

## about the author

Nazlı Develi is a food designer, an inventive, aesthetically minded hands-on chef and artist with an eye for details, an award-winning author and the founder of GREEN & AWAKE: Plant Food Design Studio based in southern Sweden.

She specialized in healthy plant-based and raw cuisine, restaurant consultancy, recipe development, workshops, chef training and creative concepts, all rooted in food expression with nature as a core.

Obsessed with art, design, health, travel, wellness and experimental flavours, she's strongly committed to spreading awareness about plant-based food as the most sustainable and necessary alternative for the planet.

Instagram: @gurmevegan I @greenandawake
Website: www.gurmevegan.com
www.greenandawake.com

www.ingramcontent.com/pod-product-compliance
Ingram Content Group UK Ltd.
Pitfield, Milton Keynes, MK11 3LW, UK
UKRC031011141026
15625UKWH00082B/648

* 9 7 9 8 9 8 7 8 5 3 6 2 7 *

9 798987 853627